ALCOHOLISM
A Practical Treatment Guide
Second Edition

Edited by

Stanley E. Gitlow, M.D.
Clinical Professor of Medicine,
Mount Sinai School of Medicine,
New York, New York;
Chairman, Committee on Alcoholism,
Medical Society of the State of New York;
Former President, American Medical Society on Alcoholism,
New York, New York

Herbert S. Peyser, M.D.
Visiting Consultant Psychiatrist,
Smithers Alcoholism Center,
St. Luke's-Roosevelt Hospital;
Chairman, Committee on Mental Health,
Medical Society of the State of New York;
Associate Attending Psychiatrist,
Assistant Clinical Professor of Psychiatry,
Mount Sinai School of Medicine,
New York, New York

1988

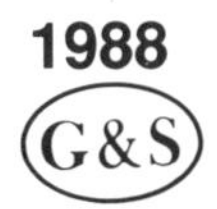

Grune & Stratton, Inc.
An Imprint of W. B. Saunders Company
Harcourt Brace Jovanovich, Inc.

Philadelphia, San Diego, London, Toronto, Montreal, Sydney, Tokyo

Library of Congress Cataloging-in-Publication Data

Alcoholism: a practical treatment guide.

Includes bibliographies and index.
1. Alcoholism. I. Gitlow, Stanley E. II. Peyser, Herbert S. [DNLM: 1. Alcoholism—therapy. WM 274 A3543]
RC565.A4452 1988 616.86'1 88-5106
ISBN 0-8089-1912-1

Grune & Stratton

Philadelphia, PA 19106

Library of Congress catalog Number 88-5106

International Standard Book Number 0-8089-1912-1

Printed in the United States of America

88 89 90 10 9 8 7 6 5 4 3 2 1

Contributors

Richard A. Baum, M.D.

Clinical Associate Professor
Department of Medicine, Division of Gastroenterology
University of Maryland School of Medicine
Baltimore, Maryland

LeClair Bissell, M.D.

Researcher, Author, Consultant
Sanibel, Florida

Marvin A. Block, M.D.

Emeritus Associate Professor of Clinical Medicine
State University of New York at Buffalo Medical School
Buffalo, New York

Marvin D. Feit, Ph.D.

Associate Professor
Norfolk State University School of Social Work
Norfolk, Virginia

Robert D. Fink, M.D.

Clinical Associate Professor
University of Tennessee, School of Health Sciences
Memphis, Tennessee

Vernell Fox, M.D.

Medical Director of Alcoholism Treatment
Pomona Valley Community Hospital
Pomona, California
Associate Clinical Professor of Psychiatry
University of California at Los Angeles
Los Angeles, California

Stanley E. Gitlow, M.D.

Clinical Professor of Medicine
Mount Sinai School of Medicine
City University of New York;
Committee on Alcoholism
Medical Society of the State of New York;
Former President, American Medical Society on Alcoholism
New York, New York

Lynne Hennecke, Ph.D.

Chairwoman, Alcoholism Task Force Women in Crisis
New York, New York

Frank L. Iber, M.D.

Departments of Gastroenterology and Liver Diseases
Edward Hines Jr. Hospital
Hines, Illinois

James A. Knight, M.D.

Professor of Psychiatry and Medical Ethics
Louisiana State University Department of Psychiatry
New Orleans, Louisiana

David H. Knott, M.D., Ph.D.

Clinical Professor of Psychiatry
University of Tennessee at Memphis
Memphis, Tennessee

Jack C. Morgan, M.D.

Clinical Associate Professor of Psychiatry
University of Tennessee at Memphis
Memphis, Tennessee

Robert D. O'Connor, M.D.

Medical Director, Conifer Park–Mediplex
Scotia, New York

Herbert S. Peyser, M.D.

Visiting Consultant Psychiatrist
Smithers Alcoholism Center
St. Luke's-Roosevelt Hospital;
Chairman, Committee on Mental Health
Medical Society of the State of New York;
Associate Attending Psychiatrist
Assistant Clinical Professor of Psychiatry
Mount Sinai School of Medicine
New York, New York

Joseph A. Pursch, M.D.

Family Care Clinic
Newport Beach, California
CPC Hospital of Laguna Hills
Laguna Hills, California

Frank A. Seixas, M.D.

Former Medical Director
National Council on Alcoholism
Clinical Associate Professor, Public Health
Cornell University Medical College
New York, New York

Gerald D. Shulman, M.A.

Addiction Recovery Corporation
Waltham, Massachusetts

Joseph J. Zuska, M.D.

Medical Director
Family Recovery Services
St. Joseph Hospital
Orange, California

Preface to the Second Edition

Since the publication of the first edition in 1980, the field of alcoholism and other drug dependencies has grown explosively. Public awareness, once the primary effort of Marty Mann and a small band of cohorts who united under the banner of The National Council on Alcoholism, now seems so largely achieved that the major effort remaining is often directed from the public toward tardy and inattentive legislative officials and medical personnel. As with any rapid advance in understanding, some confusion must be expected: the concept of drug dependence as disease, the effectiveness of treatment, the variation in treatment modalities, cost effectiveness, and the interface of this illness with a rapidly changing process for payment of medical care and for socioeconomic support systems in general—represent just some of the more critical issues.

Therapeutic effectiveness, a concept long accepted by the self-help community (Alcoholics Anonymous and others) and understood by occasional professionals with extensive clinical experience or their own clinical recovery from alcoholism, was embraced by the health care industry: a startling number of rehabilitation centers and employee assistance programs (EAPs) resulting in ever increasing availability of in-patient and out-patient counselling and therapy. Despite some questionably-designed scientific studies to the contrary, therapeutic intervention clearly led to substantive savings in health care cost and human suffering. Less well understood by the scientific community have been those elements responsible for treatment success within a widely diverse assortment of programs. Their eclectic nature as well as their involvement with spiritual, moral, and ethical values have responded with resistance to scientific dissection.

These same factors have brought a flood of new workers to this field: counsellors, nurses, paraprofessional therapists, social workers, psychologists, and physicians specializing in addiction medicine. Organizations of these people have sprung up, setting standards in training and fellowship and formulating certification and credentialing procedures. Some of the latter have resulted from the activities of private groups (e.g., The American Medical Society on Alcoholism and Other Drug Dependencies or AMSAODD) and others from the efforts by individual states to organize and/or control professional behavior. Largely as a result of the enormous increase in the numbers and complexity of the treatment personnel, educational activities within the general field of drug dependencies have increased to the point that one need not be deprived of some conference, seminar, or meeting on the subject in one state or another during almost any week of the year. Verbage in the form of a multitude of proprietary and professional journals has perhaps outstripped the availability of new and pertinent thought.

More important, there has been a healing of those wounds which resulted many years ago from disproportionate support of treatment and educational efforts by various governmental agencies in the fields of alcoholism versus narcotics dependence. Mixed drug dependence, once affecting no more than a third or less of the alcoholic population, now involves the majority. In 1950, one would occasionally encounter the alcoholic simultaneously dependent upon barbiturates and rarely one actively using amphetamine derivatives. In 1987, the cornucopia of drugs available for the achievement of decerebracy includes not only the old standbys of alcohol and narcotic analgesics, but a host of other soporifics, so-called minor tranquillizers, cocaine, hallucinogens, and other substances which any garage chemist can offer for the pickling of the exquisitely precise functions of the human brain. It has become more than ever apparent that one cannot hope to cope with "the drug problem" without learning about the entry drug, alcohol (or more precisely, beer). Our children have learned from us,—not just which drug to use, but the basic desirability of achieving a reversibly dysfunctional brain. As with all other generations, they have gone us one better: they have found drugs that do it better (worse!). We do not have "a drug problem" or an "alcohol problem," but rather an age-old problem with how we cope with life: do we deal with issues that threaten us or run away. Although Linus (from "Peanuts") believed that there was no problem so large that one could not successfully run from it, the magnitude and complexity of our drug problem in the United States has perhaps reached that point at which we will be forced to deal directly with the more basic issue.

Although A.A. has attempted to steer a course around this issue, more and more metropolitan groups welcome and support members with mixed drug dependency. In other areas, such subjects are treated at P.A. (pills), D.A. (drugs), C.A. (cocaine), etc. In the same vein, The American Medical Society on Alcoholism (AMSA) became AMSAODD a few years ago.

In the present edition of this text, the contributors strove to weave the complexity of multiple drug use into the diagnosis, evaluation, and treatment of the alcoholic. On the other hand, street narcotic use must remain the subject of a separate book. Obviously each substance to which man can become dependent may give rise to its own treatise on epidemiology, toxicology, diagnosis, and treatment. Nonetheless, the sedatives and stimulants yield a common enough clinical picture and therapy so as to permit publication of the present text under the general heading of alcoholism.

Beside multiple dependency, dual diagnosis—addictive and psychiatric—has also become of primary concern to the therapist undertaking the care of the alcoholic. Some of these issues are presented in the initial chapter and a totally new one added on clinical psychiatry and alcoholism.

The chapters on medical complications, women, and psychotherapy have each undergone extensive revision. Not the least of the changes, however, is that of our new less expensive soft-cover format. More than ever there is need for broad distribution of clinical material to the large number of treating people who have entered this field but recently. In a basically clinical and empirical field, where mathematically precise conclusions and objective data are at a premuim and perhaps even ultimately unobtainable—as with psychotherapy in general, the editors again turned to some of the most experienced practitioners of this art in order to share their many years of clinical experience. Sound clinical judgment, careful individual observation, long-term follow-up, and detailed outcome knowledge have always offered major guidance in the study of disease, and alcoholism should be no exception. Thus, this text contains the same basic message concerning the treatment of alcoholism that was true, useful, and even fruitful eight years ago. Some details have changed, and they must be noted, but the fundamentals—as in all good medicine—abide.

Stanley E. Gitlow, M.D.
Herbert S. Peyser, M.D.

Preface to the First Edition

This volume is intended to assist the practitioner in detecting and treating one of the most common illnesses currently challenging the art of medicine. Despite the often noted difficulties of treating the alcoholic, specific lay and professional efforts have succeeded in attaining impressive recoveries. What follows is a distillation of experiences of some of the foremost practitioners of this art. As a pragmatic guide, it avoids detailed references to scientific studies. No attempt is made to achieve the status of a reference text, of which there are currently many fine examples.

Throughout this text, the masculine gender has been used to refer to the patient with alcoholism, and the consort has been assumed to be feminine. Rather than a sexist bias, this reflects only a desire to achieve a convenient style. The reader should bear in mind that at least 30 percent of the alcoholics are women (see Chapter 11).

The editors wish to express their gratitude to the individual contributors whose experience and expert knowledge permitted the formulation of such a treatment guide. Lucy Robe offered great assistance in achieving a useful format, and Shirley Miller worked hard and long in transcribing material that could at times only be kindly described as disorganized.

If this text helps the clinically oriented practitioner to bring relief and recovery to some of those patients suffering from alcoholism, all of our efforts will be rewarded.

Stanley E. Gitlow, M.D.
Herbert S. Peyser, M.D.

Contents

1 **An Overview** 1
Stanley E. Gitlow

2 **Diagnosis and Recognition** 19
LeClair Bissell

3 **Motivating the Alcoholic Patient** 36
Marvin A. Block

4 **Initial Treatment of the Alcoholic Patient** 54
Richard A. Baum and Frank L. Iber

5 **After Detoxification—The Physician's Role in the Initial Treatment Phase of Alcoholism** 67
David H. Knott, Robert D. Fink, and Jack C. Morgan

6 **After Detoxification—The Rehabilitation of the Alcoholic** 78
Gerald D. Shulman and Robert D. O'Connor

7 **Long-Term Management** 98
Joseph J. Zuska and Joseph A. Pursch

8 The Medical Complications of Alcoholism 124
Stanley E. Gitlow and Frank A. Seixas

9 Alcoholism and Clinical Psychiatry 142
Herbert S. Peyser

10 Implications of the Disease Model for Psychotherapy and Counseling 156
Herbert S. Peyser

11 The Woman with Alcoholism 172
Lynne Hennecke and Vernell Fox

12 Problems Peculiar to Patients of Low Socioeconomic Status 181
Marvin D. Feit

13 The Family in the Crisis of Alcoholism 190
James A. Knight

Appendices

A. Sedative-Hypnotic Drugs 209
B. Criteria for the Diagnosis of Alcoholism 211
C. AMA Guidelines for Alcoholism: Diagnosis, Treatment and Referral 226
D. Antabuse 231

Index 236

1

An Overview

Stanley E. Gitlow

The practicing physician, steering his personal course through life, suffers at least the common adversities that beset people forced to cope with the overwhelming forces that tend to swamp their frail vessels. This is so despite the physician's own reputation, and perhaps even an intimate need for being able to control the frightening events that modify one's course to the final harbor. While attempting to exercise such precarious and fragile control, the physician encounters patients who fail to respond to assistance as well as those who, through noncompliance, appear to aid and abet their natural enemies. These enemies—infection, trauma, and neoplasia—even appear to be courted by lifestyles at variance with the medical optimum. Sadly, the physician, who might well embrace the medical discipline for the purpose of sharpening an ability to control such unpleasant fates, is thrust face to face with those very patients who thwart his desire to control disease and delay death.

This circumstance might explain in part the reticence with which today's physician approaches any chronic and recurrent illness. The special reticence with which the medical community has approached alcoholism, however, demands a greater endeavor for its understanding. Hospitals treat the medical complications of alcoholism but almost routinely fail to possess even a rudimentary treatment program for alcoholism itself. The term alcoholism is rarely applied as a discharge diagnosis from an acute medical care facility to those very patients for whom the control of alcoholism represents a primary requirement for the adequate treatment of their hepatic cirrhosis, primary myocardial disease, or tuberculosis. Even those physicians working in hospitals with alcoholism treatment programs fail to refer such patients for appropriate care. Why? Can it be that in contradistinction to the other chronic illnesses, alcoholism makes specific and special demands upon the physician since drug therapy plays so small and insignificant a role in its care? Is

ALCOHOLISM:
A Practical Treatment Guide
ISBN 0-8089-1912-1

it simpler to label these patients as "untreatable" rather than invest the time and personal involvement required in order to achieve therapeutic success? Was alcoholism the subject when we were taught "for every problem there is an answer—quick, easy, and wrong"? Does alcoholism, through its societal and moral implications, somehow awaken discomfort, perhaps even fear, within the physician? Or is it simply that we were taught so blessed little in our medical training that we can only approach this patient with a sense of foreboding, frustration, and futility?

The callous and uncaring attitude masquerading as "scientific" by the primary care physician has failed to convince the now cynical lay public of our motives. Those of us with many years of clinical experience do not require consumer advocates to convince us of the serious errors inherent in medical school curricula that result from "power plays" by departmental chairmen without regard for the health needs of the public. Exposure to the patient with alcoholism during the first 8 weeks of medical school revealed that the student's preoccupation was with such issues as "why does a person drink," "what is this person's life like," "how does his family relate to the problem," and "how does he feel," rather than the 4th-year student's fixation with the SGOT and even less important esoterica.* It takes us four long, hard years to eradicate the student's humanism, all the while missing an enormous opportunity of allowing him to care for and empathize with the millions suffering from this common but treatable illness. Not only does alcoholism offer overwhelming numbers for the developing physician, but here he can study the intricate interrelationships of somatic complications, psychic and societal impacts upon disease, paramedical roles in disease treatment and prevention, and the import of his own attitude upon the outcome of treatment efforts.

This text has been planned in answer to the need for a simple and straightforward method by which the physician may conceptualize alcoholism, the patient's suffering from it, and those therapeutic modalities that experienced therapists have used for its treatment. Though perhaps succumbing to the stylistic problems inherent in multiple authorship, the book capitalizes on this circumstance by reflecting viewpoints of many of the experienced and authoritative experts in this country today.

At this juncture, the disease concept of alcoholism will be briefly examined in order to permit the student of medicine to approach this illness within that rational framework of study commonly applied to other human ailments.

DISEASE CONCEPT OF ALCOHOLISM

Alcoholism is a disease characterized by the repetitive and compulsive ingestion of any sedative drug, ethanol representing but one of this group, in such a way as to result in interference with some aspect of the patient's life, be it health, marital status, career, interpersonal relationships, or other required societal adap-

* Experience with course on "Perspectives in Medicine" at Mount Sinai School of Medicine.

tations. As with any other illness, alcoholism represents a dysfunction or maladaptation to the requirements of everyday life. The key aspect of the definition rests in the recurrent return to the use of a soporific *despite* the subject's definitive best interest. No mention need be made concerning the specific volume of alcohol consumed nor the frequency with which such consumption takes place. Indeed, there are patients with this illness who ingest nothing stronger than beer, and there are those whose alcoholic intake is limited to but once or twice per year. Many, if not most, patients with this disease make substantive efforts to control the frequency or volume of their drinking, thereby achieving the status of what is commonly called "a periodic." The essence of the diagnosis rests in their need to control their drinking as opposed to their inability to do so. Normal subjects do not need to control their drinking any more than patients with alcoholism need to control their intake of carrots, beets, or cauliflower.

Unfortunately, inadequate clinical experience has led to some semantic abominations that lie in wait to entrap the unwary student. Our federal legislators notwithstanding, just what is "alcohol abuse"? Does it include repetitive injury to the individual's life? If so, the name is alcoholism, and if not, we need no special term. Similarly, the DSM-III, our standard reference work for psychiatric nomenclature, refers to "alcohol dependence (alcoholism)," without apparent appreciation that the disease known as alcoholism does not equal alcohol addiction (physical dependence) for a number of reasons: (1) one may have alcoholism but no longer drink; (2) physical dependence signifies that discontinuation of a drug results in objective physiologic derangements that may, at least in part, be relieved by the drug's readministration. In that sense, the elevated psychomotor activity (agitation) that follows the sedative action of ethanol represents the addictive phenomenon; it can be relieved by further sedative ingestion (only to reappear, even worse, later). It has been clearly established by clinical pharmacology, as well as by animal studies, that such evidence of addiction to sedative drugs starts and can be demonstrated objectively with as little as a single modest (social or therapeutic) dose. We must therefore conclude that despite the quantitative differences in the degree and frequency of ethanol addiction in the social drinker versus the alcoholic, alcohol dependence is nonetheless not synonymous with alcoholism. Similarly, the attempt to artificially differentiate alcohol abuse from alcohol dependence (presumably alcoholism) in DSM-III rests entirely upon the issue of physical dependence, a phenomenon that is measurable following even minimal soporific administration to any mammal. Since the effort to classify alcohol abuse as distinct from alcoholism lacks scientific basis, one can but assume that this nosologic slight of hand fulfills some inner need of the medical/psychiatric community or society at large. Along with the use of other euphemisms (problem drinker, alcohol misuse, etc.), this phenomenon usually earmarks the presence of denial.

The student of medicine might well consider alcoholism within that framework of disease that permits some variation in its expression without necessarily resulting in overwhelming diagnostic difficulty. Thus, instead of labeling typhoid fever as alpha, beta, or gamma in type, we simply accept that in any typhoid epidemic there will be patients whose disease results in minimal dysfunction, enormous and prolonged disability, numerous complications, or even death despite the best of medical care. Similarly, lupus erythematosus may at times run a reasonably benign course involving only certain tissues, whereas in other patients it may involve other tissues and result in a rapidly progressive and downhill picture.

The term *disease* signifies only the absence of comfort, but more detailed definitions demand that the ailment be specific or particular and that it possess characteristic symptoms or causes (a dysfunctional state with characteristic form). Thus a *symptom* is a phenomenon of disease, and the ultimate decision regarding classification of any illness as a disease rests upon whether or not the signs and symptoms commonly associated with it suffice to describe a specific entity. Any morbid entity can only be so evaluated by determining whether or not its associated symptoms, signs, etiology, distribution, complications, prognosis, and therapy are similar among the majority of patients so as to warrant the term *disease* as opposed to *symptom*. Differing social, ethnic, and racial factors result in variability in the expression of many illnesses, a circumstance that does not ordinarily detract from the use of the term *disease*. Those who have worked with patients suffering from alcoholism have had little question but that the histories, symptoms, and signs of this illness form a recognizable pattern. Indeed, there is little or no difference of opinion concerning this illness during its period characterized by substantive addiction. Rather, the nosological problem arises with the patient who has successfully completed detoxification. Even then, however, the student of this disease sees patterns of behavior that remain remarkably consistent and result in therapeutic and prognostic issues possessing similar consistency. The complications of this illness, though varied, are nonetheless similarly reproducible. Confusion has often resulted from the mistaken belief that one cannot have a disease if it is "self-induced" (the obese diabetic or hypertensive notwithstanding), if it is associated with patient denial (tuberculosis, cancer, and venereal diseases are all denied daily), or keynoted by self-loathing or depression (present with almost all chronic or recurrent illnesses).

Perhaps the circumstance that has caused the greatest misunderstanding, namely the nature of the premorbid personality of the patient suffering from alcoholism, may be viewed best from the vantage point of the full-blown clinical illness. Though the alcoholic's illness may begin from quite diverse psychological origins, once the disease of alcoholism has been grafted upon this personality structure, it dominates the clinical picture and eventually becomes the major determinant in both choice and efficacy of therapy. Thus, a patient's neurosis, character disorder, sociopathy, or affective disorder—each posing singular and somewhat specific problems—all present a clinical picture and therapeutic needs of great similarity once alcoholism has appeared.

It is hoped that we have passed the era in which functional disorders of the brain, whether of demonstrated biochemical nature such as phenylpyruvic oligophrenia or of unknown etiology such as schizophrenia or alcoholism, required the use of a term lesser or other than *disease* simply because 19th-century pathologists had difficulty observing a defect in the gross anatomy of the organ.

Application of such a term permits the dignity and right to obtain medical attention. It fixes the responsibility for the clinical care of the alcoholic and for research into the nature of the alcoholic's suffering upon physicians and their paramedical and basic science partners. Finally, it is in the best interest of our patients since it is associated with the lowest rate of recidivism.

ALCOHOL ADDICTION

As a "lumper" rather than a "divider" of medical entities, it was natural to coin the term *sedativism* a few decades ago when it became apparent to this writer that, to most of his patients with alcoholism, it mattered little whether they ingested ethanol or any of the other somnifacient medications listed in Appendix A of this text. In fact, it seemed that chloralism, bromism, barbism, valism, or paraldism would have been the logical name of this illness had these other sedatives simply appeared prior to alcohol. These soporific drugs act upon the brain in an almost identical manner. They elicit short-term, large-amplitude sedation, followed by long-term, low-amplitude agitation (Fig. 1-1). The exact temporal relationships of these asynchronous effects vary with the soporific in question, just as the rates of absorption and catabolism of the various drugs also vary. Approximately twofold tolerance can be achieved to the various soporific drugs, and when such tolerance has been achieved to any one drug of this group, it is simultaneously present for the remaining. Thus, patients with alcoholism reveal cross-addiction and cross-

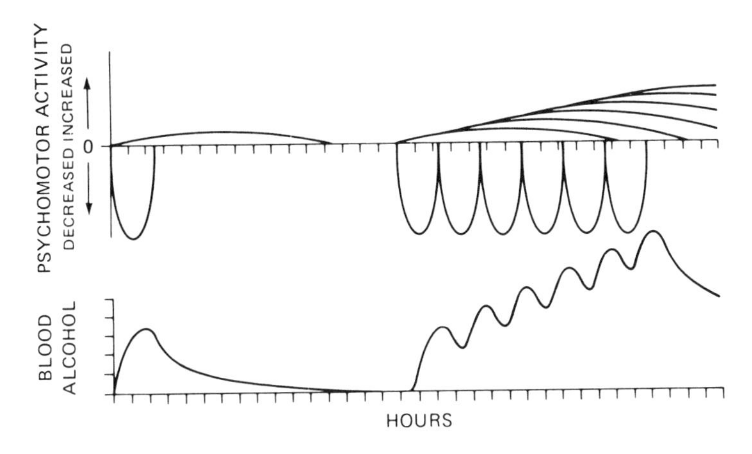

Fig. 1–1. Schematic representation of asynchronous relationship between short-term, large-amplitude sedative effect of ethanol and its long-term, low amplitude agitating effect (left). Repeated doses of ethanol result in summation of its agitating effect (right). [Reprinted by permission from Gitlow SE: Alcoholism: A Disease, in Bourne PG, Fox R (eds): *Alcoholism: Progress in Research and Treatment*. New York, Academic Press, 1973.]

tolerance among all of the agents that are classified as somnifacients (see Appendix A). It is not unusual to hear patients describe Librium as just "the very driest of martinis." Over 50 percent of the alcoholic patients in my own community have had addictive problems with one or another of the solid sedative compounds. The benzodiazepine addict, though missing the malodorous breath, florid facies, protuberant abdomen, and some of the other organic complications of alcoholism, nonetheless presents a clinical picture and a therapeutic problem almost precisely the same as those of the patient whose only soporific has been alcohol. This circumstance is stressed at this point in order to prevent the physician from offering the patient assistance out of the frying pan of alcohol use and into the fire of solid sedatives. Rarely does a therapeutic response result from the outpatient administration of tranquilizers or other sedatives to the actively drinking alcoholic, despite the patient's deep conviction and desire to learn what medical/drug techniques the physician might offer to enable him to continue drinking in his usual manner.

The major tolerance to sedative drugs results from central nervous system (CNS) adaptation; that is, a new balance is set up between the agitation remaining from yesterday's sedatives and the sedation resulting from today's sedatives. When the latter is discontinued, the agitation appears in full and the patient is said to be suffering from a withdrawal syndrome. Such CNS adaptation is the reason why one may occasionally observe active and mobile alcoholic subjects with what would otherwise represent lethal levels of blood alcohol (0.5 percent–0.7 percent).

A second type of tolerance, of much more modest clinical importance than the first, results from biochemical differences in ethanol metabolism by the drinking subject. There may be individual, sexual, or ethnic variations in the ability of a patient to catabolize ethanol. Each might lead to a slightly different blood alcohol concentration (BAC) following a standard ethanol dose. This type of tolerance would also vary with changes in the secondary ethanol-catabolizing system, the Microsomal Ethanol Oxidizing System (MEOS). Such changes occur in response to a multitude of drugs, including warfarin, most of the hypnotic/somnifacient drugs, the benzodiazepine tranquilizers, certain antibiotics, quinidine, phenylbutazone, phenytoin, isoniazid, and tolbutamide, through a mechanism known as enzyme induction. Chronic use of ethanol or any other of these substances might lead to a fractional increase in the catabolic rate for all such materials. Since these agents share in part a catabolic pathway, an acute simultaneous dose of two or more may result in an unexpected prolongation of turnover time. An apparent reversal of what had appeared to be elevated tolerance might then terminate in a degree of synergism adequate to elicit a demise.

A third critical variation in tolerance appears to result from increasing age. Thus, most older patients with this illness will grudgingly confess that less alcohol results in intoxication, a shorter period of pleasure, and a more prolonged and disagreeable agitation than had been noted previously. This phenomenon appears to parallel the ability of the CNS to tolerate other untoward incidents as well. The boxer at 40 years of age cannot tolerate head trauma as well as the boxer at 20 years of age. Superficially, this appears to be distinct from whatever

CNS injury the drug itself might have produced on a chronic basis, since teetotalers or modest drinkers can also detect this change with age.

The sedative effect of alcohol rarely persists longer than 2 to 5 hours, agitation appearing coincident with the peak blood levels of this drug (usually at the end of the second hour after its oral administration). The term *withdrawal syndrome* is in that sense a misnomer. Thus, the same blood ethanol levels on the uplimb and downlimb of the blood concentration curve are associated with sedation on the one hand and agitation on the other. Whereas the sedative effect of ethanol is of short duration but large amplitude, the agitation following it is more subtle (lower amplitude) and of much greater duration. These diphasic and asynchronous psychomotor effects occur with each of the soporific drugs, though precise amplitude and duration of each effect may be specific to the individual agent. Though alcohol ingestion results in a varying psychological response, the desired effect is always concomitant with the sedative effect of the drug. It may be casually observed that no one imbibes for the effect noticed the morning after. It is more than a little intriguing that the agitating actions of these compounds that make up the so-called withdrawal syndrome bear no relationship whatever to the rate of excretion or degradation of the soporific substance. Thus, the temporal and sequential relationships between sedation and agitation in the human and the mouse are precisely the same despite the fact that the rodent catabolizes alcohol tenfold faster. Apparently the pharmacologic effect is specific to neural tissue rather than the metabolism of the drug. An analogy may be made to head trauma with a hammer: the speed with which the hammer is removed from the scalp bears little relationship to the extent or duration of the CNS dysfunction following the blow. The phenomena associated with the agitation can be temporarily controlled by the sedative action of any of the soporific drugs, but each would add its own agitation to the eventual problem. The withdrawal syndrome would appear most mild in that youthful subject who drank the smallest amount for the shortest period of time and who was otherwise in good health. As the quantity and duration of sedative administration increases, the severity of this syndrome similarly increases from simple tremulousness, insomnia, palpitation, diaphoresis, and a vague sense of foreboding to the extreme of amnesia, hallucinations, and delirium tremens. At all levels of this syndrome, there is an increased tendency to grand mal seizures.

So much then for a brief description of the addiction to alcohol, a circumstance that can be reproduced in any normal volunteer. What must be kept in mind, however, is that such an addictive state in a volunteer is far from the disease called alcoholism. It is unlikely that any volunteer who once had experienced acute alcoholic hallucinosis or delirium tremens (DTs) replete with seizure activity would be likely to revolunteer for a similar experience. On the other hand, the patient with alcoholism "volunteers" over and over again, somehow unable to learn that each time alcohol ingestion begins, the stage is set for repetition of the enormous discomfort and personal danger associated with the withdrawal syndrome. Some psychoanalysts may well believe that this "inability to learn" stems from some purely functional quirk of the personality structure. It is so simple to assume that temptation affects us all and that we must all control our appetites equally. Moral turpitude would then seem the essential ingredient in alcoholism. How pompous and self-indulgent a conclusion when some, perhaps most, of us require so little control. Is it not equally possible that *excessive need* represents the problem rather than *deficient resistance*? One is reminded of the congenitally obese rodents who fail to control their abnormally large appetites until given nalorphine to counteract their excessive endorphin synthesis. Similarly the genetic data of Goodwin, Shukit, and others should give us pause to consider the possible organicity of this disorder. Though it is tempting at the present time to embrace either a medical, psychiatric, or societal model for alcoholism, should we not use all of these in order to maintain an open mind today concerning the nature of this disease that few understand and nobody knows?

THE DIAGNOSIS OF ALCOHOLISM

It has long been obvious that in the teaching of medicine no one learned the characteristics of a disease without the opportunity of intimate clinical contact. Since most of those patients with alcoholism with whom a young physician has contact have not recovered from the illness, and since denial and deception represent so great a part of its expression, little can be learned about alcoholism from such patients. It is therefore essential that in order to sharpen one's diagnostic skills as well as to conceptualize a clinical picture of the illness adequate enough to permit the later development of a dialogue with such a patient, young physicians or students must attend at least a dozen open meetings of Alcoholics Anonymous (A.A.). With but rare exception, they could not obtain as much clinical material through a visit to some other "epidemic." The diagnosis of alcoholism first requires, then, a clinical awareness of the nature of the illness. Second, a high degree of suspicion should be maintained whenever a patient presents multifactorial dysfunctional elements within his life. This patient can be likened to the Little Abner cartoon character who possessed his own personal raincloud that followed him wherever he went. Marriage, career, health—all seem destined to fall into a disrepair beyond this patient's ability to change. Yes, one may legitimately hypothesize that some other personality problem might be responsible for such dysfunction, but in today's society, alcoholism still represents the bet to beat. More specifically, the tremulous, flushed, diaphoretic patient who appears thyrotoxic but who tests negatively is most likely alcoholic. So, too, is the patient who arrives for a physical examination one morning replete with alcohol on the breath; the patient with multiple burns especially on the fingers and chest; the patient with protuberant abdomen, thin legs, dilated venules over the nose and malar eminences, and unhealthy gingival tissues; the patient whose peptic disease, hypertension, or tuberculosis seems impossible to control consistently; the patient with adult-onset generalized seizure activity; the patient with otherwise unexplained hepatomegaly or hepatic dysfunction; the adult patient with bilateral parotid enlargement; the patient with conversion and psychosomatic symptoms, including headache, gastrointestinal dysfunction, low back strain or muscle spasm, chronic fatigue, and recurrent palpitations; the patient with decreased attention span, diminished ability to concentrate, and reduced memory for recent events who also notices secondary insomnia and agitation; and those with other appetite disorders such as gambling, bulimia, or dependence upon other drugs. In the 1950s, about a third of my patients with alcoholism were also dependent upon other soporifics, usually barbiturates. A few used such drugs to the exclusion of ethanol. Still fewer used "ups and downs" (amphetamine derivatives and sedatives). These often revealed the more bizarre behavior, replete with paranoia and sudden swings in affect (differing from other psychiatric disorders, especially in the timing and periodicity of such events). More recently, these patients have been replaced by those with the ups and downs of cocaine and sedatives (benzodiazepines, ethanol, or others). The song is the same but the music is louder. Worse, by the 1980s fully two-thirds of my alcoholic patients are dependent upon more drugs than alcohol alone. Sudden and rapid changes in affect should still be the major warning signal, but the complications of psychedelic use (cannabinoids, LSD, PCP, or "designer drugs") will often confuse even the more astute psychiatrist attempting to differentiate alcoholism (that form with multiple drug use) from some premorbid primary psychiatric illness. To detect the cocaine user, we must avoid the naiveté of looking for no more than the hole in the nose of the coke snorter; rather, look for the pulmonary problems of the free-baser, the acute cardiovascular catastrophies of the crack user, and the tachyarrhythmias, strokes, or seizures accompanying this most positively reinforcing of all dependency-producing drugs. All of these represent clues for the alert physician, but none are as rewarding as a carefully taken history in which intimate personal behavior and relationships are examined in a warm and friendly fashion. The ultimate diagnosis of alcoholism, then, requires a sympathetic confrontation, revealing to the patient those very circumstances discovered while taking the history. One might be unable to establish a definitive diagnosis at the moment of initial contact with the patient, but a relationship should be established that would eventually permit an intimate and candid discussion. The physician must be trustworthy, credible, and nonjudgmental in order to achieve such a relationship. Rather than reflect on how big a liar the patient is, bear in mind that his denial of the problem remains proportionate to a sense of hopelessness in dealing with a compulsion, the nature of which he cannot understand and the magnitude of which has invariably dominated an ability to cope rationally with the problems of life. This is not the only illness associated with denial. Very few years ago, a brilliant colleague of mine who taught clinical internal medicine for many decades died after failing to detect his colonic carcinoma despite a change in bowel habits and blood in his stools.

Those patients who seek your care for reasons apparently unrelated to their sedative ingestion but whose real diagnosis is alcoholism reflect the size of their denial by the magnitude of the problems or symptoms that they are attempting to ignore or blame on unrelated circumstances. The physician can thereby gauge the fear with which the patient approaches the possible need to stop drinking. Most patients are usually quite convinced that you should leave their drinking alone and simply deal with their symptoms. Should you do that, you assist in the eventual destruction of your patient. Should you alternatively attempt to correlate his alcohol ingestion and somatic difficulties, you may alienate and, despite all the tact you can muster, lose further contact with the patient. A prolonged opportunity for your patient to ventilate, interspersed with sympathetic and understanding comments of your honest concern may, however, serve as a bridge over which you may be able to carry your most unwelcome and frightening message. Should you fail in this confrontation, this patient and this particular illness will not be the first to leave your good office in order to find an easier-to-accept opinion from a colleague. It is hoped that your colleague will also be honest, knowledgeable, and tactful, but it may be many years before this patient will confront you with gratitude for the role that you played in his recovery.

TREATMENT OF ALCOHOLISM

Having established a diagnosis of alcoholism, what next? Treatment of all illnesses is aimed at improved function. This is true in dealing with a broken limb or with congestive heart failure. It is also true for alcoholism. We have heard much about abstinence representing an aim in treatment of this disease. This is an error. Abstinence is not an aim but rather a means to an end. The end is simply that of improved function. For the patient with alcoholism, this aim cannot be consistently attained without abstinence, the reasons for which are threefold:

1. *To diminish the elevated psychomotor activity associated with alcohol ingestion.* Classically, the alcoholic prefers the minimally sedated state. In fact, it is not unusual to hear such a patient claim that it was only after the first drink that he felt "normal; like everyone else, for the first time." If the patient's normal psychomotor state is almost untenable, if a moderately sedated condition is more agreeable, and if each and every sedative drug eventually results in prolonged agitation, how then will this patient adjust to the continued or intermittent use of soporific durgs? The pharmacology of these agents serves to explain the reason for the A.A. view of "one is never enough but always too much." The clinically naive consider that this so-called medical model of alcoholism requires uncontrollable drinking to follow any single ingestion of alcohol or other sedative. This is simply not true. Rather, the alcoholic can never be certain which initial drink will eventually result in loss of control and substantive self-destructive behavior. The issue, then is that any rational and healthy person who could not anticipate which drink would lead to eventual injury would avoid drinking in the first place. The alcoholic is unable to accomplish this consistently. Use of the soporific results in the variable agitation described earlier; it represents the "hook" of the addiction and as such is enormously uncomfortable for the alcoholic.
2. *To control organic pathology.* Almost every complication of alcoholism requires abstinence for a maximal rate of improvement. In almost every instance, medical therapy in the presence of active drinking fails to achieve a satisfac-

tory recovery. Similarly, a minimal therapeutic effort is usually followed by maximal recovery when abstinence is achieved. Hence, the physician, from no matter what discipline, should focus firmly on the requirement to achieve abstinence since this and this alone appears to achieve the greatest likelihood for recovery from the organic complications of this illness.

3. *For psychotherapy.* It is as impossible to develop insight for the actively drinking alcoholic as it is to perform psychotherapy on one of the active contenders in the midst of a prize fight. Just as the internist must realize that the organic dysfunction associated with the withdrawal syndrome has a concomitant defect in cognitive function, so, too, must the psychiatrist realize that sedative drugs modify brain function in such a manner as to markedly interfere with the development of insight. I am reminded of the patient who quipped, "It's hard to learn to navigate from the deck of a sinking ship." Numerous alcoholics, including alcoholic physicians and psychiatrists, have volunteered their experiences relevant to the impossibility of achieving psychotherapeutic results during the use of alcohol. In fact, the development of insight during psychotherapy tends to be quantal in nature rather than a continuum. The patient need only drink periodically, at those times during which insight might otherwise develop, for the psychotherapeutic effort to be largely cancelled.

Thus, abstinence becomes our means to the aim of improved function. Therapy itself is roughly divided into three parts: achieving motivation, detoxification, and definitive care. These tend to blend together just as establishing the diagnosis and confronting the patient will very often blend with the act of motivating the patient. During the period of detoxification, the able physician is setting the stage for the patient's definitive course.

Accomplishing any of these three elements of treatment requires the willingness on the part of the physician to treat both the patient and the disease. This willingness can be determined by asking three questions:

1. *Does the physician believe that he has something to offer?* Every physician, with perhaps the singular exception of the pathologist, treats the alcoholic. Unhappily, the majority are probably unaware of the diagnosis their patients present. But whether it is the pediatrician who treats the abused child of the alcoholic parent, the obstetrician who delivers the infant disabled by the fetal alcohol syndrome, the surgeon who operates on the mangled trauma victim destined for DTs, or the ENT surgeon who resects the laryngal cancer, each, directly or indirectly, is treating the alcoholic. Thus, every physician should have something to offer. In truth, however, only the physicians who feel they can help, do help. For this, they must have acquired personal experience with recoveries achieved by other patients who had suffered equally or greater from their alcoholism.
2. *Can the physician give the necessary time?* The diagnosis and confrontation of the alcoholic requires at least an hour and sometimes a number of separate hours of intimate contact with the patient. Motivating the patient can usually

be accomplished during that period. Under the best of circumstances, most physicians should be able to accomplish this much: making the diagnosis, confronting the patient, and motivating the treatment. The patient's further care through detoxification and definitive therapy may well tax the physician too much and require areas of expertise that he might not possess. The chapters that follow go into considerable detail concerning the methods for referral of such a patient.

3. *Can the physician identify with the patient?* There is some reason to believe that when the ratio of patients to physicians is too great, when the patient's appearance or other qualifications differ too greatly from that of the physician, or when the patient elicits personal fear or possibly frustration in the physician, the quality of medical care suffers. This is true in epidemics, major disasters, and circumstances wherein the physician may differ greatly from the patient in religion, race, and ethnic origin. The problem of "overidentification" also must be noted, since a physician might well require, for himself, a patient's recovery. The physician's personal drinking habits, as well as his attitude toward drugs and chemotherapy in general, may well determine the ability to treat an alcoholic. It is of more than casual interest that, until a few years ago, a training psychoanalyst would examine in detail the physician-patient's attitude toward love, money, sex, family, and so forth, but almost uniformly fail to evaluate attitudes toward the use of social-psychoactive drugs—despite the estimated 10 percent incidence of alcoholism and other drug addiction among physicians.

Having determined the willingness of the physician to treat the alcoholic, how can he motivate the patient to enter into treatment? At the outset, it should be apparent that the need to be motivated may be estimated from the characteristics of the patient's initial presentation. For instance, if the patient comes to the physician's office primarily because drinking has resulted in a loss of control of his life and those aspects of it that he most values (home, job, and health), it implies that major steps towards recovery have been taken; the patient recognizes that alcohol and/or other sedative ingestion plays a major role in the illness, that he is powerless in controlling it, and therefore requires professional assistance in combating it. The patient has quite apparently, though perhaps temporarily, abandoned some of his denial and may possess, with little effort on your part, that motivation necessary to initiate rehabilitation. If, on the other hand, the patient seeks your assistance primarily because someone else demands that he speak to you concerning his drinking, there is still active denial. His appearance at your office implies suspicion that he might indeed have a drinking problem, and it also permits immediate discussion of those personal events in his life that led to the displeasure and concern of a significant other. His appearance also implies that he continues to possess circumstances in his life that maintain substantive meaningfulness to him; otherwise no coercion would be possible.

Finally, the patient may seek your assistance for a reason that seems to him to be unrelated to alcohol use. Whether physical (headaches, gastrointestinal disturbances, hypertension) or emotional (marital discord, anxiety over job, insomnia, or agitation), the patient fails to formulate any connection between the drinking and the problem. The immensity of the denial can best be estimated by the magnitude of the symptom that is ignored or blamed on unrelated circumstances. The physician can thereby gauge the fear that the patient has concerning the possible need for giving up alcohol. In approaching this most difficult problem, the physician must bear in mind that the patient has attempted to relinquish his particular method of dealing with life's problems by substituting some alternative scheme for coping—to no avail. Hence his conviction that you should leave his drinking alone and simply deal with his symptoms. Foremost, he would prefer that you exert all of your professional skill in developing a plan whereby he can continue to drink without further difficulty. If you are unwilling or unable to accomplish this, the patient is at least certain that: (1) having lived with himself for innumerable years, he is much more cognizant of his personal problems than you could possibly be; and (2) he knows a great deal more about drinking than you possibly could. Sometime during the interview, it will be incumbent upon you to disabuse him of this concept. With great tact and allowing ample opportunity for the patient to describe his problems, you may intersperse sympathetic and understanding comments of your concern for his pain and suffering. Your generally supportive and sympathetic attitude may lead to the formation of that fragile relationship that would permit development of courage for a therapeutic effort.

What specific techniques may the physician use?

1. Reflect to the patient those critical factors by which alcohol is adversely affecting the patient's preferred self-image: The patient who claims a desire to continue an intimate relationship with his wife and children, but whose drinking has seriously compromised an ability to fulfill this; the patient whose financial and career needs are in jeopardy, but who continues to drink despite warnings from his superiors; the patient whose career and intimate personal pleasures are dependent upon sound cognitive function, but whose continued use of soporific drugs damages the CNS—all of these require a sympathetic confrontation concerning the exact role played by continued drug (ethanol) use.
2. Offer the dignity of the disease concept of alcoholism. Numerous studies have revealed an inverse relationship between acceptance of the disease concept and recidivism. Physicians who fail to appreciate or understand this view would do well to embrace it if only for the benefit to their patients.
3. Offer hope. The despairing patient must have restored belief in his recovery. This circumstance must be supported by the physician's previous experiences with treatment of this disease, or a personal exposure to the recovered members of A.A.
4. Impress the patient with your personal knowledge concerning this illness. Obviously, the patient's faith in your diagnosis and therapy, as well as in the hope that you hold out for his recovery, is totally dependent upon his faith in your expertise and general knowledge of the illness. Quite apparently this knowledge is unlikely to result from that degree of clinical contact and instruc-

tion offered by the majority of medical schools today. Visits to A.A. meetings, alcoholism treatment centers, and rehabilitation facilities will be necessary in order to gain a conversant and even facile level of awareness by means of which the patient may be reassured.

5. Educate the patient about the nature of alcoholism. It is imperative that the patient realize how little he knows about his own illness. In describing the compulsion to drink, the author has often used the analogy of a bullfight wherein the determination to resist drinking is likened to locking horns with the bull. The lack of success inherent in such a circumstance is easily imagined, but the singular act of learning the nature of the bull—how and when it charges, and how it moves its horns—enables the patient with a cape to make the bull look remarkably like a jackass. Considerable time must be spent with the patient pointing out the pharmacology and pathophysiology of sedative ingestion in order to verify the likelihood that knowledge and understanding might lead to recovery. The patient will often be confused about a more recent loss of tolerance, unaware that tolerance to sedatives decreases with age. He will have noted but not understood the relationship of ethanol's sedation to its inevitable agitation. He may have recognized but never openly admitted to himself that his drinking resulted in memory defects and loss of ability to concentrate. Now is the moment for the patient to see the dead end of that alley down which he has been progressing.
6. While offering sympathy for the patient's suffering, present a specific method for therapy. Although flexibility might marginally increase the number of patients who can fit into any therapeutic scheme, it is quite critical that the physician remain unyielding in the application of those therapeutic methods that he knows by experience are vital for recovery.
7. Exert leverage when available and necessary. Confrontation in and of itself will often represent as much leverage as the patient may require for the initiation of therapy. On the other hand, some patients require somewhat more of a crisis and, for them, loss of a job, a consort, or a professional license might offer that leverage that is required to initiate the meaningful treatment regimen. The subtleties inherent in applying such leverage at the appropriate moment require great clinical judgment and are discussed at greater length in the chapters that follow.
8. Relieve pain during detoxification. Your willingness to appreciate the patient's physical and psychic discomfort during detoxification increases the patient's belief in your personal interest. Such an intimate relationship may go far toward motivating this patient to continue in a program for rehabilitation following the treatment of his withdrawal syndrome.

Having motivated the patient to comply with your therapeutic suggestion, your concept of his treatment requirements necessitates that you define the degree of his illness and resources, and that you set a legitimate therapeutic goal. Does the patient require acute hospital care for the treatment of the withdrawal syndrome, for the organic complications of alcoholism, or for physical protection from excessive sedative use? Do the patient's resources still include intimate relationships, emotional stability, and private finances? Is his status such that one might legitimately aim at nothing less than complete recovery, or has there been enough physical and mental damage so that a therapeutic compromise must be anticipated?

Having defined these circumstances, the physician can more rationally determine the need for in-hospital detoxification, the potential length of time for treatment of the withdrawal syndrome, and the need for long-term care and rehabilitation. Relapses (slips), though possible at any time in the course of treatment of the alcoholic, tend more frequently to occur shortly after discharge from an inpatient facility (within 1 month of initial treatment), approximately 3–4 months after initiation of treatment, and again about 10–11 months after beginning such therapy. Recidivism diminishes appreciably if consistent sobriety has been maintained within an active therapeutic program for 24 months. A small but definite relapse rate continues indefinitely thereafter. Clinical improvement in cognitive function appears to be greatest during the first few months of abstinence but increases progressively to an asymptote at approximately 24 months. It is remarkable that the functional improvement in career and interpersonal relationships of the alcoholic bears such a specific temporal relationship to recovery from brain injuries following stroke, trauma, and infection. Should it appear to the physician that the patient does not have the personal resources, strength, and support mechanisms that would permit an early return from an acute care facility to his usual environment, then a prolonged stay at a rehabilitation facility offers both the education and duration of abstinence that might make definitive recovery more likely. These factors usually become clear to the physician immediately prior to or during detoxification. The patient who has stopped drinking himself or has been discharged from a treatment facility now requires definitive assistance in combating the illness within the confines of his own environment. The major precept to be followed by the physician at this juncture is to avoid the Timothy Leary concept of "better living through chemistry." The care of the patient at this stage in treatment should be without the use of drugs, with the major exception of Antabuse (Appendix D). The use of any solid sedatives or tranquilizers at this stage in the patient's care will markedly increase the likelihood of relapse. More appropriately, one should offer a directive, confrontative, and supportive type of therapy, the principal aim of which is to break the patient's isolation. Extensive clinical contact has substantiated the author's belief that isolation is pathognomonic of this illness and that therapy is successful only in proportion to its ability to change this specific circumstance. The physician's relationship with the patient may often be the initial opportunity for the patient to relate to another human being on a deep and intimate level. As noted by Dr. Kenneth Williams, the isolation may have started with the anomie experienced in the patient's childhood, a circumstance aggravated later by the aberrant use of alcohol in a society in which 90 percent of its drinking members are not forced to drink covertly or excessively. The physician's successful relationship with the patient may enable him to eventually formulate relationships with others. This often requires a peer group with whom the alcoholic may identify. Alcoholics Anonymous offers such peer group support as well as educational and other mechanisms for ongoing recovery. It is not uncommon for the family members of the alcoholic to require similar support and treatment. Long-term sobriety and recovery of the patient's health, career, and interpersonal relationships often result in marked improvement in self-esteem; this in and of itself supports continued therapeutic success. Successful interference with the problem of isolation and inadequate self-esteem may be more difficult in the socioeconomically deprived or female patients (Chapters 9 and 10).

At any time during therapy it may become apparent that "A.A. is not working": the meetings are inconvenient to get to, the A.A. members are not "my kind of people," the discussions are boring and repetitive, and "I never feel like drinking except when I go to a meeting." Such announcements might only surface if the therapist is alert and active enough to inquire. They reflect the early part of reisolation, step 1 in the return to drug use (a slip). Step 2, that the patient is handling some intimate relationship in a manner so as to lose self-esteem, is usually almost concomitant, and step 3 (the drink) may follow hours or weeks later. Unfortunately, the patient's failure to attend a session with you is commonly followed so closely by drug use that it is too late to prevent the slip. Instead, the effort to reintegrate the patient into A.A. must be made early. The "rule of 10" might be helpfully presented to the patient by a sponser, group members, or you:

1. Attend at least one and preferably more meetings daily. At least some should be "beginners" or "step" meetings.
2. As soon as you have found two or more groups that you prefer, arrange to attend their meetings without fail (so much so that the other members would be certain that they had come on the wrong day, were you to be absent). Travel and other personal commitments must not interfere with attendance.
3. Arrive before all others and leave last.
4. Always sit in the first row.
5. If there is a stranger seated nearby, introduce yourself.
6. Raise your hand to enter a discussion at least once in each meeting (even to ask a question), and qualify promptly at 90 days.
7. Explain to the chairperson that you require that a task be assigned to you (chairs, basket, coffee, or whatever).
8. Never leave a meeting without sharing a discussion and/or beverage with another member (especially a stranger).
9. Never leave a meeting without requesting someone's company for further dialogue.
10. Whether classified formally as a sponsor or not, arrange for regular social contact with a successfully abstinent member of the group.

When the impact of this commitment registers, the usual question is, "How long must I do this?" The reply, "until you like it." Obviously not every patient will need or respond to such a confrontative approach, but by one means or another the stark difference between therapeutic involvement and life on the one hand and return to drug use on the other must be drawn clearly. That person who embraces magical thinking (my improved job, love life, or venue will replace the need for a commitment to A.A.) usually suffers an early relapse. Although a slip in and of itself may teach one more than it appears to cost, bear in mind that an associated sudden accidental demise might preclude all further treatment. Moreover, a single slip is much more costly to an intimate relationship with a spouse than continued drinking prior to the onset of treatment and the hope of recovery. Similar anger, despair, and hopelessness may be experienced by an employer.

About 2 percent of the patients under treatment for alcoholism will also need treatment for a complicating major psychiatric problem, such as schizophrenia or a bipolar affective disorder. Such a diagnosis requires a period of absolute abstinence from soporific drugs in order to make a bona fide evaluation of the patient. It has been assumed, somewhat naively, that the rate of recovery from a drug-induced neurologic injury must be directly related to the turnover rate of the substance and/or its active metabolites. As we have seen with alcohol, the two issues are almost unrelated if the drug induces an injury. It is quite clear that many of the dependency-producing drugs may indeed cause functional and structural damage to the brain. It should therefore not surprise us to find that recovery from such drug use might require abstinence for many months, even years, and might even on occasion remain incomplete. Long-term evidence of such dysfunction (anxiety, panic, and somatic symptomatology) is especially common after extensive use of benzodiazepines. The assumption of a primary psychiatric diagnosis other than drug dependency within a month or two of the onset of abstinence is fraught with danger. Only continued abstinence and supportive therapy will permit the gradual disappearance of the symptomatology and the avoidance of a diagnosis by an overanxious physician that is nothing more than a self-fulfilling prophecy. Readministration of an addicting soporific/tranquilizer will induce a temporary improvement followed later by increasing evidence of anxiety or panic. At that point, the physician's diagnostic error is compounded by his certainty.

Some of the patients with premorbid personality deficits can be treated without recourse to psychotropic drugs. The use of tricyclic antidepressants, lithium, or phenothiazines should be eschewed when possible, since they markedly complicate the care of the alcoholic. On the other hand, those few patients for whom such drug therapy is imperative must be individually supported in order to avoid alienation from such support mechanisms as Alcoholics Anonymous.

The chapters that follow are complete with numerous details that will serve to shed light on many of those issues to which I have alluded. An old Talmudic quip notes that "for the man who doesn't know where he's going, any road will take him there." Though the past 3 decades have often emphasized the wisdom of that ancient scholar, it has become progressively clear that those physicians who have worked extensively with patients suffering from alcoholism are in far greater agreement about the nature of the illness and its treatment than the pertinent scientific literature would suggest. I can only trust that this text will encourage all physicians to detect and confront the patient with alcoholism and some physicians to join us in the treatment of these seriously ill patients. Not only will the patients benefit, but the physicians will experience extraordinary rewards.

BIBLIOGRAPHY

Boston Collaborative Drug Surveillance Program. Clinical Depression of the Central Nervous System Due to Diazepam and Chlordiazepoxide in Relation to Cigarette Smoking and Age. *N Engl J Med* 288:277–280, 1973

Castleden CM, George CF, Marcer D, et al: Increased sensitivity to nitrazepam in old age. *Br Med J* 1:10–12, 1977

Chappel JN: Attitudinal barriers to physician involvement with drug abuse. *JAMA* 224: 1011–1013, 1973

Cregler LL, Mark H: Medical Complications of Cocaine Abuse. *N Engl J Med* 315:1495–1500, 1986

Gitlow SE: Alcoholism: A disease, in Bourne PG, Fox R (eds): *Alcoholism: Progress in Research and Treatment.* San Diego, Academic Press, 1973

Gitlow SE: Considerations on the evaluation and treatment of substance dependency (Bond Symposium). *J Subst Abuse Treat* 2:175–179, 1985

Gitlow SE, Hennecke L: Etiology of Alcoholism: A New Theoretic Mosaic. *Semin Adolescent Med* 1:235–238, 1985

Goodwin DW: *Is Alcoholism Hereditary?* New York, Oxford University Press, 1976

Hamerman D: Primary care—is it here to stay? The implications for medical education. *Bull NY Acad Med* 55:540–550, 1979

Macy Foundation: Medical Education and Drug Abuse: Report of a Macy Conference. Josiah Macy Jr. Foundation. Report of a joint conference on instruction in the problem of drug abuse. New York, William F. Fell Co, 1973

Main TF: The ailment. *Med Psychol* 30:129–145, 1957

McQuarrie DG, Fingl E: Effects of single doses and chronic administration of ethanol on experimental seizures in mice. *J Pharmacol Exp Ther* 124: 264, 1958

Pace N: The Cornell medical student's field trip through the world of alcoholism, in Seixas FA (ed): *Currents in Alcoholism*, New York, Grune & Stratton, 1977, pp 233–242

Petursson H, Lader M: *Dependency on tranquilizers.* Oxford, England, Oxford University Press, 1984

Reidenberg MM, Levy M, Warner H, et al: Relationship between diazepam dose, plasma level, age, and central nervous system depression. *Clin Pharm Ther* 23:371–374, 1978

Schukit MA, Goodwin DS, Winakur G: A study of alcoholism in half siblings. *Am J Psych* 128:1132, 1972

Spalt L: Alcoholism: Evidence of an X-linked recessive genetic characteristic. *JAMA* 241:2543–2544, 1979

Wilkinson, DA (ed): *Cerebral deficits in alcoholism.* Toronto, Addiction Research Foundation, 1984

2

Diagnosis and Recognition

LeClair Bissell

Virtually every physician who treats older adolescent or adult patients is already seeing people with serious drinking problems. If asked, however, whether or not he is treating any alcoholics, the doctor will frequently say no. Since only a relatively small number of physicians report that they see alcoholics, and since alcoholism is not a particularly difficult diagnosis to make, one is forced to question why this situation exists. There is little reason to believe that alcoholics seek treatment only from the minority of physicians quick to recognize them. They do in fact distribute themselves rather impartially among us.

WHY DOCTORS AVOID DIAGNOSIS

While it has been claimed that the physician does not want to look into the drinking habits of patients because of a reluctance to examine his own, and while this may at times be true, I think that for most of us the difficulty lies elsewhere. Doctor and patient are often products of the same culture, a culture that has groomed us from childhood to believe that alcoholism is not really an illness but is instead a sign of weakness. We then feel that we are not making a diagnosis of a disease but are accusing the patient of something. We are embarrassed and a little bit afraid of how our patients will react. They may get angry or defensive and certainly will not greet the diagnosis with delight, not only because they then have to face the need to learn to live without their accustomed drinking but also because they must accept an illness that still carries with it a degree of social stigma.

ALCOHOLISM:
A Practical Treatment Guide
ISBN 0-8089-1912-1

To make the diagnosis of alcoholism, then, is going to involve the physician in what he fears may well be an uncomfortable and awkward discussion with a patient, who, most likely, is going to deny its accuracy and is going to insist that the real problem is something else altogether, usually some difficulty—real or imagined—that lies beyond the ability of either of them to control.

Physicians face an additional problem. Like anyone else, they like to feel competent, to know what they are expected to do and how to do it. They are told that alcoholism is a disease and not a symptom of something else and that they are expected to know how to treat it. Since they may well have received less than an hour of education about alcoholism in their formal medical training and since they may have been taught little or nothing about what to say to an alcoholic when actually faced with one, they will then have to rely on what they have observed their colleagues doing with their alcoholics. This kind of role model teaching usually has been a demonstration of denial that alcoholism exists, an attitude that even if it does exist little or nothing can be done about it, and, in any case, that it is up to the patient somehow to find the motivation to change and devise a cure.

THE ALTERNATIVE DIAGNOSIS

The physician's role, then, is usually seen as limited to dealing with the late medical complications of drinking, with perhaps a warning to patients that alcohol is hurting their bodies and, if they continue to drink, will doubtless do increasing harm. Social consequences of the drinking behavior may be left to others or totally ignored. That patients may well have been attempting unsuccessfully to control their drinking and may be trying desperately to understand the predicament in which they find themselves is often not considered. That being an active alcoholic is a painful experience and that a desire to escape that pain can provide motivation toward recovery for an alcoholic, as for many another patient, may be forgotten.

Clearly, then, if to diagnose alcoholism is simply going to mean that the doctor is faced with an embarrassing confrontation with the patient, at the end of which nothing constructive will have occurred for either of them, and if, in addition, the physician is going to be left feeling inept, incompetent, and uncomfortable, the easiest way to handle the situation is to pretend that the disease isn't there at all. The patient doesn't really want to hear the diagnosis, his insurance coverage will sometimes specifically exclude reimbursement for alcoholism if it is honestly diagnosed rather than masked by a euphemism, and the doctor doesn't want to be faced with the expectation of treating an illness that he doesn't know how to treat.

COMPROMISE BY REFERRAL

A frequent compromise is to acknowledge that the patient appears to be drinking too much but to assume that he must be self-medicating for an underlying emotional problem. Recommending consultation with a psychiatrist makes the referring physician feel much better and shifts the responsibility to another physician. Many psychiatrists, however, are reluctant to diagnose or treat alcoholics for the same reasons as the rest of us.

Another compromise by referral occurs when the patient needs other forms of help: with employment, housing, planning for convalescence, or making contact with family members. The physician recommends that the patient see a social worker or clergyman. This avoids discussing the drinking problem yet offers the hope that a professional in another discipline will deal with it. If things go well, the doctor is vindicated. If things do not, at least the responsibility is shared. Meanwhile, the doctor/patient dialogue has been restricted to less threatening topics than the drinking problem.

Instead of pushing or pretending it away, we should be willing and able to diagnose alcoholism, but we must know enough about it to feel reasonably comfortable discussing it with our patients so we can convince them that this is indeed their problem. Sensible patients, alcoholic or otherwise, will not cooperate with treatment plans for a disease they don't think they have. Our attitude toward the patient, our knowledge about the disease, and our willingness to communicate candidly with the patient represent the initial requirement for motivating recovery.

FURTHER IMPEDIMENTS TO RECOGNITION

Once physicians are willing to recognize an alcoholic and once they are able to accept that the stereotype of what an alcoholic is like may be interfering with their abilities as diagnosticians, they are almost ready to find alcoholics.

One-line definitions of alcoholism are not really very helpful. Nor are demands for simplistic statements about etiology. With alcoholism, we are dealing with a disease of complex etiology where many factors—mental, physical, genetic, and environmental—all combine in one individual to make him fall victim.

Just as there is no single etiology for this illness, neither is there any one symptom that every alcoholic has or that only an alcoholic has. Sometimes what appears to be vagueness about definition or causality is used as an excuse for avoiding the treatment of the alcoholic patient. One senses the basic discomfort attached to making this diagnosis not only in the fruitless arguments about etiology that also serve as delaying tactics but also in the long theoretical discussions that concern themselves with the difficulty in diagnosing very early, subtle, and perhaps equivocal cases of alcoholism. Since there will be no shortage of obvious alcoholic patients once we are committed to finding them, we must address our attention initially to the easy-to-identify cases and move on to the more obscure ones as experience and diagnostic acumen improve.

Alcoholism is a progressive illness that in the majority of cases takes from 5 to 20 years to develop. Not only do physicians have to guard against reluctance to diagnose, but they must also become aware that they have been taught by social attitudes and tradition to think of alcoholism only in terms of its late stages. They are going to be uncertain and uncomfortable when faced with it in its early stages.

They may feel vaguely guilty, as if they are becoming prudish or judgmental, a kind of culturally induced ambivalence more likely to leave them indecisive than in the face of other addictions such as cigarette smoking or opiate abuse. Meanwhile, patients are likely to minimize their drinking. The classic statement by the recovered alcoholic patient looking back on early contacts with physicians, when the diagnosis might well have been made but was missed, is, "I didn't volunteer the facts and no one really asked." Dr. Stanley Gitlow has said, "Alcoholism is the disease that keeps telling the person who has it that he doesn't." Conscious of what they're doing or not, alcoholics don't want to hear their problem discussed, and because of fear, embarrassment, or some other reason they're not at all sure they want their doctor to know.

Most of us think about alcoholics in stereotypes: usually male, middle-aged, perhaps a bit shabby, certainly hedonistic and irresponsible on some level, often unemployed or in low-status jobs. The underlying assumption is that only a certain type of person becomes alcoholic. If doctors defer to this myth, they may not even consider the diagnosis in a young, attractive, wealthy, responsible career woman whose presenting complaint will include no mention of drinking, whose dress will be meticulous, and who is highly unlikely to smell of alcohol at her eleven a.m. appointment.

If alcoholics are viewed as somehow different from the rest of us, it will be doubly hard to recognize the illness in our patients, our colleagues, or in ourselves until it is far advanced.

DIAGNOSIS

Diagnosing alcoholism is basically the same as diagnosing pneumonia, except that it can be a lot more challenging. A disease may be conceptualized as a state of altered or diminished function. Although commonly related to aberrant physiology, biochemistry, or anatomy, its precise cause may be unknown. In the case of pneumonia, the infectious microorganism might be a common pharyngeal inhibitant that would not therefore represent the complete etiology in itself. The ultimate proof of diagnosis, the morbid anatomy, is obviously rarely demanded, but instead the clinician accepts a conglomerate of subjective and objective findings in order to establish a diagnosis sufficient to support rational therapy. The ultimate aim in formulating any diagnosis lies in the desire to restore function. To that end, the recognition and treatment of the patient with alcoholism parallels all other illness. Although alcoholism, especially in its early and uncomplicated form, may not offer the objective handle many clinicians prefer for diagnosis—elevated blood pressure, a pathogenic bacterium, elevated BUN, or Gaucher cells in the bone marrow—it is nonetheless readily recognized by a rather specific history and pattern of behavior. The accuracy and reliability of diagnosis, rarely achieving perfection in any branch of medicine, does not differ substantially in the case of alcoholism.

The patient's denial system, representing a major and frequent impediment in the diagnosis of alcoholism, is not peculiar to this disease alone. One might but consider cancer, tuberculosis, and venereal disease, a few others commonly minimized by suspicious patients. Fortunately, diagnosis of these illnesses is rarely complicated by a denial system within the physician as well.

It is crucial to realize that patients will not find it easy to give an accurate history; in fact, they may find this next to impossible. It may appear to the doctor that patients are deliberately lying. Perhaps they are, but usually they first lie to themselves. Therefore as they see it, they're telling their physician the simple truth. Noting the tremendous gap between what alcoholic patients report and the reality of their situations, it may seem incredible to the physician that patients can be so steadfast in their denials. If the physician is naive about alcoholism and uncertain about the diagnosis, the patients' unruffled airs of sincerity can often convince the unwary professional that he is the one who has the problem, that he is being unfair and overly suspicious, or that concerned friends and family are exaggerating reports of trouble.

Simply, one is looking for patients who repeatedly ingest a sedative drug (perhaps ethanol) despite their own definitive best interests. The diagnosis is inherent in the fact that the subject compulsively uses sedation (ethanol) despite its interference with job, home, health, or interpersonal relationships.

Diagnostic clues are available from history, physical examinations, and the laboratory. Certain signs will relate quite simply to alcohol itself, either because too much of it is present in the patient or because the patient shows signs of withdrawal from physical dependence on alcohol.

Simple drunkenness and alcoholism are not the same thing. One sign may be useful, however: alcoholics often demonstrate a very high tolerance to alcohol, particularly in the early years of their drinking. A male patient will often report this significant bit of history with actual pride, saying that after the unpredictable adolescent learning-to-drink experiences, he was the one who didn't get sick, didn't get drunk, didn't have hangovers, could take a tremendous amount of alcohol, "drink them all under the table and drive them all home." And he probably could. (Later, as the disease progresses, this early high tolerance will become unpredictable and then be lost, so that he eventually gets drunk on amounts that previously didn't affect him.)

The physician should be suspicious if a very high blood alcohol level—one that would normally result in serious impairment—is noted in a patient who continues to function well. For example, a recovered alcoholic physician recalls his drinking being questioned by a senior physician after a house staff party. Full of pride, the alcoholic countered that he'd been the only doctor to report on time the following morning, make rounds, tend to all his patients, and complete his charting. "True," said the senior man, "but that takes a lot of practice. Better think about it!"

Amount Patient Drinks

Asking alcoholic patients at the start of their interviews to declare exactly how many drinks they take, or in what form, places the doctor in an unnecessary power struggle. Since this is the very line of questioning that alcoholics expect and are prepared to resist, they are unlikely to give accurate answers.

We don't need a signed confession from our patients, nor arguments we cannot win—it only puts the patients on the defensive and makes them conceal the truth from the beginning. Just as we don't need to know the number of acid-fast bacilli in a person's lungs to diagnose tuberculosis, we don't need to know how many ounces a patient drinks to diagnose alcoholism.

The amount consumed is not nearly as important as the effect it has upon the drinker, whether the drink be vodka (under the misguided notion that vodka isn't detectable on the breath), whiskey, wine, or beer. Many an alcoholic will insist, however, that one "can't be an alcoholic on just beer." Look for the coexistence of alcohol and trouble, not for the amount consumed or the volume of fluid in which it is diluted.

Patterns of drinking (solitary, periodic loss of control) and attitudes (purposeful, medicinal) about it can be revealed when we take the patient's history. A change in style of response can yield a good clue, such as the patient who tells you the exact number of cigarettes smoked and cups of coffee drunk. If, however, when asked about alcohol, the same patient shifts from precise and quantitative answers to "I drink socially" or "I take a few," this should make you wonder why.

Avoid a change in your own style of questioning when shifting from such innocuous subjects as family history to that of ethanol ingestion. A joking tone or judgmental phrasing or inflection of your voice can close out any significant or truthful response by the patient. You may use, "Do you smoke or drink?" followed by, "How much?" "Do you have some every day?" or "Just on weekends or holidays?" or "More than one or two?" Integrate the drinking history with the less threatening discussion of other substances (coffee, cigarettes, etc.).

Withdrawal Symptoms

We can assume that by the time a patient is in full-blown delirium tremens, most physicians will know what is happening. However, other signs indicative of physical dependence are often overlooked or misunderstood.

A first grand mal seizure in an adult should always make us think of alcoholism, particularly if it occurs during the 72 hours following a marked reduction in drinking while the secondary hyperirritability that follows the initial depressant action of alcohol is still having its effect.

Another indication is intention tremor following a drinking bout, intensified if the patient is self-conscious. An example is the alcoholic trying to control his hands enough to sign his name while being watched.

Less obvious indications of alcohol withdrawal are mild hypertension, tachycardia, slight elevations in temperature, mild diaphoresis, and occasional atrial premature contractions. Laboratory work commonly will reveal an elevated blood glucose and a slightly subnormal BUN. If the patient also has an abnormally elevated SGOT, no matter how mild, that returns to normal almost at once after admission to a hospital (and cessation of drinking) and if, in addition, the patient diureses 1–2 kg (2–4 lb) in the first three hospital days while the initial minimal proteinuria and low BUN return to normal, this is strong evidence that alcohol in quantity has been present.

Although we have not yet done a formal study of this phenomenon, it is my impression that nearly half of the male Smithers Center Rehabilitation Unit patients have been told of hypertension or glucose intolerance and are often being medicated for these problems. After 28 days of abstinence, however, most show no evidence of hypertension (even under considerable emotional stress) or evidence of diabetes.

Personality Change

Seizures, tremors, and peripheral neuropathic and cerebellar signs are often reasons to refer alcoholics to neurologists. Less commonly, a patient's family reports a marked and sudden personality change during an evening's drinking and they wonder if this could be a form of epilepsy, especially since the patient had no previous history of this kind of behavior.

The change is usually from pleasant to extremely hostile, belligerent, even violent, or to helpless, whining, and maudlin. The behavior seems out of proportion to the amount of drinking observed by the family. In actuality, the alcoholic may be concealing the true extent of his drinking or combining alcohol ingestion with other sedatives. His own behavior is often frightening for the alcoholic, if descriptions of it are believed or if the altered behavior is remembered. The alcoholic has heard the phrase "in vino veritas" and is afraid of really being the nasty person who appears so unexpectedly.

Blackouts

Another frequent but little understood phenomenon is the "blackout." This must not in any way be confused with "passing out." The alcoholic blackout is a period of total amnesia in a drinking setting during which the drinker may or may not appear to others to be under the influence of alcohol.

Pilots have reported cross-country flights and surgeons successful operations during blackouts, yet they were not recognized by others as being impaired. The alcoholic's spouse frequently feels that the drinker remembers what happened but doesn't want to admit it. The psychiatrist assumes that the patient thought or did something guilty or anxiety-provoking during the blackout and now unconsciously refuses to remember it. The neurophysiologist speculates on reduced RNA synthesis when blood alcohol levels are high.

(I wonder if blackouts are a form of chemically induced retrograde amnesia caused by belated drinking in an individual episode. Perhaps the person who did not appear drunk to family or colleagues was in fact not drunk at the time but can't remember because of getting very drunk later.)

Occasionally nonalcoholics experience blackouts, particularly early in their drinking when learning by trial and error what they can tolerate. Most of us, however, were we to experience such a frightening event—a real period of time in which we walk and talk and make telephone calls and do business and park the car, yet cannot remember doing so—would go at once to a physician for an explanation.

Not so alcoholics, who sense that blackouts are part of their drinking, the part of life that they don't want too closely examined. They will adapt to blackouts, learning ways to cover up their occurrences, and will continue to drink in spite of them. This willingness to tolerate repeated blackouts as part of one's method of living rarely if ever occurs in the absence of alcoholism. The diagnostic clue, then, becomes the patient's equanimity in the face of repeated blackouts.

Physical Examination

People familiar with alcoholism notice physical signs without even touching or talking to the patient. Obvious characteristics can be spotted on the street or in a social situation.

I recall a medical seminar on the treatment of the public inebriate where one of the physicians present was obviously in trouble with alcohol himself. We all discussed the disease of alcoholism in the abstract, avoiding our colleague who was so clearly very ill and sat with shaking hands, slightly bloated and plethoric facies, telltale parotid swelling, and a Cushingoid look. (This facial resemblance to Cushing's disease, coupled with a story of personality change, hypertension, and glucose intolerance, has inspired many an eager house officer to start collecting 24-hour urine specimens or to order ACTH stimulation tests, while instead a waiting period for the patient of three to four days without alcohol might make all of these symptoms disappear.)

One might draw attention to another look-alike, that of the thyrotoxic. The tremulous, nervous, sweating patient with mild systolic hypertension, tachycardia, and an occasional arrhythmia who fails to reveal objective measurements of hyperthyroidism may simply reflect the hyperadrenergia associated with ethanol dependence.

Examination not only of an alcoholic's face but of the skin may yield other clues. The perifollicular hemorrhages on the inner thighs of a scorbutic derelict are discussed ad nauseam, but small bruises on the alcoholic housewife are far more common. When she drinks, she bumps into doorknobs and furniture; sometimes she falls. Her bruises are not usually massive ones, but they're found in different places and in variety of colors, depending on when they occurred.

Cigarette burns on fingers, chest, legs, or pajamas or nightgown may imply dependence on alcohol or other drugs.

Physical examination will also indicate whether or not other sedatives are involved. The patient using only alcohol can usually be roused from sleep by pain or by vigorous stimulation. However, if decubitus ulcers or blistered skin from remaining too long in one position are evident, it is wise to suspect other drugs.

Severe peridontal disease is another clue. Alcoholics as a group do not neglect physical or oral hygiene. Rather, in my experience, typical alcoholics are usually clean and neat, especially on visits to the doctor. They may frequently brush their teeth to disguise their breath, just as they take extra vitamins in hopes of protecting their livers. Nonetheless, Vincent's gingivitis and pyorrhea are, for reasons still not fully explained, common in alcoholics; teeth relatively free of caries are often lost while the patient is still fairly young.

Secondary Diseases

Every pathology textbook describes the physical complaints stemming from body systems damaged by long-term exposure to the small, toxic alcohol molecule itself. Although diseases secondary to chronic alcoholism were thought initially to result from malnutrition and alcohol toxicity, more and more they are revealed as inducible by alcohol alone. Lieber and Rubin demonstrated that alcohol itself can cause fatty liver and proximal myopathy in normal, well-nourished, vitamin-supplemented medical students[1-3] as well as actual cirrhosis in some primates.[4]

Alcoholism should be regarded as a probable cause or concomitant factor until proven otherwise in the following: cirrhosis, fatty liver, pancreatitis, initial grand mal seizure in an adult, and peripheral neuropathy. Less obvious alcoholism-related illnesses include antibiotic-resistant tuberculosis in an adult, carcinoma of the head and neck, and lung abscesses not related to malignancies. Significant impairment of the T cell immune system by alcohol was demonstrated by Lundy et al.[5]

Casual observations of abnormal liver functions (elevated SGOT, SGPT, GGTP, etc.), abnormal serum lipid profile (Fred. type IIA, IV, etc.), elevated serum uric acid, hyperglycemia, or hyperosmolality should raise the suspicion of alcoholism, although none of these findings is diagnostic per se. Similarly, an alcohol level in a bioligic aliquot should raise a diagnostic suspicion but cannot serve as proof unless it is extremely elevated in conjunction with a clinical state demonstrating tolerance. These biochemical measurements must be evaluated in conjunction with the clinical circumstances in order to establish the diagnosis of alcoholism. A blood alcohol level of 0.10 percent may establish drunkenness for purposes of motor vehicle operation but does not necessarily or absolutely make the medical diagnosis of alcoholism. Lieber and colleagues have developed a test of amino acid metabolism that may similarly indicate heavy or persistent ethanol ingestion, but it remains to be seen if it will successfully separate the chronic heavy social drinker from the alcoholic while still managing to detect the so-called "periodic" alcoholic. For more detailed laboratory data, see Appendix B, "Criteria for the Diagnosis of Alcoholism."

Detection in General Hospitals

Approximately 70 percent of all adult Americans are drinkers. Somewhere between 5 and 10 percent of these are or will become alcoholics, with the urban dweller and those at the two extremes of the educational ladder most at risk. Alcoholics, or patients whose illness is alcohol-related, occupy between 20 and 60 percent of the adult beds in acute general care hospitals. Careful studies bear this out even in hospitals not located in areas with heavy concentrations of alcoholics.

Just because alcoholism is diagnosed less in one specialty than in another does not mean that it is unusual in any group. The tendency to diagnose more alcoholism in ward areas than in private and semiprivate sections is misleading; it usually reflects physician attitudes and social expectations rather than reality.

More men than women are alcoholic (ratio of 3:1, approximately[6]), and since the disease is most common after the age of 30 years, alcoholism rates are usually low on obstetric floors and in adolescent units; however, both women and young people are showing an increase in alcoholism rates.

By contrast, thermal injury treatment units have many alcoholics. Unless there is preexisting nerve or vascular disease, stroke, or some other very clear-cut explanation, almost all freezing injuries will be found in alcoholics, particularly in urban populations.

Many fire deaths are alcohol-related. A study of third degree burns showed over 40 percent to be alcohol-related, usually women who fell asleep while smoking as well as drinking and using other sedative drugs.[7]

Trauma floors are excellent areas to seek alcoholics: victims of automobile and pedestrian accidents, falls, fights, private aircraft, snowmobile, home injuries, and drownings and near-drownings, particularly late afternoon boating accidents. Assaults in the home are common in conjunction with alcohol; thus we must consider alcoholism in an assaulted patient's spouse or in the parent of a battered child.

Psychiatrists often find alcoholics admitted for attempted suicide. Because many are in conflict with family members, it is important to find out if different perceptions of the patient's drinking pattern form a part of that conflict.

We must learn to ask about drinking behavior in a variety of settings. For example, suppose we note a chest film on display in an emergency room corridor x-ray viewing box. The film depicts a male with the mild degenerative bone changes of early middle age. If there is evidence of old rib fractures in different stages of healing and in different parts of the rib cage, one accident could not possibly account for them. Suppose there are signs of old tuberculosis and metal clips from old gastrointestinal surgery visible in the epigastrium. Here is a person with evidence of multiple traumatic episodes and a history of ulcers and tuberculosis, who uses a hospital emergency room rather than a private physician. The chances that this person is an alcoholic are excellent.

OBTAINING PATIENT'S HISTORY

While it may not be difficult to relate heavy drinking to a particular argument or injury, to a single episode of aspiration pneumonitis, or to an impulsive overdose, the confusion of cause and effect in chronic alcoholism may require deft questioning to untangle. Most alcoholics are as naive about their disease as their physicians. If we realize that this is a progressive illness that changes and develops through the years, we can begin by asking questions that do not seem particularly threatening.

What we are after is a story of alcohol use through time, as perceived by the patient himself or by those close to the patient. Understanding the epidemiology of alcoholism will prove useful. More fundamental is familiarity with the way in which the disease usually develops in an individual.

While there is still debate about the role of genetics in alcoholism, there is no question that this is a familial illness. If there is alcoholism in a patient's family, that patient is more at risk than if there is not. Less well known is the fact that 30 percent of the wives of alcoholic men will have had an alcoholic parent.[8] Since heavy drinking in young people shows a strong positive correlation with both peer group pressure and use of alcohol and other drugs by parents, a quick family history is certainly in order, including current and preceding generations.

This information is usually offered quite freely by the alcoholic. For example, a male alcoholic may relate a history of problem drinking in his parents' home to his own difficult childhood because it makes his own drinking understandable. His wife's family history may explain what he perceives as her unreasonably critical attitude toward his drinking. His son's use of drugs could be a worry that makes him likely to drink. With all of these woes, small wonder that the patient drinks, and small wonder that he appears anxious and depressed!

The physician's impulse is to respond with sympathy, understanding, and the offer of yet another mood-changing drug as a substitute for alcohol. Physician, stay thy hand! What if the boss complained, the wife left, the money went—and the child as well—because of the patient's drinking? What if the problem has been for years that this person seeks chemical answers to human problems? Is the answer really a change of drug?

Attitude of Physician

How much a patient is likely to admit will depend on the attitude of the questioner. A hostile, angry, or harried interviewer whose line of inquiry shows that he understands little or nothing of the patient's situation will not get far.

If, however, the questioner is knowledgeable, interested, comfortable, and nonjudgmental, he can often at the end of a thorough history-taking ask: "Do you feel you've been having a problem with your drinking?" He can then go on to: "Do you think you might be an alcoholic?" A surprising number of patients will answer "Yes," while many others will say, "Maybe a little bit," or, "I don't know. How do you tell?"

Sedative–Hypnotic Drugs

Personal history should include queries about use of other drugs to alleviate the tension or insomnia caused by alcohol. If, however, aware of self-prescribing in a way that might provoke criticism, the alcoholic may not give accurate answers.

A blunt question such as, "Do you take pills?" will often produce the same evasion as, "How much do you drink?" It is better to start by asking about the symptoms for which medication is likely to be used. Then ask if a doctor has ever been seen about these problems. Follow with a sympathetic, "And what did the doctor give you to help?" This will at least identify the drug, although generally not its quantity.

Many of us are unaware that alcohol is a member of a large family of sedative–hypnotic drugs. All of them act in much the same way. All can be substituted for one another, allowing for differences in strength and speed and duration of action.

This is an era of widespread use of sedatives and "minor" tranquilizers, potentially the cause of far more trouble than the so-called "major" tranquilizers (see Appendix A).

Many an alcoholic who would never drink in the morning or smell of alcohol at inappropriate times is drugged 24 hours a day by taking an alcohol substitute in tablet or capsule form. The subject may walk quite steadily, make reasonably good sense, and have no alcohol on the breath (although he probably takes extra care with mouth deodorants and gargles) and may appear to be fairly normal, particularly to someone who doesn't know him well or to someone who sees the alcoholic infrequently enough to be unaware of gradual change. The alcoholic may show a subtle decrease in mental alertness, personal sensitivity, and appropriateness of response; diction may seem more deliberate and careful, with extra spacing between words, and the alcoholic's eyes may lack sparkle.

Alcoholics are unaware that alcohol initially sedates while later heightening tension, irritability, mood swings, and insomnia. They assume that they drink to relieve these very things. If they decide to cut down on their drinking, or to cut it out, they may take tranquilizers or sedatives to deal with their discomfort. Tranquilizers or sedatives, however, usually produce the same symptoms that were caused by alcohol. Alcoholics will take them in gradually increasing amounts, either to supplement their drinking or, at times, in lieu of it. They are still chemically dependent alcoholics but now may use alcohol rarely if at all.

Women use minor tranquilizers and sedatives more often than men, although this probably reflects more frequent contacts with doctors, physician attitudes, and subsequent prescribing habits more than any intrinsic difference between the sexes.

(In my experience, patients who use illicit narcotics tend to exaggerate the amount they use, while patients obtaining pills from physicians or pharmacists usually minimize.)

It is my personal feeling that warning against the casual use of minor tranquilizers and sedatives is the single most important educational job to be done by those treating alcoholics today, since many alcoholics become dual addicts through well-meaning but uninformed physicians.

REASONS FOR DRINKING

Whether on a psychiatric floor, in a surgical area, or in the internist's private office, a hallmark of alcoholism is the use of alcohol as a mood-changing drug instead of as a beverage.

Patients reporting that they drink to calm nerves, to sleep, to give courage or confidence, to relieve anxiety or depression, or for nightcaps, are not social drinkers; they are self-medicating to alter feeling states. Patients often sense this and become uneasy, particularly if they are sneaking drinks.

Conflict with self or conflict with others around the use of alcohol is a sign of trouble. The patient can more easily acknowledge trouble than the fact of alcoholism.

Patients admitted to a psychiatric floor may actually prefer to be labeled mentally ill rather than alcoholic. There is less social stigma. Also, they hope that if they cooperate with treatment, gain insight, and engage in attempts to understand the reasons for their drinking, they may not have to abandon it.

They will therefore oblige with a history containing much that is accurate but featuring a reversal of cause and effect—stories of conflict with fellow workers, unreasonable employers, and lost jobs; divorce, separation, or conflict with spouse or lover; disappointment in children, who may be in trouble with drugs; tangled finances; a career that initially showed high promise but has inexplicably gone into a decline.

OBSESSION WITH ALCOHOL

As alcohol becomes increasingly important to alcoholics, it exerts a subtle influence on lifestyles. Alcoholics begin to avoid people and places that do not permit drinking. Freed from self-consciousness about their own alcohol consumption, they can then honestly report that they don't drink any more than their current friends. Questions that explore hobbies and activities may therefore be revealing, for alcoholics may be unaware that they have gradually selected their friends and activities for drinking purposes.

For example, a cellist who regularly plays chamber music with a group of European friends is far less likely to be an active alcoholic than is a jazz musician performing at resorts where drinking is an important part of the social scene and where performance is often rewarded with a bottle of whiskey.

As alcohol becomes more necessary and used more as a drug than a beverage, the drinker will start to feel uneasy about it. His discomfort will heighten when his behavior differs from that of peers. The drinker may need a drink before going to a party or may turn away from guests to take an extra drink, unobserved, in the kitchen. The alcoholic will usually down the first drink a little faster than do others present, feeling impatient at their leisurely pace.

The need for additional alcohol and the need to conceal that need provoke anxiety, discomfort, and rationalization. The drinker is no longer merely participating in a social custom with peers; he is a deviant.

Alcoholics may encourage others to drink more with them to conceal their need for increasing amounts.

CONTROLLED DRINKING

Alcoholics may decide to prove to themselves that they don't have drinking problems. They may try control by limiting themselves to wine or beer, to drinking only in certain places or at certain times, by substituting other drugs for all or part of their alcohol intake, or even by going on the wagon.

Most alcoholics are in some control of their drinking most of the time. Almost all can stop altogether for periods of time. What typical alcoholics find difficult is to drink limited amounts on a regular basis without at least periodically exceeding the amounts they planned to drink. They may find themselves getting drunk when they'd firmly decided that they wouldn't. They may stop drinking only to start again impulsively.

This means that the alcoholic is losing the ability to keep promises made privately to himself about drinking. Breaking promises made to other people is less significant, since the alcoholic may never have intended to keep them in the first place.

It is vital for the physician to realize that normal drinkers have no big problem controlling their drinking. When patients report that they regularly swear off drinking, or that they're trying a variety of maneuvers to regulate their intake, they're saying that they are already in trouble. Only alcoholics need to control alcohol intake.

RESISTING ABSTINENCE

An addiction, any addiction, should not be considered in terms of physical dependency alone, or only in the context of the patient's entire life situation being in a shambles. Instead, the strength of an addiction should be measured in terms of the amount of pressure a person is prepared to resist in lieu of relinquishing use of the drug.

A man or woman who is willing to live in constant conflict with the self or with others rather than stop drinking is in trouble. So is the person who is willing to give up physical health or a valued job rather than the bottle.

He or she has developed a new value system that no matter how it's rationalized indicates that freedom to drink is more important than health, work, and human relationships. This state of affairs is alcohol dependency—an integral part of the illness, whether or not the patient shows physical withdrawal symptoms.

It is also an uncomfortable situation for the patient, even though it may appear irresponsible, pleasurable, and hedonistic to an unsophisticated observer.

Denial

If abstinence is too painful for the patient to face, the way to avoid self-confrontation is obvious: deny the problem.

The patient reverses causal relationships by shifting the blame to someone or something else. Thus marital discord is not caused by drinking but becomes the reason for it. Dejection over the multiple problems caused by alcohol becomes the depression that one drinks to relieve. Insomnia and anxiety are not caused by withdrawal, but are the reasons why alcohol is needed to relax. An employer's prejudice explains failure to gain promotion. Alcohol provides a justified escape from a nagging spouse and mounting debts.

Since alcoholism is not usually seen by the patient or the doctor as a disease in its own right but is instead regarded as a symptom of something else, both parties may embark on a search for an explanation of the drinking.

Extreme care must be exercised that a quite valid effort to uncover the psychodynamics of the patient's illness does not result in an alliance aimed at supporting the patient's denial. The latter often results in continued although temporarily modified use of the addicting drug—to be followed at a later date by return to the full-blown expression of the disease.

The alcoholic patient has every motive to minimize or explain away his drinking and to deny it as a primary concern. It won't take long to find plausible excuses: virtually every adult human being has a set of present problems and a history of at least one or two genuine tragedies. If the physician joins the patient in explaining away the illness, the patient may be lost.

Most people, however, face painful life situations without turning to chemical solutions to the degree that the solution becomes a problem in its own right. Only with some effort can the physician establish that heavy drinking actually preceded most of the events presented as having caused it.

A history of accidents or injuries is usually not too hard to elicit. It pays to ask if there had been drinking at the time of traumatic episodes. We don't need a confession that the patient was actually drunk or how much was consumed—enough that alcohol and trouble are occurring together.

DENIAL BY FAMILY

Denial is not the exclusive property of the alcoholic. Spouses and children cover up for their alcoholics. They worry that medical reports may get back to employers or that the alcoholic may view them as disloyal or be angry if they divulge too much.

The family unit may present a deceptively normal exterior to the world, closing protectively around the alcoholism that is destroying it. I am repeatedly surprised by the ability of alcoholic families to preserve a facade that when it finally crumbles has concealed a truly agonizing situation for all concerned. The fear of change and of exposure evidently outweigh the pain of continuing to live with the familiar.

If the alcoholic has accused family members of being the cause of his drinking, repeatedly cataloguing their inadequacies, they will feel entirely culpable. Also, they may believe in stereotypes about families: the understanding wife and the virile husband supposedly have contented marriage partners, not rejection through alcoholism. The truth is an admission of failure.

Sometimes alcoholism will present not in the person of the alcoholic but as part of the illness of the spouse. If we make a habit of searching beyond the identified patient for clues to illness and puzzling behavior in the surrounding environment, a casual mention that a spouse drinks a lot may take on diagnostic significance.

For example, wives of alcoholics may be reluctant to accept a needed hospitalization for fear of what might happen at home if they aren't there to protect the children. They may request that no visitors be permitted so that the alcoholic can't arrive drunk and make an embarrassing display. They may receive constant phone calls from home.

As outpatients, spouses of alcoholics are often nervous, upset, and likely to request tranquilizers or sedatives for themselves. Symptoms may be vague, responding poorly to treatment. They cannot follow instructions to rest, or avoid stress, if the home is in a state of constant chaos, nor can they buy prescribed medicine if the paycheck is spent in the bar rather than at the drug or grocery store.

SOBER ALCOHOLIC/PHYSICIAN RELATIONSHIP

Successfully sober alcoholics report that many doctors refuse to believe they are alcoholics.

Perhaps for the physician the subject doesn't look like an alcoholic. He isn't drinking. He's likely to be a member of Alcoholics Anonymous, whose members urge each other to inform their physicians about their alcoholism. He is doing just that, hoping for understanding, encouragement, and, more importantly, that the physician will never prescribe alcohol-containing medicines or inappropriate mood-changing drugs.

Too often this patient discovers that the doctor is uncomfortable with the entire subject, however. The doctor may even argue that the patient can't really be an alcoholic—that he was probably talked into this by ill-advised and possibly fanatic friends. If the patient is still fragile in his new-found sobriety and ambivalent about the need to remain abstinent, the naive white-coated authority's observations can result in disaster.

If patients say they are alcoholics, believe them.

To diagnose and to recognize alcoholism, then, requires us to suspect it not only in our patients but also as the reason behind unexplained illness in others. It can be seen by the sophisticated observer in social settings and in friends and colleagues as well as in those labeled as ill. It affects directly 1 out of every 20 adults and indirectly easily twice as many more. Although the urban dweller and those at the two extremes of the education ladder are most at risk, no population of drinkers is exempt. This chapter has mentioned some clues to making that diagnosis. There are many more. The National Council on Alcoholism has collected and set down in tabular form many of them in an interesting attempt to establish more precise criteria for diagnosis[9] (see Appendix B).

Alcoholism will remain invisible unless and until one is able to become willing to see it. As this occurs, the physician will become aware that much that was formerly puzzling becomes explainable and obvious. Simple truths are too threatening to be heard easily. Our society is too uncomfortable and too ambivalent about drinking for mere facts to be convincing. The scars left by prohibition were deep.

The fanaticism of wet versus dry still stirs unpleasant feelings.

To search one's own feelings and attitudes and to examine one's own drinking and that of others is hard and not always pleasant work. When that is done, one is comfortable with one's own choice to drink or to abstain in a drinking world. One can differentiate between the disastrous drinking of the alcoholic, the moderate use of alcohol in appropriate social settings, and the often excessive and irresponsible behavior of the heavy drinker. When our inner ambivalence is resolved, we can then speak clearly and comfortably about alcohol with our patients.

REFERENCES

1. Rubin E, Lieber CS: Alcohol-induced hepatic injury in non-alcoholic volunteers. *N Engl J Med* 278: 869–876, 1968
2. Lieber CS: Liver adaptation and injury in alcoholism. *N Engl J Med* 288: 356–362, 1973
3. Song P, Rubin E: Ethanol produces muscle damage in human volunteers. *Science* 175: 327–328, 1972
4. Lieber CS, DeCarli L, Rubin E: Sequential production of fatty liver, hepatitis, and cirrhosis in subhuman primates fed ethanol with adequate diets. *Proc Natl Acad Sci USA* 72: 437–441, 1975
5. Lundy J, Raaf JH, Deakins S, et al: The acute and chronic effects of alcohol on the human immune system. *Surg Gynecol Obstet* 141: 212–218, 1975
6. Cahalan D, Cisin IH, Crossley HM: *American Drinking Practices: A National Study of Drinking Behavior and Attitudes*. New Brunswick N. J., Rutgers Center of Alcohol Studies, 1969, p 260
7. MacArthur JD, Moore FD: Epidemiology of burns, the burn-prone patient. *JAMA* 231: 259–263, 1975
8. Bullock SC, Mudd EH: Interrelatedness of alcoholism and marital conflict. *Am J Orthopsychiatry* 29: 519–527,1959
9. National Council on Alcoholism: Criteria for the diagnosis of alcoholism. *Ann Intern Med* 77: 249–258, 1972.

BIBLIOGRAPHY

Diagnostic and Statistical Manual of Mental Disorders, Third Edition-Revised (DSM-111-R). American Pychiatric Association, Wash., D.C., 1987

3

Motivating the Alcoholic Patient

Marvin A. Block

Having diagnosed the patient's alcoholism, the physician must now present the problem to the patient. If the physician in charge is a specialist in the field to whom the patient had been referred by a another physician, the problem is comparatively simple. When patients are aware of their illness or have been diagnosed as alcoholic by their own physicians, or when they have full knowledge that the physician to whom they have been referred specializes in the field of alcoholism, there is apparently some recognition on their part that they have the problem. This does not necessarily mean, of course, that such patients are well motivated. What it does mean, at least, is that the subject of alcoholism has already been introduced and that the patients might be prepared to discuss it further. Some patients may be inclined to deny the existence of the problem in their cases—as a defense against a possible diagnosis to that effect—but at least the first step has been taken. For the generalist, or for the physician who first suspects alcoholism, particularly if the patient has presented for any one of a number of other reasons, the problem of motivation is often greater.

It is important to remember that it is in the course of the history-taking and the reviewing of the diagnostic considerations that the motivation—particularly the early motivation—of the patient is determined. As the physician takes the history, he will be observing the patient's existing motivations as to the drinking problem and also will be looking for areas that will aid in further discussions with the patient. Motivating the patient is determined to a greater degree by what is going wrong with the patient's life due to alcohol and the other sedatives. The patient may have, for example, physical difficulties or disturbances at home and in inter-

ALCOHOLISM:
A Practical Treatment Guide
ISBN 0-8089-1912-1

personal relationships, or perhaps problems functioning at work. While taking the history and determining the diagnosis, the physician must keep in mind the following questions: What is it that the patient wants in life, in the way of thinking or doing or receiving? How is that interfered with by the alcohol? It is this leverage that the doctor will use when embarking upon the process of getting the patient to see what is wrong and what must be done about it.

Each patient is an individual, and the approach to his illness must be eclectic. What constitutes excessive drinking for one patient may not for another. Necessarily to be taken into account are the patient's age, weight, mental stability, background, social environment, and various other specifics to which his individual life is tied. It must also be at all times borne in mind that the early stages of alcoholism are extremely difficult to pinpoint and that the definitions and classifications of the disease covered by the term are spread over a wide range of drinking patterns.

It is not always the best technique to make a definitive diagnosis at the first consultation. Only if patients have already been told that they have drinking problems—or that their use of alcoholic beverages has awakened suspicion—is immediate diagnosis even advisable. More than one session may be required for the physician to reach a warranted conclusion. Also, it isn't always easy to get a patient to accept a positive diagnosis without protest.

Unfortunately, there is still attached to the term *alcoholism* a kind of stigma that makes mere mention of it repugnant to patients as a whole. The terms *alcohol dependence* or *problem drinking* appear to be far more acceptable to the average patient, at least during early interviews. It should be noted that some people might feel this to be ducking the issue, and they would urge quick confrontation with the use of the word *alcoholism*. It is a matter of one's own strategy and technique, but many workers in the field have found it useful not to confront people at once in such a manner that might cause them to run away. Patients must often be prepared more slowly to face the issue.

EARLY RECOGNITION BY THE PHYSICIAN

Few persons come to the specialist in the incipient or early stages of alcoholism. Most appear at a time, later on, when a correct diagnosis can be made by almost anyone—by family members in particular. Generalists are nevertheless in a position to uncover alcoholism in its very earliest stages—provided they take time to elicit accurate histories from their patients regardless of the reason given for seeking medical help. Many incipient alcoholics are missed because physicians fail to develop full or accurate enough histories. There are no early physical signs of alcoholism, and the diagnosis in most cases depends upon careful history-taking. Where such symptoms as gastric distress, headaches, gastrointestinal disorders, lack of appetite, insomnia, depression, etc., are present, alcoholism should be at least suspected as a possible cause. Again, where other signs or symptoms of toxicity are manifested or are complained of by patients, careful and extensive histories must be taken. Many early alcoholics volunteer no signs or symptoms that can be effectively diagnosed. Thus only a detailed history will provide the needed indications if these exist.

Many questions have been designed to expose the early stages of alcoholism. Some that have been in use for several years, effective as they may be in revealing later stages of the disease, do nothing to help unearth its beginning stages.

Such questions as the following have been used in the belief that affirmative answers would point to the existence of incipient alcoholism:

1. Does the subject drink to calm his nerves or to sedate himself?
2. Does he become increasingly irritable while drinking?
3. Does he frequently drink until he becomes quite drunk?
4. Does he drink a steadily increasing amount of alcohol?
5. Does he hide his source of alcohol?
6. Does he lie about his drinking?
7. Does he take a drink the first thing in the morning?
8. Does he miss work or shirk his duties because of drinking?
9. Does he neglect his family?
10. Does he experience periods of blackout or amnesia?
11. Has he been hospitalized for drinking?
12. Has he lost his job because of drinking?

Recent studies suggest, however, that the information developed through use of the above questionnaire relates to the later, rather than the earlier, stages of alcohol dependence. It is now recognized that such questions as the following are better geared to the search for signs of incipient alcoholism:

1. Is the *desire* for a drink a frequent occurrence, the key word being "desire?"
2. Is there a *need* for a drink at a certain time of the day, the emphasis on "need?"
3. Is there anticipation of drinking in the evening, as the day wears on?
4. Is alcohol used to induce sleep?
5. Does frequent drinking go *beyond* ritual socializing?
6. Is there a desire to get *high* and to maintain that feeling through drinking?
7. Does the absence of drinks at a restaurant or party produce *disappointment*?
8. Is the patient's drinking *criticized* by a friend or anyone who cares?
9. Does the subject resort to a drink to relieve discomfort or tension of any kind?
10. Does the care taken to keep a supply of alcohol *on hand* "just in case" sometimes amount to more than a modest consideration?
11. Is there a tendency to prefer the companionship of those who exhibit a drinking pattern similar to one's own and to *shun* as far as possible the society of nondrinkers?

12. Does the subject resent the remarks of others concerning his drinking habits?

Helpful as the above questionnaire might be, negative answers can nevertheless be misleading, but recognition of an early problem with alcohol cannot but follow from the display of any adverse effect whatsoever following the ingestion of alcoholic drinks. This is a more broadly recognized definition—a more reliable clue—in that it exposes not only physical and psychological symptoms of disorder but those of social involvement as well. Should the ingestion of alcoholic beverages, however, result in a sociologic problem, family disruptions, or serious arguments of any kind—particularly at home or at work—this could well point to an alcohol-related problem. If in such a situation a more temperate drinking pattern is not swiftly established, failure to cut down or stop the use of alcohol would be a strong indication of a developing drinking problem and a sign of the incipient disease.

Again, the point of reviewing this diagnostic information is that as each issue is examined to determine the diagnosis, one is also determining the motivational approach. For example, the patient who is suffering from gastritis and complains vigorously about inability to tolerate the symptoms invites one to discuss the alcoholic etiology of the disorder. Again, if the patient uses alcohol to calm nervousness or to relieve psychological symptoms, it would be in order to point out that the addiction may conceivably help temporarily or initially but that very soon the alcohol will result only in increased agitation requiring more alcohol (in the morning, for instance) to relieve that. Indeed, much of the agitation may be due to the alcohol and will be relieved merely by detoxification.

It could further be pointed out how alcohol interferes with social life, sexual functioning, or work and career, or how it encourages the development of character traits such as resentment, argumentiveness, lying, deception, neglect, or irritability toward people who are needed, worked with, or held dear. All this could be done while the physician is going through the above questions. Perhaps the subject has lost the companionship of friends he liked, or the esteem of others he has respected, or perhaps he has caused difficulties at home.

As one goes into the second set of questions particularly, one can also bring out to patients the progression of the degree of dependency on alcohol and get them to appreciate how much control over themselves and their lives they have lost or are in the process of losing.

RECOGNITION BY FAMILY AND FRIENDS

It is a well-known fact that the alcoholic is the last person to recognize his illness. Family members are sure to become aware that a person is drinking to excess long before the patient himself faces up to that fact. Patients may deny it, of course, quite as almost every person is likely to deny being drunk when a lack of sobriety is obvious to others. A longer period may be required for an employer to recognize an employee's excessive drinking, mainly because contact between the two may be limited to working hours, during which the worker may be careful not to expose a proclivity to alcohol. But immediate families, seeing alcoholics at close range when their guards are down, are sure to detect their drinking patterns long before anyone else. When those who live with and care for alcoholics seek help, it is often because the alcoholics themselves will do nothing about their problems; they may not even be aware of them. This does not necessarily mean that nothing can be done. If a patient refuses to see the physician when begged or advised to do so, the next best thing is for the doctor to interview the drinker's spouse.

It is possible that one may involve other significant persons—co-workers, relatives, friends—if patients somehow conceal their alcoholism at home and reveal it elsewhere—at work, in other social situations, etc. If the spouse is ignorant or negative and obstructionistic, one may derive from such people the data needed to confront the patients with their illness or other inadequate coping mechanisms. Usually, however, the spouse is the most useful person to involve at this point, since there may be, despite the patient's denial, threats to job and career that one may learn only from the spouse. The alcoholic might, for example, be in danger of losing his auto license, or the marriage might be imperiled, or sexual functioning might be impaired, yet he denies or minimizes it. Thus the doctor may have to involve a parent, a sibling, a co-worker, a superior, a lover, or a friend; but the most important person in the overwhelming majority of instances is the spouse.

Not only may the spouse represent one of the most important factors both in the diagnosis and in the patient's motivation to recover from alcoholism, but the spouse may even represent an etiologic factor in the disease. Often enough an alcoholic's spouse misjudges the situation and wrongly assumes that the patient drinks excessively from sheer perversity. Overlooked is the fact that a serious progressive disease is involved and that the drinking is anything but misbehavior whose purpose is to agitate and annoy. Often the alcoholic partner is suffering from a mental problem or depression and resorts to the sedative of alcohol in order to mask an underlying psychological illness. In other instances, the alcoholic husband or wife may find in this readily available and socially acceptable drug a means of making life more tolerable when problems are too difficult with which to cope. Once the nonalcoholic spouse has had these conditions explained, an attitude of whining and nagging irritation may well give way to one of sympathetic understanding.

PHYSICAL EXAMINATION

Having taken a complete history, the physician has now come to the conclusion that the patient might have a drinking problem. A complete physical examination is now in order. Such a physical examination will rarely reveal any abnormalities related to excessive alcohol ingestion unless the problem of drinking has been of long duration. When overt physical manifestations are apparent, such as enlargement of the liver, evidence of capillary dilatation around the areas of the nose and cheeks, inflammation of the larynx, excessive palmar erythema, or other signs of long-standing alcohol ingestion, one can suspect alcoholism in its rather late stages. Laboratory procedures must be completed in order to determine if there have been any other ill effects from the ingestion of alcohol. A complete liver study and x-rays of the gastrointestinal tract may be indicated. Again, these findings supply useful information for discussion with and for motivation of the patient to give up alcohol for the sake of physical well-being. The implications of the laboratory data and the results of physical examinations must be pointed out to the patient.

It is important to note that the usefulness of the different areas where alcoholism is causing difficulties varies considerably. One person may not at all be moved—for whatever reasons—by the physical harm experienced but may be moved instead by the fear of loss of the spouse. Another may not be fearful of that but may respond to threats to a career. This why no overly simple "cookbook" approaches suffices. One must try here and there, feeling out the patient and getting to know him, and then try whatever tack proves most fruitful.

DENIAL OF ALCOHOLISM

Where such positive evidence of alcoholism does not exist, however (and this occurs in the majority of early cases), the patient may not readily accept the diagnosis of alcoholism as made by the physician. Since denial is a characteristic of patients suffering from alcoholism, they may refuse to admit that they have lost control of their drinking and insist that they "can take it or leave it," even though they may admit readily that they have been drinking too much. They are sure they can control their drinking and reduce the amount to what is known as social drinking—a drink or two per day. Under these circumstances, a physician is confronted with the problem of motivating patients to cease ingestion of alcohol altogether, as is the wise decision indicated for any case of alcoholism. How does one convince the patient, however?

One approach is to question patients for their definitions of an alcoholic. Most often patients will describe an advanced case—the skid-row bum or the public inebriate. There is general agreement that such a case is definitely alcoholism. "Do you think he was born that way?" is a good question to ask. Without exception, patients will agree that he was not. "What do you suppose he was like ten years before you describe it?" The patient will describe a less severe case. "What about five years before that?" The description becomes less definite. The picture is now not quite as positive. By gradually going back into the development of the disease from its late stage, easily recognized, to its earlier stage, not so easily recognized, patients begin to see that their own patterns of drinking could be forerunners, if not actually early stages, of alcoholism—portrayed so definitely by the skid-row alcoholic. This technique has awakened many patients to the fact that the early stages of alcoholism are not as easily apparent but that they could develop into the full-blown disease that is so obvious at the late stage.

Where denial is still present, it is often wise to suggest to patients that tests be made of their ability to control their drinking. Such tests may be to take no more than two drinks per day and no less than one drink per day. A 3-week test of this procedure will often be very enlightening. The importance of being honest in this test must be explained, and if it is presented in a nonjudgmental way, it will usually produce the desired cooperation.

After 3 weeks of such a test have passed and the patient comes in to report on the experiment, it is usually found that on one or two occasions, or perhaps more, he has exceeded the quota that was agreed upon. Any number of excuses may be given for the breach. Nevertheless, the patient must recognize that the test has failed, since the agreed upon amount was not adhered to. This in itself will sometimes shake a patient's confidence about controlling drinking. Rationalization under these circumstances is extremely common, and patients may want to be tested again. By sheer willpower, such patients are often able to control their drinking as suggested. Over a period of time, however, the alcoholic, regardless of the stage in which he is found, will usually be unable to control drinking and will have to admit over a period of time to going beyond the agreed-upon amount.

Even though the term *alcoholism* is used and patients may admit it is possible that they are alcoholics, it does not necessarily mean that they are willing to accept abstinence. They often will intellectually accept the fact that they are suffering from alcoholism, but emotionally it is very difficult for them to do so, and on occasion they may test themselves to prove that they are not alcoholic. The test consists of taking one drink and not drinking any more. Having done this on several occasions, patients will be convinced that they are not alcoholics. It is only a matter of time until they begin to drink excessively again. This can be spelled out to patients in advance if the therapist wishes to do so. On the other hand, over a period of time, in reporting to the physician patients may often discover these things for themselves.

If one has convinced the patient that he is alcoholic, and this may take some time to do, the patient's desire to stop drinking must be tested. Often such patients will profess their desire to stop drinking after having been convinced that they are suffering from alcoholism but will quibble about the necessity for complete abstinence. Since alcohol is an addictive drug and alcoholism is a true addiction, it must be explained to such patients that as with any other addiction the drug to which an individual is addicted cannot be used with impunity. Eventually the patient will return to the excessive use of the drug. This is the story of every addict who attempts to use his drug moderately.

Each patient feels that his case is different and he, unlike the others, will succeed in drinking occasionally without drinking excessively. When asked why it is worth taking the risk, the patient will give any number of answers, not the least common of which is feeling uncomfortable in the presence of others who drink when he does not. Such patients feel that they are being isolated from the group and that failure to drink with others is a point of notice by them. Their wish is to drink the way others drink, a drink or two, which would be satisfactory.

Upon careful questioning, however, as to whether or not one or two drinks would be sufficient, the alcoholic patient will usually admit that one or two drinks will not result in the desired effect and that the object in drinking at all is to attain a desired state regardless of the number of drinks it takes to obtain that state.

This is the alcoholic's objective in drinking. Alcoholics do not drink for social purposes, although this is what they prefer to believe. They actually drink for drug effect, and if carefully questioned they will admit this. They must therefore drink enough to get this effect. With the alcoholic, even in the early stages, this amount is usually more than the average drinker requires. The patient will generally recognize this fact once pointed out. It is apparent from past history that the desired state is not achieved by one or two drinks and that to cease after one or two drinks is something that the patient cannot do reliably. Such discussion often illustrates to the patient the fallacy of rationalizing.

DISULFIRAM

How do we evaluate the motivation of the patient who, at that point, professes willingness to accept abstinence? Here is one place where the use of disulfiram (Antabuse) may serve a distinct purpose. Patients are offered the pills with the warning that if they have consumed anything with alcohol in it in the previous 24 hours it would be unwise to take these pills, since they might become severely ill. Many patients who come to the physician with the express desire to stop drinking will demur when offered the pill, even though they have told the therapist that they have had nothing to drink for several days. Upon being presented with the pill, however, and admonished about not taking it if they have drunk in the previous 24 hours, they will admit to having had a drink or two very recently. This again is one way of determining the motivation of the patient as well as the patient's honesty.

Some patients who profess a desire to stop drinking and are then offered the pill will give any number of reasons why they do not want to take the pill immediately or feel that taking it is unnecessary and that they do not wish to use a "crutch," which the pill represents. Having professed a desire to stop drinking and having been offered a method of preventing drinking over a period of time, practically guaranteeing abstinence, and their refusing such an offer, they will often have proven to themselves that the professed motivation is not sincere. Many patients, after having refused the disulfiram (Antabuse) and had this brought to their attention, will reconsider their original statements of the desire to stop drinking and recognize the insincerity of those statements. After thinking about it for several minutes, some of these patients who are truly well motivated will change their attitude and accept the use of disulfiram (Antabuse). Such a test has proven to be very valuable in changing the minds of many individuals when they discover that their original intentions were not honest. Confronted with the evidence of the frequency of the problem and the necessity for doing something about it, they often change their minds and accept the drug as a method of attaining abstinence (see Appendix D).

APPROACHES TO MOTIVATION

Some of the patients are indeed quite ambivalent. They would like to stop drinking, but other forces within them push them to continue—physiological, psychological, social factors. Thus they may be driven to deny, to minimize, or even to defend the alcohol use so as not to have to come to terms with the decision they must ultimately make to give it up. This denial and minimizing must be confronted.

Convinced that the patient before me is alcoholic and detecting in that patient a hesitation concerning the diagnosis, I have found certain procedures very valuable. If the patient has a child ranging from 6 to 10 years old, they are more effective. If there is no such child, I usually present the patient with a hypothetical problem. "Supposing you had a 6-year-old child who is found to have juvenile diabetes, a very serious condition, as I am sure you know. How would you go about convincing your 6-year-old child that he can go to all the birthday parties with the other children but must not eat the candy, the cake, or the ice cream that all the other children can have? Your child looks at you and says, 'Why not?' and you answer that he has been found to have a serious illness requiring that he refrain from having these 'goodies' of which he is so fond. Your child looks at you and asks, 'Who says I have this illness?' You reply, 'the doctor.' 'The doctor doesn't know what he is talking about. I feel fine, there is nothing the matter with me, and I like candy and cake and ice cream,' the child replies, with what seems to him perfect justification.

"How," I ask the patient, "would you go about training the child to desist from eating those things that he must not have?"

As a rule, a kind of perturbed look comes over the face of the patient, and by far the vast majority will answer, "I don't know, I don't know what I would do." I then respond to that by saying, "You know it must be done for the child's sake and for his health and his life. How would you go about it?" Again, the patient looks at me and answers, "I don't know what I would do." I look straight at the patient and say, "This is the job I have with you. You must believe that my diagnosis is made with the utmost sincerity and for your benefit. You must take my word for it that abstinence is the only answer to your problem, and to learn to live without alcohol is your job. My job is to teach you that." It is astounding how this technique will affect the patient. For the first time the alcoholic recognizes what the problem is, how difficult it is to explain to the patient, and what must be done. I have found this approach very effective.

Another situation with which I have been confronted on many occasions is the patient in whom the diagnosis of alcoholism has been made and who feels that he cannot stop drinking completely. On so many occasions patients suffering from alcoholism do not wish to abstain but wish to be able to drink on occasion, infrequently in most instances, when they feel the overwhelming desire to have a drink or when they feel that abstinence would mark them as alcoholics among other drinkers who are not so afflicted. Since alcohol is an addictive drug, most in the field agree that attempting to accomplish this feat of an occasional drink will lead only to disaster over a period of time. It is possibly true that certain individuals might be able to take a drink now and then and by sheer willpower refuse to drink more. However, in the long run, particularly when they find that one drink has not produced any severe adverse effects and does not immediately lead to excessive drinking, the occasional drink becomes more amd more frequent until the patients are back in the pattern that originally brought them to their alcoholic conditions. To many such patients, the idea of not being able to drink at all represents a horrible prospect. After some discussion of this situation, my usual statement to them is, "I could take you to any hospital in this city, and to any bed in that hospital, and there isn't a patient in that hospital who would not trade places with you if all he had to do were to give up drinking in order to achieve a recovery." Almost without exception, the patients will admit that this could very well be true. Then I add, "Here you have an illness that has an answer. All you must do is sacrifice alcohol. Is that too great a sacrifice to retain or regain your health?" I have had only one exception to the affirmative response. That 33-year-old man stated that he would rather live only to 58 and drink than to achieve the accepted three score and ten years alloted to us if had to sacrifice his drinking. At 33, he thought he could take that risk. Unfortunately, he did not stop drinking, and his life ended at 41. I often cite this to my patients as an example of what alcohol can do to the person who refuses to recognize its dangers, particularly after a diagnosis of alcoholism has been made.

Another common problem that I have encountered stems from patients who ask, "Why me? What have I done to deserve this?" I responded by calling to the attention of the patient the fact than anyone who contracts a disease of any kind asks, "Why me?" I then add, "Do we have a choice as to what disease we may have? Illnesses occur in people without their asking for them and without their choice of illness. The mark of maturity is to accept these problems as they come and meet them in the best possible way. No matter what the illness, whatever must be done to recover from it must be followed through with conscientiousness and it will usually result in success. For those who continually repeat the question "why me," I refer them to the book by Bill Gargan with the title *Why Me?* Bill Gargan had a laryngectomy for cancer. For years, he went about the world lecturing on the subject and teaching people who had similar conditions to learn how to speak with the air swallowed into the stomach and expelled through the esophagus. *Why Me?* has been an inspiration to many people afflicted not only with cancer but with other serious diseases as well.

Speaking of cancer, I have used this as well as other diseases to induce people with alcoholism to refrain from drinking. "If you were to have a cancer in your body that I assured you would never get any worse if you ceased to drink alcohol, but if the cancer would continue to grow if you continued to use alcohol, would you give up drinking?" Without exception, under these conditions, even the most reluctant patients have stated that they would give up drinking. I then draw the similarity between the progressive disease that cancer represents and the progressive disease that alcoholism represents. This also clarifies for the alcoholic patient certain inevitabilities if the proper steps are not taken to control the illness.

I also compare the severe diabetic patient with the alcoholic patient. Each of such patients must refrain from ingesting the materials enjoyed. On occasion, a well-informed patient will challenge me with the fact that insulin may be used for diabetics, whereby they can continue to eat the various foods that they enjoy without any particular harm. My response to that is, "If it were possible for us to produce a drug that would neutralize the effect of alcohol so that it would not be harmful and would not produce the effects that alcohol does in the body, would you then be satisified to use alcohol under those conditions? Bear in mind that you would feel no effect of the drug at all. It would just be a matter of swallowing the alcoholic beverage with no effect to be felt." After giving some thought to that statement, the patients will usually look up at me in consternation and say, "There would be no point in drinking under those circumstances." "Exactly," I reply. "This calls to your attention the fact that it is the drug effect for which you are looking, and it is the drug effect that makes you the alcoholic who requires that drug effect." I also use this procedure in discussing the problem with those who insist that they drink because they enjoy the taste—also a rationalization in most cases.

There are many such approaches toward motivating individuals to stop drinking. However, for the most part, patients will not respond properly unless they themselves can see the damage that the alcohol has produced. In severe cases—where cirrhosis of the liver has produced hemorrhage from the varicosities at the base of the esophagus, or where edema is the result of that cirrhosis—there is no doubt that patients are aware of the effects of excessive drinking. Even among such patients, however, I have found those who were not convinced that they were alcoholic. Many of these patients are self-destructive in their tendencies and—regardless of any reasoning or logic being used—are bent upon destroying themselves. Such patients—and very often these represent cases of depression—require deep psychiatric therapy to relieve their conditions. For the most part, however, if the patient has any intelligence to which to appeal, many of the discussions that I have described will bring about the proper motivation for abstinence.

Even with success in achieving abstinence for many patients, it must be borne in mind that slips will occur. This does not necessarily spell failure, since slips can be used advantageously as a lesson when applied properly. It is human for people to begin to doubt the diagnosis when after a period of abstinence they feel no particular desire to drink. Curiosity is then aroused as to what a drink might do. Many believe that it is impossible that they cannot take one drink and stop. This conflict in their own minds as time goes on—whether or not they are alcoholic, particularly when they have no desire to drink—continually haunts them. "What kind of an alcoholic can I be if I don't even feel like having a drink? That can't be alcoholism. Alcoholics are supposed to crave drink. I not only do not crave it, I don't even desire it. How can I be alcoholic?" They mull this over in their minds week after week until they feel they cannot go on without making sure that they either are or are not alcoholic. "How do I prove it? Simple—I take a drink. If I continue to drink after that, there'll be no doubt about the alcoholism and I must stop forever." Thus the conflict and argument in their minds goes on until at last they decide they must experiment. And so they do. "Take a drink, and nothing happens. Well, now I feel much better. There you are—I took a drink, I didn't continue drinking. I don't even want another drink."

The following week the same temptation returns and the experiment might be repeated. No harm, no continued drinking. The following week, the same thing. "Well, now, I'm normal just like anyone else. I can take a drink now and then and that's all." And so they take the drink now and then, but the now and then becomes more and more frequent, until they are drinking on a daily basis. Now it is Bill's birthday. "Let's have another drink." "Not me, I'm a one-drink man." "Oh, come on, don't be a spoilsport, have another drink." The thought runs through the "exalcoholic's" mind, "I've had not more than one drink every day for weeks now; I'm not going to make a habit of this, but on an occasion like this, a second drink is not going to hurt me." Thus such people yield to the temptation and take another drink. Nothing happens. The next time a special occasion arises for a second drink—why not? "I did it a few weeks ago—nothing terrible." Thus again the occasion is repeated. Two drinks, and then back to one drink the following day. The two-drink occasions arise more frequently, however. Now the patient is taking two drinks a day. It is only a matter of time before the original condition of excessive drinking returns.

I have repeated this story to numerous patients, all of whom looked at me and said, "I have been through that several times." We then go back and go over the ground again. It is these approaches, these discussions that can motivate patients not only to believe that your interest in them leads you to the diagnosis of alcoholism but to finally face up to the fact that the diagnosis is correct and that their best interests lie in complete abstinence.

THE THERAPIST'S ROLE

All too often patients feel that the therapist's attitude is toward children who have abused their toys; since they have abused their toys or broken them, they are taken away as punishment. "You have not treated them properly, so now we are going to take them away from you. You don't deserve to have toys." A tremendous number of patients have this feeling about drinking. They feel that because they have abused alcohol we are denying it to them as punishment. This must be explained very carefully in a nonjudgmental way; that punishment has nothing to do with the treatment. This is strictly a matter of health, and we are asking them to refrain from taking the very material that is injuring their health. One does not deprive diabetics of certain foods, particularly sugar, because they have taken too much sugar in the past; they are deprived of the sugar because it is injurious to them, and they must refrain from certain foods because they tend to increase the risk of illness. The same goes for abstinence regarding alcoholism.

Of course, these discussions and all the questions and answers and explanations cannot be accomplished in one session. It requires session after session of deep involvement with the patients and their lives. Very often it is a matter of teaching individuals how to live without using a drug for escape. Motivation takes time to develop in some patients and requires great persistence and patience on the part of the physician. One must not give up too easily and write a psychological funeral oration. As long as there is contact with the patients, and as long as they give the doctor a chance, one must persist, no matter how endless the rebuffs seem.

Many patients will ask me what my program is. My statement to them is that this is a reeducational program, where they can unlearn many things that they have learned in the past and can learn to live in a complex and often difficult world without resorting to a drug to escape from problems. A favorite expression of mine in discussing instances with patients is that one gives an anesthetic to do away with pain, but that this does not do away with the problem that has produced the pain. Alcohol is used as a rule as an anesthetic for many alcoholic patients to do away with the pain of living in a world that to them is often unhappy and difficult. One can allay this pain by using alcohol, but the problems that have brought about the desire for such oblivion and anesthesia have not been solved. As one would teach a child to live in a complex world and meet its problems in a mature way, one must learn to live in this complex world and learn to meet one's problems the same way. It is very often advantageous to discuss the alcoholic patient's problems as a parent would discuss it with a child. Parents particularly understand this, especially if they have had difficulty with children.

FEES

Another problem that confronts physicians, particularly those in private practice, is the matter of payment for services by alcoholic patients who are already concerned about financial matters. All too often by the time patients reach the physician for help with an alcoholic problem, they have already become financially embarrassed. One of the most common dodges when the matter is discussed is patients claiming they cannot afford the fees that the doctor commands when they are already in financial trouble. Where insurance policies cover the care of alcoholic patients, this problem, to some extent, is alleviated; however, for those patients whose policies have already lapsed or who do not have that kind of protection, the financial burden represents a problem.

Poorly motivated patients will often use this excuse as a method for not continuing treatment. Their rationalization tells them that the doctor who is not to be paid will no longer be as interested in pursuing treatment of the patient. With a conscientious doctor, of course, the financial returns are secondary, the main interest being the welfare of the patient. When I encounter such a patient, I use the following technique: "You are already in financial trouble and here am I trying to help you, while at the same time adding to your burdens and difficulties. Can you see the position in which this puts me? Still, I feel it is worth it because I know that if you follow my advice and take the treatment seriously and stop drinking, you will eventually recover your health and be able to increase your earning capacity to where you will be able to pay, not only for your treatments with me, but to get rid of your other debts as well. But I expect to be paid. If you are conscientious about your treatment and your response, I will bear with you and will accept partial payments while you are under my care. If there is a balance after you are fully recovered, I will expect you to pay that balance when you can. I do want you to know that I appreciate the fact that your financial burdens are being increased by coming here. There is one important fact, however, that I would like you to know. Doctors rarely can guarantee anything in the treatment of a patient, but with you, there is one thing that I can guarantee—and that is that *it will cost you less to come here than to continue drinking*."

SYMPATHY AND EMPATHY

All of these techniques are advantageous, and one could not possibly enumerate all the possible approaches one could use. A few that I have given may help the therapist to induce the somewhat reluctant patient to a motivation that will result in abstinence. Over a period of time, with patience and understanding, this can be done. Certainly, one must apply both sympathy and empathy for the patient and identify with the patient and with his problems.

An important part of the motivation is the overcoming of denial. Denial can be expressed as "they do not like me"—which manifests itself as isolation. Although alcohol is used by many patients initially to overcome shyness (through its disinhibiting function), inevitably shame and guilt over the alcoholic's behavior will result in even more withdrawal and isolation.

One can counter this by giving patients recovered alcoholics with whom they can identify—whose background or gender or occupation or social standing or alcoholic history is like theirs. These persons can tell their own stories, take the patients to *appropriate* Alcoholics Anonymous (A.A.) meetings, and introduce them to others. Then their defensive shyness can diminish, their relationships spread out, and their sense of isolation decrease.

The physician must have contacts in the community of A.A. or the local National Council of Alcoholism group to find such people to "Twelve Step" the patient. The same thing can be done for the family through Al-Anon and Alateen.

Do not become too critical if patients slip. Understand that they have not done this to annoy you, nor should it be considered a failure if they do slip. Encourage them to try again. Use the slips as proof of what you have discussed with them. Your sympathy, your empathy, and your understanding will encourage them to go on.

It is comparatively easy to diagnose and treat alcoholic patients who wish to get well and are perfectly willing to give up drinking without protest once the diagnosis has been made, but for the alcoholic patients who feel that they are being discriminated against, who feel that the fates have worked against them, who feel that in overcoming a sense of inadequacy they can by forcing the issue continue to drink and succeed in drinking without getting drunk, bringing about motivation is a most difficult task. It can be *done*, and it can be done successfully in the vast majority of cases. It takes patience, understanding, and a desire to help unfortunate human beings who have been caught up in a web of dependence upon this socially acceptable and readily available drug.

The demonstration of the understanding of the patient's problems, and the addition of those problems that the therapist is making, often brings about in the patient an appreciation of the physician as well as a willingness to cooperate. Based on past experience the patient also appreciates that the guarantee that the doctor describes is a reasonable one, and this often marks a turning point in patient attitude and provides for additional motivation.

Every practicing physician should study the early psychological symptoms as I have listed them earlier in the form of telltale affirmative answers to questions. If any of those questions are answered in the affirmative, the patient should be admonished regarding a developing drinking problem, and a record should be kept by the doctor. If at any future time those same questions should be put to the patient and those same affirmative answers obtained, there can be no doubt that the illness has more or less firmly established itself and is to be watched, studied, and pursued. If the patient has not changed drinking habits and is continuing to drink excessively, either by his own admission or as confirmed by family, friends, or employer—with patient permission, of course—it must then be pointed out in no uncertain terms that the patient has lost control of his drinking. If, on the other hand, the patient has been able to control his drinking and the questionnaire elicits only negative answers, then and only then is it appropriate to wait upon further reports to ascertain whether or not the patient has successfully passed the test and escaped the suspected early stages of alcohol illness.

There is also a difference between understanding patients and allowing sympathy for them to lead to permissiveness. Many physicians, perhaps because of their own drinking patterns, fail to suspect alcoholism where it is definitely present and will allow patients to consume one or two drinks a day on the theory that that much alcohol can be metabolized without damage to his physiology. This is fallacious. One must always bear in mind that alcoholism is a drug addiction no different from other drug dependencies and that the use of any drug upon which a patient has to any degree become dependent will eventually lead to its excessive use.

FINAL THOUGHTS

Prognosis

There is no guarantee that every patient who comes to the physician with the problem of alcoholism will completely recover. Too many factors are involved in the life of an individual for a single therapist to contend successfully with a particular alcoholic's every possible need. With patience, medical knowledge, and understanding of the victim's physiology and psychology, however, the therapist is in a position to be of great help, and in most cases the prognosis is bound to be favorable, if not excellent. As with any disease, the earlier alcoholism is recognized, diagnosed, and treated, the better will be the results.

Misdiagnosis

Let me put a word in here regarding the possibility of a misdiagnosis. Suppose that the patient who is being diagnosed as an early alcoholic really is not. Of what have we deprived this person? Were alcohol a necessity to life, then we should be grossly remiss, I believe, in setting such a patient down as a definite alcoholic before checking and double-checking our diagnosis for accuracy. But alcohol is not a necessity of life, and it is a drug that can lead to dependency. Should an individual have displayed some indication of having a problem as a result of that drug's use, surely to deprive that person of its further use in no way cuts him off from anything critical! Many persons who have chosen total abstinence live full and happy lives. As much can therefore be said of anyone who is deprived of alcohol, even though it can be shown that it never in any way disadvantaged or caused that person harm.

Working with the Spouse

A final word as to the value of promoting the alcoholic's motivation to seek help through interviewing—and sometimes even treating—the spouse. The most common question put by workers in the field of alcohol disease is, "What can be done if the patient who is obviously alcoholic denies the problem and refuses to seek treatment for it?" The answer I regard as most appropriate is, "If the victim will not seek help, the spouse should do so." One can motivate the patient indirectly through the spouse's own treatment—either psychotherapy, other forms of counseling, or Al-Anon.

In many instances, failure of the nonalcoholic spouse to understand the other's problem with alcohol gives rise to a relationship that threatens the very marriage itself—and thus through countersuggestibility, born of hostility, causes the victim of alcoholism to be all the more stubborn in refusing to seek treatment. If anything, the alcoholic's view of the total situation leads to denying alcoholism, refusing to modify drinking habits, and seeing no reason for treatment.

Where such a chaotic relationship exists, an interview with the alcoholic's partner—wherein the nature of alcohol involvement is carefully explained—will often result in a changed attitude on his or her part. Understanding the character and cause of the sick one's suffering, relief from which is sought in a readily available drug, may well alter the attitude of the well partner and replace hostility with sympathy. This in time may lead the alcoholic partner to become more accommodating and cooperative—often to the point of voluntarily seeking help, or at least advice, even though not personally feeling the need for such resort. This gives the therapist an opportunity to discuss the problem with the patient who otherwise might never have appeared in the office.

Although the primary goal of treating the nonalcoholic spouse may well be the spouse's own benefit, this in turn may also influence the alcoholic indirectly through the withdrawal of the secondary rewards of drinking. For example, as the spouse acquires increasing distance from the alcoholic's illness and develops a detachment and separateness from the situation, the purpose of the alcoholic's drinking (such as revenge through humiliation and embarrassment) may well lose its effectiveness. Furthermore, the growing separateness and possible loss of the spouse—a threat now not merely words but a real possibility—can push the alcoholic into treatment. (It is crucial that these threats—loss of job, spouse, etc.—be deeply meaningful and actual, not just empty words that have no effect and might even reinforce the drinking.)

It is a common occurrence that such leapfrog interviews in the end motivate the victim of alcoholism to submit to treatment. Denial, one of the characteristics of alcohol disease, is a factor to be carefully investigated and overcome—and that denial well may be overcome through attempting to modify the attitude of the victim's spouse.

The Physician Himself

One other point is to be mentioned: what goes on in the mind of the physician himself. As noted, doctors must be patient. They must not have the alcoholic's cure at stake for their own purposes, for self-aggrandizement or for reassurance as to their ability as doctors, for then they would not be able to tolerate the patient's resistances and denial or recidivism without getting angry and taking it personally. Physicians must be patient, tolerant, and persistant and must be convinced themselves of what they are doing and the correctness of it. Only thus can they tolerate, for example, a patient's anger should that form of defense and resistance occur. Doctors must not fear that; it is part of the illness itself. If discussion has really frightened the patient, that anger towards the physician might conceivably be instrumental in the patient's working out his own particular path to recovery, using another helping area—A.A. or another physician.

The doctor, as noted, must have solved his own problems with alcohol and alcoholism and must be convinced of the seriousness of this disorder and the temptations and dangers in a society that minimizes its harmfulness, jokes about it, and even encourages it. The physician must be willing to tolerate the anger and even oppositional and obstructionistic behavior in family members and others who regard the diagnosis as a disgrace or who have some hidden stake in the patient's being ill. Again, Al-Anon or counseling or even psychotherapy here might be necessary for the relative if that person is important in the patient's life situation. (One example is the husband or wife whose alcoholic spouse is always home, drunk, but who, now on his or her way to sobriety, is frequently out at A.A. meetings and elsewhere, exposed to others of the opposite sex; the nonalcoholic spouse's latent jealousy and fears now flare up, and the spouse might much prefer the alcoholic to be back home, drunk again, in a controllable situation once more.)

Physicians therefore must be convinced that alcoholism is a disorder, an illness, a disease, and not just a weakness, a nastiness, not just someone's fault. They must not become punitive or judgmental, certainly not toward the patients and not even toward family members, etc., whose help they may be able to use and on whom the patients may be very dependent. Here too physicians must have resolved their own problems over their own feelings of dependency. They must not despise dependency as a weakness and must not be punitive toward or rejecting of the dependency feelings and behavior on the part of patients—especially in the relationship when the patient may desperately need gratification of such needs. A doctor might well permit it, might even encourage it in order to have some influence over patients to guide them and get them to stop drinking and begin on the road to recovery—even a path to recovery that at first exists for the sake of the dependent relationship with the physician.

On the other hand, as the relationship develops, the therapist must avoid luxuriating in patient dependency and must encourage patients to take their own paths away from the doctor. Between the beginning game and the end game—as it were, in the middle game—no matter what area of the patient's life is being worked on, the doctor must always keep in mind the primacy of the alcohol problem and must always keep an eye on the patient's motivation as to that. It is always the first and foremost consideration. The physician must thus wend his way carefully.

Motivating an alcoholic patient is a matter of perspicuity and judgment. The approach must be eclectic and suited to the individual involved. A few techniques have been described, but many more can be added through experience and observation as one treats more and more victims of this prevalent illness.

REFERENCES

Forman, R.F. *The use of metaphors in substance abuse counseling*. Vol. 1, #6, Alvernia College Addictionary, Havertown, Pa., 1985.

4

Initial Treatment of the Alcoholic Patient

Richard A. Baum
Frank L. Iber

The alcoholic patient presents a spectrum of clinical and diagnostic problems to the physician among which are management of acute intoxication and subsequent withdrawal. The difficulties inherent in acute drunkenness include lack of cooperation on the part of the patients, denial of the problem, unreliability in keeping appointments and inconvenient time of meeting with family and client seeking relief of an intolerable situation; all may limit initial goals to providing shelter, securing safe withdrawal, and identifying intercurrent illness. The frequent occurrence of mixed drug-alcohol habits, including some unknowingly produced by physicians, the variable syndromes mimicking chronic brain damage in the elderly, and the denial of the drinking by family members may compound the problems. On the other hand, many alcoholic patients are alert, cooperative, and desirous of assistance. In all of these persons, ongoing alcoholism treatment should begin with a thorough health check-up.

INITIAL ASSESSMENT

The initial assessment of an alcoholic or potentially alcoholic patient must be tailored to each patient and should accomplish three things: (1) establish a therapeutic relationship, (2) assess urgent health needs, (3) formulate a plan of action for the alcoholism and its related problems. The initial relationship must be based on a clear statement by the doctor of the existence of an alcohol or alcohol-

ALCOHOLISM:
A Practical Treatment Guide

ISBN 0-8089-1912-1

drug problem, and the offer of compassionate assistance. The degree of alcohol use (and other drug use if appropriate) as well as malnutrition and alcohol-related health problems should be inventoried. Thorough historic and physical examination as well as appropriate laboratory testing will reassure the patient of your concern and will allow the identification of conditions that require prompt treatment. Urgent management problems, as well as less urgent subacute or chronic ones, are identified and incorporated into the ongoing management plan. The subacute and chronic problems may be ignored for a few days while the therapeutic relationship is established. Recognition of problems requiring immediate attention is based upon knowledge of what these are and how they are manifest, coupled with the thorough examination. Occasionally the patient is obtunded or unable to provide a history but the essential minimum information may be obtained from the family, a companion, or a coworker.

In patients appearing ill, intoxicated, or uncommunicative, certain features of the physical examination are to be emphasized. Obtundation or severe agitation and mental confusion have many causes besides drunkenness or alcohol withdrawal. The obtundation of drunkenness reaches a maximum within 90 minutes of the last drink and should decrease noticeably within an hour or two of reaching a peak. If blood levels of alcohol or breath alcohol determinations are available, levels should be in excess of 300 mg/0.3 g/dL in persons who are obtunded but not comatose. If the patient can be aroused, has no focal neurologic signs, and the cranial nerves are intact, observation may be safely extended for an additional few hours. If there are convulsions or focal neurologic signs, close observations and admission to an observation area are indicated with prompt neurosurgical assessment.

Alcohol withdrawal of life-threatening severity requires continuous and heavy drinking for more than 2 weeks and is more likely to occur if the drinking has been continuous for many months. The initial withdrawal symptoms occur about 6 hours after the last drink and there is worsening for an additional 48 hours. All sedation may lessen the withdrawal signs. Thus, a clear drinking history, including the time of the last drink and other medicines and drugs, is important. Trauma of all forms, particularly including head trauma, is more common in alcoholics, even among those who do not recall the trauma. The history allows one to assess the probability of withdrawal. Patients tend to have stereotyped clinical courses in subsequent withdrawals so those patients with a history of convulsions, hallucinations, or large requirements for sedation may be appropriately managed. The history should define the nature of previous withdrawals, the presence or absence of convulsions, and specific allergies to medicines that might be used in treatment.

Physical examination should stress those conditions requiring immediate intervention or those that are potentially life threatening (Table 4-1). Death in the acute alcoholic is generally due to head trauma, untreated pulmonary infection, untreated withdrawal, or overdosage (especially with solid sedatives). Occasionally, meningitis or peritonitis, cardiac arrhythmia, alcoholic pancreatitis, or bleeding or perforated ulcer are present and life threatening. When these conditions are

Table 4–1
Necessary Physical Examination

Life-threatening problems
Vital signs
Consciousness and neurologic status
Ability to be aroused
Movement, reflexes, and gross sensation in all extremities, head, and trunk
Inspection and palpation for head injury
Cranial nerves II, III, IV, VI, VII, IX, XI, and XII
Chest, for infection and adequacy of respiration
Heart, for rate and rhythm
Abdomen, for ileus or peritoneal signs
Withdrawal
Agitation
Irritability
Disorientation and/or hallucinations

severe, they are usually apparent on careful evaluation of a completely undressed conscious patient. Rarely, additional diagnostic tests are required to rule out these serious complications; most often additional hours of observation documenting improvement will render serious conditions very unlikely. Most life-threatening abnormalities are apparent on physical examination and usually alter the level of consciousness and vital signs; such patients need additional observation and the diagnosis of withdrawal as the cause should be made cautiously and somewhat reluctantly. Thus, temperature elevation greater than 101°F or 38.3°C is usually due to infection or aspiration and should not be attributed to withdrawal. Similarly, a respiratory rate greater than 24, or pulse rate greater than 120 or pulse irregularities require further evaluation. Skin lesions, signs of malnutrition, and abrasions, lacerations, and possible fractures are common in the alcoholic, but can usually wait a few days for definitive evaluation. Mental and neurological examination and detailed evaluation of the chest and abdomen are much more important.

The interaction of the patient with the observer and the environment, regarding the level of consciousness, is of great importance; small changes observed in either direction are significant. Ideally, the same person should make the initial and follow-up observations over the first 2 to 4 hours. Intoxification rarely leads to unconsciousness or loss of deep tendon and corneal reflexes; if this is found, preparation for respiratory support should be made until the situation reverses itself because drug overdose or CNS trauma are likely. Drunkenness watched 1 or 2 hours will usually show a clear increase in responsiveness to mild stimuli and improved orientation, making head injury of a type requiring urgent action unlikely. Although many alcoholics have confused speech and somewhat slowed thought processes, they are usually cooperative and retain acute memory. Withdrawal produces a flood of mental content that is accurate but may seem jumbled as one skips from one logical sequence to another and then back again. Momentary

Table 4–2
Stages in Alcohol Withdrawal

1. *Earliest: patient sensations*
    - Sensation of internal uneasiness
    - Consciousness of visceral function, nausea, churning, tightness
2. *Minimal: discernable by observer*
    - Fidgits; many unnecessary movements
    - Agitation
    - Chain smokes, drinks many cups of coffee
    - Pulse increases to 20+ beats/min.
3. *Moderate*
    - Severe agitation
    - Pulse increases to 20–50 beats/min.
    - Difficult to keep patient in bed
    - Short spells of lapse of attention
    - Involuntary tremor may be marked
4. *Severe*
    - Hallucinations: auditory, visual
    - Irrational fears, sensitive to noise
    - Extreme agitation
    - Usually unable to cooperate
    - Pulse increases to 50 beats/min.
    - Muscular hyperactivity
    - Severe diaphoresis
5. *Extreme*
    - All of stage 4 symptoms and signs
    - Totally irrational
    - Extreme diaphoresis
    - Extreme tachycardia
    - Convulsions

lapses of attention with return to clarity in a fraction of a second may occur. Motor hyperactivity and inability to keep the limbs quiet is more a feature of withdrawal than drunkenness. Table 4-2 lists common findings in alcohol withdrawal. Hypertension during alcohol withdrawal is very common and may persist into the third day. If the patient is nearly coherent, is a reasonable historian, did not have severe withdrawal symptoms or convulsions in the past, has no alarming findings on physical examination, and now does not have substantial agitation or restlessness, then further close observation or urgent treatment is not necessary. Such a patient may return home in the care of another person.

If the level of consciousness is depressed or there is a great deal of agitation or restlessness, further observation for 3–5 hours is essential for safety. Unconsciousness secondary to alcohol will not persist beyond 3–4 hours after the last drink. Failure to brighten mentally during this period suggests the possibility of

Table 4–3
Common Changes in Usual Laboratory Tests in Alcoholics

Test	Change
WBC	May not rise if folate deficient
Hematocrit	Often depressed 3–7 percent
Blood sugar*	Often wide swings accompanying poor carbohydrate intake and stores
Electrolytes	Increased anion gap due to lactate
Potassium and phosphorous	Often quite low
Uric acid	Elevated for 2–5 days
Alanine aminotransferase (ALT) aspartate aminotransferase (AST)	25 percent abnormal
Gamma glutamyl transpeptidase (GGTP)	Elevated in most

Note. All return to normal in 1 week of abstinence and normal eating.
* Requires 1 week of adequate carbohydrate intake to become normal. Occult blood in stool: positive in 10–20 percent for 3–4 days.

other longer-acting psychotropic drugs, head trauma, or a postictal state. Withdrawal symptoms alarming to physicians begin in the first 12–24 hours after drinking stops and close observation in this period is essential.

INITIAL LABORATORY EVALUATION

Although laboratory abnormalities are common in recently drinking alcoholic patients (Table 4-3), very few of these are helpful in management of the acute situation. Blood alcohol levels and drug screens for prescription and street drugs are very valuable in patients with disorders of consciousness and may occasionally identify a diagnosis in patients denying drug or alcohol use. A patient obtunded from alcohol alone usually reveals a blood alcohol level in excess of 300 mg/dL (0.3 g/dL). A level above 100 mg/dL indicates the ingestion of four to six drinks in the last 4 hours, or greater quantities if ingested previously. Seriously ill patients may require laboratory tests for treatment, but in most patients who appear healthy, it is better to delay laboratory tests for 1 week to allow many tests that would be borderline to normalize. Abnormalities persisting after 1 week in liver tests, stool occult blood, uric acid, and hemogram indicate conditions that merit further diagnosis and treatment.

Disorders of consciousness or first occurrence of convulsions usually require head CT scan for thorough evaluation and may require EEG to determine whether chronic treatment of an epileptogenic focus is indicated. Tachycardia or arrhythmia require ECG evaluation, and fever or cough require chest x-rays.

Patients who have not had significant fever or obtundity are usually given no testing initially. After 2 weeks, SGOT, albumin, alkaline phosphatase, and hematocrit are obtained. If the patient has failed to gain weight in 2 weeks of abstinence, a chest film or skin test for TB is obtained and stool samples for occult blood are requested. The common nutritional depletions are noted in MEDICAL COMPLICATIONS (Chapter 8).

MANAGEMENT OF ALCOHOL WITHDRAWAL

Alcohol withdrawal is a state of CNS hyperactivity and irritability produced upon cessation or sharp reduction of alcohol intake. The cardinal features are agitation and autonomic hyperactivity characterized by diaphoresis, tachycardia, and restlessness often with tremor. The syndrome begins 6–24 hours after stopping drinking, reaches a peak by 36–48 hours (occasionally later but rarely if ever after 96 hours) and then subsides. This time course is dependable and of value in diagnosis. Fever or major intercurrent infection can accelerate the course and increase severity of withdrawal, and any form of sedation can ameliorate the symptoms and signs. Seizures may occur after 12–36 hours, whereas auditory or visual hallucinations or acute psychosis rarely occur prior to 24 hours or start later than 96 hours. Full DTs with acute psychosis and extreme irrational agitation has a mortality of 5–15 percent but can be prevented by prompt early treatment. Table 4-2 indicates diagnostic signs of withdrawal. Recognition of the earlier and milder stages using the time occurrence and the typical findings offer ample time for successful management to prevent the later more severe stages.

All the symptoms and signs of alcohol withdrawal may be exacerbated by sensory stimuli, unfamiliar people, unknown surroundings, or confrontational behavior. Successful therapy of alcohol withdrawal requires an environment that calms, reassures, and does not alarm the patient. Some of the components that should be considered are listed in Table 4-4, which emphasizes that the patient should be surrounded with familiar items and people similar to those in their home, rather than stimulating, threatening ones such as are occasionally encountered in the hospital. Restraints, intravenous infusions, and bedsides should be avoided in almost every instance.

Alcohol withdrawal may often be accomplished at home if the patient is motivated and there is a committed friend or relative with the emotional stability and expertise needed to supervise withdrawal and prevent further drinking. Home management should not require administration of psychotropic medication. Solid sedative use, substantial agitation, fever, decreasing consciousness, a seizure, or history of seizures require in-patient medical care.

We present details of withdrawal under supervision of a physician or other trained persons to illustrate important features of the process. Skilled supervision ensures that the patient will indeed withdraw from alcohol (or mixed addictions) and be protected from injuring himself in the critical initial period. The presence of a confident trained person goes a long way to allay the anxiety that accompanies the withdrawal; an institutional setting acts in a similar fashion. Both of these reinforce the concept of alcoholism as a disease and are an effective, face-saving means of enlisting the patient's cooperation in therapy.

Table 4–4
"Do's and Don'ts" in Treating Withdrawal (Sensory Withdrawal Syndrome)

	Do's	Don'ts
Visual	Lights on Familiar people Civilian clothes	Lights off Shadows
Touch	Comfortable chair Low bed Regular clothes	High bed Restraints Intravenous infusions
Sound	Light music Soft conversation with patient	Abrupt noises

General supportive care should be provided. At the time of physical examination, a bath may be in order to provide initial cleanliness and the patient may be made comfortable in loose clothing, in a bed, or in an arm chair. Almost all chronic alcoholics are overloaded with salt and water; thus intravenous fluids are not needed unless other clear indications are present. Food and/or sugar-containing beverages should be offered, with encouragement to take something every few hours. Caffeine-containing beverages should be avoided. Thiamin (100 mg) and folate (1 mg) are given parenterally to all of our patients and multiple vitamin capsule is given orally for 5 days.

Medication is useful temporarily during this difficult period of withdrawal. Nearly all patients feel better with minor tranquilizers over the first 3–5 days. We use oral doses of chlordiazepoxide (Librium) (25–100 mg per dose), or diazepam (Valium) (5 or 10 mg orally) every 2–4 hours. Intramuscular administration is ineffective. Antidepressants and phenothiazines reduce the seizure threshold and have more side-effects. Although we do not use sleeping medications, others using chloral hydrate 0.5 gm nightly for 3 or 4 days or diphenhydramine (Benadryl) 100 mg for 3 or 4 days feel they are useful. We provide symtomatic therapy for minor complaints consisting of antacids, antidiarrheals, acetaminophen, and topical skin preparations liberally. The goals of this treatment are to prevent severe withdrawal symptoms, to comfort the patient, to allow repair of the toxic and nutritional ravages of alcohol, and prepare the patient for ongoing alcoholism therapy. Total withdrawal can be completed in 3–5 days. Within this period, restoration of appetite occurs and most patients gain a few pounds by the fifth day. The healing of brain and other organ damage can be demonstrated by psychologic and detailed testing to continue for 90 days or longer. All life-threatening situations occur in the first few days; therefore, sedative therapy may not be needed after this period. If the patient has had convulsions in the past, we use phenytoin 300 mg orally daily for 5–7 days.

The ideal drug for management of alcohol withdrawal would substitute at the CNS sites for alcohol and would disappear slowly and smoothly with few or no side-effects. Useful drugs have long half-lives so that their own withdrawal would not be abrupt. A high degree of safety is also desirable because even hospital patients may not get the close supervision that patients should receive. No ideal drug exists but in general the benzodiazepines are favored because of their efficacy and high degree of general safety (Table 4-5).

Treatment of withdrawal requires prompt and continual evaluation of the patient with appropriate decisions as to the need for medication. The hallmark of therapy is individualization of management. The amount of medication required from one patient to another to control withdrawal may easily vary ten-fold. Many patients require only reassurances and comfort with little or no medication, whereas others may rarely require up to 1000 mg of chlordiazepoxide or its equivalent in the first day. Decisions regarding dose must be made by careful observation of the patient and the best withdrawal programs have the same persons making assessments every few hours in the first 2 days and ordering or withholding further therapy. Therapy is most effective when begun promptly on the recognition of its requirement. If patients are to be admitted to a special unit, it is important to shorten the admission and the evaluation process so that necessary medication can be given about 1 hour after reaching the facility. Although many patients do not require such prompt therapy, it is crucial for those few who do. The need for prompt and continual therapy coupled with the rarity of severe intercurrent illness when the initial physical examination does not reveal such abnormalities has led us to use specially trained nurses and technicians. They act as primary therapists and function under a set of standing orders to allow therapy to be both safe yet tailored to the individual's needs. Physicians provide back-up for the patient who responds unpredictably and of course evaluate all patients at some point, but do not direct hour by hour drug therapy for withdrawal. Patients who prove in retrospect to be multiply addicted to alcohol and other substances respond adequately to this treatment.

Table 4–5

Features of Drugs Used in Withdrawal Treatment

Drug	Unit Dose for Withdrawal	Half-Duration of Dose (hr)	Significant Side-Effects
Chlordiazepoxide	100 mg	24–40	None
Diazepam	10 mg	12–24	None
Hydroxazine	100 mg	10–14	None
Chlorpromazine	50 mg	12	Hypotension, spasms
Haloperidol	3 mg	12–24	Spasms, convulsions
Pentabarbital	100 mg	4	Respiratory depression
Phenobarbital	100 mg	16	Respiratory depression
Paraldehyde	15 mL	1–3	Respiratory depression, foul odor
Chloral hydrate	1 g	1–3	Respiratory depression
Clonidine	0.1 mg	12–14	Hypotension

We use a one-day regimen using chlordiazepoxide as our agent of choice because it is inexpensive, effective, and has a long half-life in all age groups. This reduces the total number of subsequent doses needed once initial calming is attained. Essentially all patients can be successfully treated with this regimen. In patients with a high suspicion of head trauma and neurologic signs, sedative drugs may be contraindicated since they can interfere with subsequent diagnosis. In such cases, we use oral clonidine (0.1 mg every 2 hours) to block the many manifestations of withdrawal. Patients with known liver disease receive the same drug regimen, but subsequent doses are given a little more reluctantly.

External environment influences therapy to a large extent (Table 4-4). Calm, well lighted surroundings, control of noise, often by soft music, and someone to talk to are often more effective than medications. It is important to avoid excitement of the patient during periods of mild confusion. Thus, confrontational interviews, bed rails, and restraints are often counterproductive at this stage, agitating the patient and leading to serious injury. When a confused patient keeps trying to get out of bed we place the mattress on the floor so that the patient is less likely to fall. These patients must also be protected from matches, cigarettes, glass, and other sharp objects. We do not permit smoking until the patient can sit and is accompanied in the room by another person.

Agitation, insomnia, nausea, and vomiting are characteristics of the withdrawal syndrome and do not require a separate treatment strategy. We have abandoned both sleeping medication and antiemetics because they do not seem to help. Nearly all patients will voluntarily ingest adequate food and fluids sufficient to avoid dehydration and hypoglycemia. Intravenous fluids are almost never required. Patients will frequently approach the doctor with a list of complaints desiring medications for each. This situation is best handled by delaying tactics, since the symptoms tend to be short lived. We offer free access to antacids, antidiarrheal agents, acetaminophen, and emolient lotions, but favor exercise, reading, and eating the food provided for nearly all other complaints.

In the subsequent management of the alcoholic, we avoid the use of sedatives, sleeping medication, and tranquilizers after the first week. Antidepressants are used only with objective evidence of depression persisting after the first 2 weeks. Other workers prefer a greater delay before attempting to make a decision regarding the presence of an underlying affective disorder. As soon as a patient is alert, they should receive counselling and be involved in planning further rehabilitation. In this period, patients tend to be depressed and need positive directive programs with reinforcement from family, home, colleagues, and friends to remain in the program. Taking responsibility for their own well-being and rehabilitation should be stressed.

Occasionally, a brief written contract including an inventory of alcohol-related problems and the patient's acceptance of a specific schedule for therapy is helpful. Accentuation of symptoms and anxiety is occasionally seen 10–15 days after the withdrawal; this agitation arises from the more realistic and perceptive interaction with the environment or to lessening amounts of therapeutic medication. Delayed alcohol withdrawal does not seem to occur, but other soporific/hypnotic drugs

Table 4–6
Criteria for Outpatient Detoxification

Low volume and duration of drinking
Previous success at efforts to withdraw self
Youth and good medical health
High motivation
Home or other caretaker support mechanism
Absence of solid sedative addiction (as opposed to ethanol or paraldehyde)
No history or current evidence of seizures or severe withdrawal syndrome
No history of severe psychiatric complications such as suicidal tendencies or paranoid states

Note: By outpatient detoxification is meant detoxification at home or in a sobering-up station without trained personnel, as contrasted with inpatient detoxification in an acute care facility, such as a hospital, or in a lay detoxification unit with trained personnel and hospital back-up. The desirable hand-off to longer term rehabilitative effort (in- or out-patient) may or may not be associated with either of these and must be considered by the physician in the disposition of the patient.

taken over a long time are often used by alcoholics and may produce prolonged withdrawal.

Outpatient withdrawal (Table 4-6) can be safely carried out in patients who appear normal on screening. An interested person to be with the alcoholic during the next 4–5 days to prevent access to alcohol and to provide the patient with some sedation is essential. We give the nondrinking helper a small number of 25-mg capsules of chlordiazepoxide with instructions to administer these to the patient under specific circumstances during the first 3 days. If it is believed that more is necessary, the helper must return with the alcoholic for further evaluation. It is unwise to offer medications directly to the patient for treatment in an uncontrolled setting.

DELIRIUM TREMENS (DTs)

On occasion, a somewhat older patient who has ingested some 500g of alcohol daily for many months or years arrives at the hospital because of an intercurrent illness. The stage is thus set for the possibility of clinical (diagnostic) obscuration and a potentially serious withdrawal syndrome. Delay and/or deficiency in the administration of adequate sedative/hypnotic therapy may be followed by confusion, picking at bed covers, and agitation during the second night in the hospital. A tendency to grand mal seizures, adrenergic hyperactivity, fever, frenetic physical activity, and delusional state with auditory, tactile, and visual hallucinations are usually evident by the next morning. Adequate sedation often requires an intravenously administered barbiturate, but preparation for maintaining an adequate airway and respiration must be completed prior to such treatment. After initial control of the delirium in this manner, the patient will likely continue to demonstrate a toxic psychosis with confusion and hallucinatory activity, but the severe agitation rarely recurs. Gradual clearing is observed during the ensuing 10 days. Although this clinical course is a common one, it is not the only one. On occasion a patient may enter DTs with little if any warning and without substantial diminution in ethanol ingestion. It is impossible for the physician to achieve uniform reliability in differentiating upon initial examination those patients destined to experience such a severe withdrawal syndrome from those who will suffer only modest discomfort. Therefore, experienced clinicians will prefer to exercise conservative judgment in the recommendation of medical treatment for the patient with a withdrawal syndrome.

INTERCURRENT ILLNESS

Alcohol withdrawal occurring in the presence of another major illness often poses unique management problems. About half of all trauma victims are alcoholics. When surgery or anesthesia is required shortly after hospital admission and withdrawal results 1 or 2 days later, the loss of patient cooperation and the violent, muscular contractions threaten wound dehiscence or fracture dislocation. Such patients are treated in much the same manner as others who develop withdrawal symptoms, but it is not unusual for the withdrawal to go untreated until it is very advanced and at that time large amounts of sedation become necessary. The extra hazards of such treatment may be avoided if emergency room personnel were routinely alert to the possibility of alcoholism and an incipient withdrawal syndrome in such patients.

Only two common diseases have produced recurrent problems if not recognized when treating withdrawal: liver encephalopathy and advanced pulmonary insufficiency. Cirrhosis eventually occurs in about 10 percent of alcoholics, producing the circumstance of a drinking patient with advanced cirrhosis who may have a confused mental state upon coming into care. Liver encephalopathy may produce confusion and obtundation, but rarely agitation. Alcohol withdrawal in a brain-injured alcoholic may feature some agitation in the presence of confusion and depression of consciousness. The usual sedation for treatment of withdrawal may result in death in advanced hepatic encephalopathy. In practice, this is rare. A careful screening examination will detect most of the patients with advanced cirrhosis who have encephalopathy and if there is reasonable doubt an electroencephalogram will separate these two conditions cleanly. The EEG in withdrawal shows hyperactivity, somewhat like epilepsy, whereas the pattern in encephalopathy is slowing of the electrical activity. Most patients with hepatic encephalopathy have elevated blood ammonia; most patients in withdrawal have a normal ammonia. If a decision must be made with lingering uncertainty, cautious use of sedation, or use of clonidine will prevent fatal errors.

Severe chronic lung disease with confusion can also be harmed by the usual sedation used for alcohol withdrawal. Sometimes the CNS anoxia results in agitation. Blood gases usually clarify this situation promptly. Again when in doubt, caution in the use of medication should be exercised.

Chronic nonurgent disease and its long-term management in the alcoholic are usually not addressed until the withdrawal period is complete. Cirrhosis, malnutrition, hypertension, peripheral neuritis, vascular disease, and tuberculosis are common chronic problems in alcoholics and can be best handled by a person knowledgeable about these diseases. We stress the relation of the chronic disease to alcoholism since compliance with the management of the chronic disease will often lead to more successful management of the alcoholism.

Alcoholic patients who present with another medical or surgical acute problem and develop withdrawal symptoms in the hospital are treated much the same as other patients but the therapy of both the withdrawal and the underlying illness must go forward, one unimpeded by the other. As this frequently requires maintenance of IV lines, catheters, and other gadgets of modern medicine, it is usually necessary to use higher doses of sedation.

ALCOHOL-RELATED DISEASE DIAGNOSED BEFORE BECOMING SYMPTOMATIC

Peripheral neuritis, gastritis, chemical liver disease, and chemical pancreatitis are commonly identified by testing at a time they do not bother the patients. Although we emphasize this early injury to the patient and the family in our inventory of alcohol-related injuries, no specific therapy is required. Abstinence and a nutritious diet will usually lead to the abnormal findings disappearing in a few weeks or a few months.

ONGOING THERAPY

The ultimate test of alcoholism programs is their success in producing sobriety and a more healthful fulfilling life. Patients should be seen by alcoholism counselors to plan ongoing treatment as soon as they are sufficiently alert for discussions, usually within the first 48–72 hours. A program is worked out progressively that involves group therapy and individual counselling when appropriate, always maintaining the clear goal of sobriety and restoration to that patient's normal life in family, home, and employment. We emphasize that drinking must cease; if slips occur we will provide access to further intensive therapy. Group therapy, Alcoholics Anonymous, family support, Antabuse, and job counselling are all provided as desired or indicated. A therapist may be a psychologist, social worker or counselor who can provide many different forms of treatment, some individually, some in groups, and some by referral. Although drinking is no basis for rejection, drinking during meetings or on a treatment unit is forbidden. If it occurs, the person is asked to leave and return sober. Frequent contact by phone and mail is used to encourage the patients to stay in therapy. Multiple types of therapy applied a few at a time are needed to encourage patients who experience failure and discouragement with one or two modalities.

SUMMARY

The treatment of alcohol intoxification and subsequent withdrawal requires some control of the environment to prevent further drinking and provide the optimal opportunity to recognize and treat withdrawal, trauma, or infection related to alcoholism, and plan subsequent therapy. Withdrawal syndromes can be controlled and severe withdrawal symptoms aborted by this plan. Compassionate comfortable withdrawal is a major inducement to the patient to continue in therapy.

BIBLIOGRAPHY

Brown CG: The alcohol withdrawal syndrome. *Ann Emerg Med* 11:276–280, 1982

Clark LT, Friedman HS: Hypertension associated with alcohol withdrawal: Assessment of mechanisms and complications. *Alcoholism Clin Exp Res* 9:125–130, 1985

Moskowitz SB, Sack HS, Chalmers T: Impact of randomized control trials on the treatment of alcohol withdrawal. *Adv Alcohol Subst Abuse* 1:101–113, 1982

Novick DM: Major medical problems and detoxification treatment of parenteral drug abusing alcoholics. *Adv Alcohol Subt Abuse* 3:87–106, 1984

Sellers EM, Kalant A: Alcohol intoxication and withdrawal. *N Engl J Med* 294:757–762, 1976

Whitfield CC, Thompson G, Matrikiaz J, et al: Detoxification of 1024 alcoholic patients without psychoactive drugs. *JAMA* 239:1409–1410, 1978

Wilkins AJ, Jenkins WJ, Steiner JA: Efficacy of clonidine in treatment of alcohol withdrawal state. *Psychopharmacology* 81:78–80, 1983

5

After Detoxification—The Physician's Role in the Initial Treatment Phase of Alcoholism

David H. Knott
Robert D. Fink
Jack C. Morgan

Whether through lay self-help groups or professional counseling, long-term management is an essential element in the therapeutic planning for the alcoholic.

Proper management of the detoxified patient who expresses some motivation for continued treatment is extremely important to the overall rehabilitation process. The physician must recognize that initial motivation on the part of the patient may derive primarily from a recent crisis situation. As the length of time between detoxification and active psychosocial therapeutic intervention increases, motivation wanes and the patient's attitude toward further treatment other than

ALCOHOLISM:
A Practical Treatment Guide
ISBN 0-8089-1912-1

medical management becomes more ambivalent. It is unfortunately common for the patient to escape from any therapeutic modality at this point, but a well established physician–patient relationship allows the clinician to expedite the patient's entry into active treatment. To accomplish this, attention should be directed toward the following:

1. Motivational considerations
2. Diagnostic considerations
3. Early treatment considerations: psychotherapy, chemotherapy, referral
4. Prognostic considerations

MOTIVATIONAL CONSIDERATIONS

The old adage, "you can't help alcoholics until they are ready to help themselves" or until "they have hit bottom" is inherently therapeutically nihilistic. Issues of motivation arise at more than one point in the course of such patients. Block (Chapter 3) referred to those techniques useful in initiating therapy; similar methods reappear at this critical treatment phase. While internal motivation on the part of the patient is important, externally motivating factors are often necessary to overcome the denial and ambivalence that are so common when the patient's physical discomfort has been relieved. A number of very effective coercive factors are useful in externally motivating the patient into initial treatment.

Legal. Alcohol-related charges such as driving while intoxicated, public drunkenness, disturbing the peace, etc., represent manifest evidence of the patient's behavioral problems with alcohol. Punishment in the form of confinement, loss of license (driving, professional, or other vocational licensure, etc.), or fines frequently coerce a begrudging individual into treatment who later may move successfully into the long-term rehabilitation process. The physician may find the judicial system extremely cooperative in this regard and should not hesitate to contact local police or courts, local and state medical societies, bar associations, or state licensure authorities within the guidelines for confidentiality.

Job jeopardy. In those instances in which the patient is referred from a business or industry that has a policy of rehabilitation rather than termination, impaired job performance secondary to alcohol abuse and the threat to job security can be strong determinants in the patient's commitment to the initial phase of treatment. A close liason with the employer without violating patient confidentiality can be established by the physician and the treatment team and is fundamental to the effectiveness of this approach. In the Armed Services, the official lines of command have developed coercive techniques for dealing with inadequately motivated alcoholics.

Family jeopardy. Alcoholism is an illness affecting all members of the family and leading to disruption and deterioration of relationships within both the nuclear and extended families. Support of the family members in terms of dealing with personal feelings of guilt, anger, and resentment and developing a willingness to set tolerance limits on the patient's alcohol-affected behavior can precipitate a "family crisis" that frequently motivates the patient toward the initial phase of treatment. Such a family crisis may consist of an imminent loss of spouse or other loved one. That person must be advised to avoid such threats without true intent, supported in his final decision, and made aware of alternate options. These options consist not only of divorce versus continued involvement in the day-to-day drama of the disease but also of withdrawal from that participation by development of a separate and meaningful life (e.g., a career).

Al-Anon may often support such intentions (see Chapter 13) and may offer pragmatic methods for avoiding "enabling" (by enabling is meant making social and job excuses, obtaining help for family or job chores left undone by patients, etc.).

Health impairment. The myriad of medical disorders associated with alcohol abuse can be emphasized by the physician's reminding the patient that further drinking behavior will result in physical destruction and ultimately death. While it is well known that patients cannot be "frightened" from drinking strictly on the basis of the tissue toxicity of alcohol, the possibility and reality of alcohol-induced physical illness does have a motivating quality, particularly in regard to encouraging the patient to enter the initial phase of treatment. Sexual function is interfered with later in the disease; this may be introduced as a factor in motivation even though the physician cannot promise return of function in many cases.

In summary, then, the following are implicit in the physician's "externally" motivating patients into treatment: (1) recognition of the patient's ambivalence toward further treatment when they are physically improved; (2) recognition that early involvement of the "significant others" (e.g., spouse, children, employer, friends, etc.) in the external motivation process is extremely important; (3) recognition that all patients have their own "bottom"—a psychosocial plateau that can often be externally precipitated; and (4) recognition that the proper use of rational authority (coercion, external motivation) by the physician is not only a valid approach but frequently is necessary to initiate early treatment and ensure long-term commitment to the after-care philosophy.

DIAGNOSTIC CONSIDERATIONS

The current confusion surrounding specific diagnostic criteria for alcoholism as a disease entity allows the physician to focus primarily on the pattern of alcohol use and to ignore psychopathology that is frequently associated (either etiologically or consequentially) with alcohol abuse. There is preliminary evidence that bona fide psychiatric disorders, such as the primary affective diseases (manic-depressive illness) and schizophrenia, occur not infrequently in an "alcoholic" population. The associated psychopathology can range from mild personality disorders to severe psychosis. A distorted psychological picture is usually evident when psychometrics are measured during the period of detoxification, but subsequent to this a psychodiagnostic approach is helpful in assisting the physician in the proper choice of medication and also the type of psychotherapeutic milieu that would be most beneficial. In addition to a mental status examination, the following tests are useful in determining the psychological status of the patient, in detecting major personality problem areas, and in defining any "underlying" major psychiatric disorder:

Minnesota Multiphasic Personality Inventory (MMPI). A comprehensive and general survey of psychopathology, this test measures the patient on ten distinct clinical syndromes and rates the extent of psychopathology existing in each syndrome. Proper interpretation by a qualified psychologist or psychiatrist is essential in order to prevent both misdiagnosis and misinterpretation.

Bender Visual Motor Gestalt Test. A brief examination to assess perceptual-motor functions for deficits associated with cerebral damage or dysfunction; this test is sensitive to organic impairments associated with alcohol abuse, which are not necessarily evident in a mental status examination.

Projective Human Figure Drawings. This series of projective drawings, interpreted by a psychologist, serves as a validity check on previously administered psychometric instruments (e.g., MMPI). This examination gives clues to the clinician for planning an appropriate psychotherapeutic regimen.

It is important to bear in mind that these psychological instruments, although easily administered, are of a preliminary or screening nature. The seriousness of psychological problems as detected by psychometrics increases the longer an individual abstains from alcohol. If serious psychopathology persists not only clinically but also as measured with psychological instruments, a psychiatric referral is usually in order. Other psychological tests such as the Wechsler Adult Intelligence Scale and such projective tests as the Rorschach may also be useful in determining the presence of organic or functional psychopathology.

The entire spectrum of personality patterns, psychiatric syndromes, and illness has been observed in the "alcoholic" population. An understanding of the psychodynamics of each patient is helpful in formulating a meaningful treatment plan and deciding on the proper referral route.

EARLY TREATMENT CONSIDERATIONS

Psychotherapy

Psychotherapy is an omnibus term and essentially involves working with patients to help them handle internal and external realities more effectively. The three essential components of psychotherapy are as follows:

Emotional support. The most important aspect of any therapy is the patient's relationship with the therapist. It is important for patients to feel understood and that with the therapist's help they can begin to manage their lives again. Understanding the patients involves gaining knowledge of the family history, of the development of attitudes and reactions in childhood and adolescence, of the problems encountered in day-to-day living, and of the situational factors and stress that may precipitate alcohol ingestion. It is important to realize that these patients' problems and discomforts are subjectively perceived and felt, regardless of how the therapist interprets the situation. Support should be offered in a nonmoralistic, nonjudgmental way.

Practical support. Intellectual insight into problems and possible solutions is not tantamount to recovery. Patients must not only learn effective problem-solving techniques but must also be encouraged to put them into action. The consequence of behavioral change may be more painful than remaining in a "familiar hell." Practical support involves defining alternative coping mechanisms from a behavioral point of view (such as abstinence from alcohol) and insisting that patients be responsible for the choice of these alternatives.

Emotional reeducation. Quite often, anxious-depressed, alcohol-dependent patients have developed defenses that protect them from admitting the extent of their problems with alcohol. It is important to be aware of and to deal with any internal or external factors in a patient's life that maintain the status quo and resist change.

Patients should begin to understand, from a mutual exploration of their responses to immediate problems, something of the personal psychodynamics and maladaptive reactions involved. The physician should try to elicit the subjective meaning patients have given to the stressful events. For example:

—Who or what is producing angry feelings?
—What does loss or threat mean to the patient and his life?
—What is the cause of the patient's ambivalent feelings?
—What role have the patient's reactions played in the excessive drinking pattern and how will this affect recovery?
—What are some different ways of coping with these kinds of stress?

On the basis of patient understanding of reactions, the therapist should help the patient learn new, more effective ways of handling himself and life situations. This may necessitate a change in friends, more rarely job, and occasionally even marriage.

Although an "alcoholic personality" does not exist as a distinct entity, there are common psychological patterns that are encountered in the initial phase of psychotherapy.

DEPENDENCY

Frequently patients with alcohol abuse problems will present with pathologic dependency. This will be expressed in one of the following ways:

The passive-dependent patient who associates being assertive with rejection and commonly employs alcohol as a vehicle for coping with unconscious resentment and anger. An effective therapeutic technique involves assertiveness training.

Inappropriately aggressive patients have "turned around" a need for dependency through the association of intimacy and interpersonal warmth with rejection. It is necessary for such persons to reject you before you have the opportunity to reject them. Their aggressiveness is a defense of their feelings of low esteem and inadequacy. Alcohol is an effective tool for maintaining this form of behavior.

Admixtures of both of these types are common. Understanding patients' dependency needs allows the physician to plan therapeutic strategies emphasizing individual responsibility while recognizing underlying disturbances in the areas of intimacy, assertiveness, and fears of rejection. Recognition that alcohol represents "a people substitute" points to the physician's role in therapeutic intervention, namely, that of establishing—either for the first time or once again—a meaningful interpersonal relationship without patient recourse to isolation or withdrawal through drugs.

OMNIPOTENCE

The alcohol-dependent patient often responds to a pathologic feeling of inadequacy and powerlessness through the psychopharmacologic effect of alcohol. This drug-induced state of omnipotence is short lived and eventually augments further feelings of powerlessness, which further perpetuate excessive alcohol consumption. The spiraling downward effect does not obviate the patient's continued drinking. The physician can play a role in emphasizing the concepts of (1) the patient's participating in his own victimization, (2) short-term pleasures for long-term suffering, and (3) pursuing alternative courses of behavior to overcome feelings of being powerless.

Psychotherapy with the alcoholic requires flexibility. There are no typical alcoholics; thus there is no typical therapy. While group and individual psychotherapy can be directed by the physician, other professionally trained persons, such as psychologists, social workers, nurses, clergymen, and alcoholism counselors, can be utilized effectively on a referral basis. Alcoholics Anonymous (A.A.) can often provide invaluable assistance to the physician. It is highly recommended that the physician learn from and cooperate with the local A.A. organization in the management of the alcohol patient.

Chemotherapy

PSYCHOACTIVE DRUGS

In selected cases, the administration of a psychotropic drug is an effective adjunct. Such drugs should not usually include the highly addicting soporifics such as barbiturates, chloral hydrate, paraldehyde, glutethimide, ethchlorvynol, benzodiazepines, meprobamate, methaqualone, and methyprylon. The phenothiazines, tricyclics, MAO inhibitors, hydroxyzine, butyrophenones, thioxanthines, and lithium can be used when there is an appropriate psychiatric diagnosis present. The manner in which such drugs are explained and offered to patients will in large part determine their attitudes and compliance. Patients need to understand that (1) no such drug can replace alcohol in regard to rapidity of action and initial euphoria, (2) the drug being prescribed by the physician is far less toxic than alcohol, (3) the drug being used is not a replacement for alcohol but rather its function is to ameliorate or remove the primary symptoms of anxiety and depression, or symptoms of psychosis, and (4) drug therapy alone is insufficient to produce effective recovery.

When depressive symptomatology is sufficiently serious to mandate chemotherapy, proper selection of tricyclic antidepressant (when there are no contraindications) can be helpful in the initial phase of treatment. Imipramine or desipramine may be more effective in retarded depressions and amitriptyline, nortriptyline, or doxepin in agitated depressions. The diagnosis of "endogenous" versus "reactive" depression in this initial phase is less helpful in making chemotherapeutic decisions than is the severity of the signs and symptoms. Patients who present with marked symptoms of anxiety and agitation can frequently be controlled with a nondependency-producing type of antihistamine drug or hydroxyzine. Extreme caution should be exercised in the use of sedative-hypnotics (benzodizepines and barbiturates), since these compounds have a high potential for abuse by persons previously addicted to alcohol. Most physicians feel their use should be limited to the detoxification period only.

ANTIDISATROPICS (AVERSIVE THERAPY)

Abstinence from alcohol is essential in the management of the patient in this initial phase. Selection of the patient for Antabuse (disulfiram) therapy should include the following criteria:

1. Does the patient thoroughly understand the rationale of Antabuse therapy?
2. Are there any contraindications to Antabuse (e.g., hypersensitivity, concomitant psychosis, severe organic brain syndrome, strong suicidal potential)?
3. What is the apparent level of the patient's motivation?
4. Does the patient understand that abstinence is a means to an end (recovery) and that its use is only adjunctive in the overall treatment process?

By emphasizing the use of Antabuse as an "insurance policy" rather than a "crutch" and stressing that a period of abstinence will allow the patient to make essential behavioral and attitudinal changes without the use of alcohol, the physician adopts a positive approach to Antabuse therapy (see Appendix D).

Referral

The multiplicity and complexity of the psychosocial and physiologic problems and needs of the detoxified patient make it nearly impossible for the physician to assume total responsibility for care. By designing an individualized treatment plan that includes other resources, the physician can appropriately direct and guide the patient into a treatment *system.*

Great care must be exercised in referring patients who have suffered repeated rejection to any other therapeutic resource. They must be reassured of your continued support, interest, and availability. Referral must not be used by the physician to justify rejection of a difficult, frequently noncompliant patient.

Selection of referral sources depends on availability and quality of other therapeutic environments and on the needs of the patient.

RESIDENTIAL AFTERCARE—QUARTERWAY HOUSE, HALFWAY HOUSE

Patients who are homeless, whose home situations are volatile and disruptive, or who suffer from significant social instability often require the type of organized therapeutic environment offered by residential aftercare. This is frequently preferable to a long-term hospital inpatient stay, since most residential programs encourage early resocialization.

COMMUNITY MENTAL HEALTH CENTERS

Most comprehensive community mental health centers offer alcoholism treatment services that include family therapy and individual and group therapy on both scheduled and nonscheduled bases. These services are designed for patients who have had previous treatment experiences and enough family and social stability not to require more protective sytems.

VOCATIONAL REHABILITATION

Job instability and unemployment are very real and pressing problems to alcoholics. Vocational rehabilitation programs, especially those with specialized services for alcoholics, can offer evaluation of individual needs, personal adjustment, prevocational and vocational training, coordination and integration of rehabilitation services, job placement and case management, and followup. Frequently it is a matter of vocational habilitation rather than rehabilitation.

The issue is a complicated one. First, there is the specific problem of the inner city alcoholic who lacks totally job skills and job potentialities (this issue is considered in Chapter 12). Second, career development, in those less deprived, represents one of the major areas in which a substantive change in self-esteem can be effected. The significance of a basic change in self-image, crucial to the development of long-term sobriety, is illustrated in Chapters 1 and 10. Physicians should be familiar with the referral guidelines of vocational rehabilitation centers in their areas and work closely with the counselors involved.

ALCOHOLICS ANONYMOUS (A.A.)

The fellowship and empathetic environment of Alcoholics Anonymous can be of assistance to many patients during the initial phase of treatment.

At no time is the patient more open and needful of the human support that can stem from a person who has recovered from circumstances similar to those currently affecting the patient. To accomplish this:

1. Choose a specific individual whom you know from your own experience will offer opportunities for patient identification in sex, age, marital status, ethnic background, socioeconomic and occupational position, personality, and alcoholic history. Such an individual would in all likelihood lead the patient to the appropriate A.A. groups. The physician out of contact with A.A. is unable to make this rational choice for a patient.
2. Discuss in depth the patient's A.A. experience, both current and past, in order to resolve those difficulties that the patient may raise to resist this therapeutic program. A specific example lies in the nonreligious patient's difficulty with the spiritual aspects of the A.A. program.
3. The physician can not only acquire necessary clinical training by attending A.A. meetings, but can influence the local A.A. membership in various medical matters. The physician may personally make the use of antipsychotic, antidepressant, and aversive therapy credible by developing a dialogue with A.A. group members.

Forming a liaison with and cooperating with A.A. can provide, in many cases, assistance to the physician in the initial and long-term management of the patient.

PROGNOSTIC CONSIDERATIONS

Once a patient is detoxified and enters the initial phase of treatment, there are certain dangers for which the physician should prepare the patient. By discovering and identifying these dangers early in treatment, the patient is more willing to deal with them on a realistic basis in the therapeutic setting. Some of the more common problems facing the patient are as follows:

The "honeymoon period." If patients achieve effective abstinence from alcohol early in treatment, they will most likely receive positive reinforcement from family, friends, employer, etc. for the behavioral change. This will continue for a few weeks, possibly 2-3 months. Then, gradually the significant others in a patient's life will begin to take this behavioral change for granted—and indeed expect it rather than hope for it. As positive reinforcement decreases, patients may interpret this as lack of support or even overt rejection. A return to the use of alcohol occurs frequently at this time. If the patients can anticipate this and if therapy can be directed toward a patient's developing an internal rather than external system of reinforcement, the sense of vulnerability can be markedly attenuated.

The problem of sexual dysfunction. The abstinent alcoholic—particularly the male—should be prepared for the possibility of some sexual dysfunction early in treatment. If this is not discussed, the patient frequently feels as if he were impotent and she were frigid, and often is extemely reluctant to broach the subject in therapy situations. The problem is usually not one of impotence or frigidity but rather a decrease in libidinal drive and depression consequent to the removal of alcohol, which had previously caused a sexually disinhibiting effect and thus an augmented libido. Reassuring the patient and talking with the patient and mate cojointly or separately concerning seeking alternative methods for libidinal stimulation will decrease anxiety and prevent the patient from feeling emasculated or frigid.

The problem of trust versus mistrust. With a dramatic change in behavior that can occur early in treatment, the patient often seeks not only positive reinforcement from significant others but also complete trust from others that the new behavior will continue indefinitely. It is important to point out to the patient that the spouse and/or employer and/or friends may view this change with some initial skepticism, and some element of mistrust should be expected. Emphasizing the destructive effect that the drinking behavior has had in the past on interpersonal relationships encourages the patient to be more realistic in what can be expected immediately from these relationships.

The problem of dysphoria associated with an increased awareness. Many patients imagine that with abstinence from alcohol, symptoms of anxiety and depression, which are normally resultant from situational stress, will no longer occur. In fact, anxiety-depressive symptomatology may be perceived more acutely by the patient without the chemical camouflage of alcohol. Prediction of this by the physician will ameliorate the pain and frustration that characterize the initial phase of treatment.

As a physician assessing the efficacy of initial treatment, it is important to keep in mind that abstinence is a means to an end; that recidivism ("falling off the wagon") does not necessarily mean treatment failure, and that specific signs of improvement should be established, such as the following:

—Does the patient have a realistic understanding of alcohol dependency in regard to her or his personal situation?
—Is the patient actively participating in a treatment program?

—Is there improvement in family and social relationships?
—Is there improvement in job performance?
—Is the patient exhibiting longer periods of effective sobriety and, if in the case of a relapse, are the drinking episodes of shorter duration and less destructive?

Alcoholism in its many guises and with its many complications is not a homogeneous disease entity but rather a disease spectrum. The medical practitioner can assume critical diagnostic and therapeutic roles in the initial phase of treatment after emergency care and medical management have been afforded. Working with other disciplines in the formulation and implementation of an early treatment plan is an essential component of an overall rehabilitation effort and will contribute significantly to the control and recovery of the patient.

REFERENCES

Barten HH (ed): *Brief Therapies*. New York, Behavioral Publications, 1971

Criteria Committee, National Council on Alcoholism: Criteria for the diagnosis of alcoholism. *Am J Psychiatry* 129(2):127-134, 1972

Department of HHS: Confidentiality of alcohol and drug abuse patient records. *Fed Register* 42 CFR Part 2, 52(110):21796-21814, 1987

Fink RD, Knott DH, Beard JD: Sedative-hypnotic dependence. *Am Fam Physician* 10(3):116-122, 1974

Flemenbaum A: Affective disorders and chemical dependence: Lithium for alcohol and drug addiction. *Dis Nerv Syst* 35:281-285, 1974

Goldfarb C, Hartman B: A total community approach to the treatment of alcoholism. *Dis Nerv Syst* 36:409-414, 1975

Knott DH, Beard JD, Fischer AA: Alcoholism—The physician's role in diagnosis and treatment, in Conn HF, Rakel RE, Johnson TW, (eds): *Family Practice*, Philadelphia, W.B. Saunders, 1972, 265-276

Knott DH, Frink RD, Beard JD: Unmasking alcohol abuse. *Am Fam Physician* 10(4):123-128, 1974

Knott DH, Thomson MJ, Beard JD: The forgotten addict. *Am Fam Physician* 3(6):92-95, 1971

McClelland DC, Davis WN, Kalin R, et al: *The Drinking Man*. New York, Free Press, 1972

B.W.: The fellowship of Alcoholics Anonymous, in Catanzaro, RJ (ed): *Alcoholism—The Total Treatment Approach*, Charles C. Thomas, Springfield, Ill., 1968, 116-127

Wallace, J. Working with the Preferred Defense Structure of the Recovering Alcoholic. In: Zimberg, S., Wallace, J., and Blume, S.B., eds. *Practical Approaches to Alcoholism Psychotherapy*. New York, Plenum, 1978, pp. 19-29.

Zimberg, S. Office Psychotherapy of Alcoholism. In: Solomon, J., ed. *Alcoholism and Clinical Psychiatry.* New York. Plenum Medical Books, 1982, pp. 213-229.

6

After Detoxification—The Rehabilitation of the Alcoholic

Gerald D. Shulman
Robert D. O'Connor

The practicing physician is likely to encounter the alcoholic patient in one of three settings: as a patient in an office practice, as a patient discovered on rounds in a community hospital, or as a patient seen in the emergency room of a general hospital. Since the situations that bring the alcoholic to the attention of the physician differ, the circumstances of the initial contact may influence the manner in which care is offered. For example, if the alcoholic is currently a patient of the physician in an office practice, there should already be established a level of trust not present when a patient meets a physician for the first time as a result of an emergency room visit. This may make a significant difference in such things as the patient's level of honesty, willingness to "hear" what the physician is saying, and willingness to act on the physician's recommendations.

After delivering whatever acute medical care might be required, whether in the office or hospital, the physician frequently admonishes the patient, saying, "Don't drink when you go home," or, "cut down on your drinking." The patient able to follow that simple advice in all probability would not have been seen by the physician in the first place. If only the symptoms and acute episodes

ALCOHOLISM:
A Practical Treatment Guide

ISBN 0-8089-1912-1

of a chronic illness are treated with no attempt to deal with the basic illness itself, then the physician has not fulfilled his responsibilities and can be assured that the patient will require treatment again. The treatment of the underlying alcoholism should be considered a specialty, requiring special skills and knowledge. For the physician who is unsure of the diagnostic criteria, or the most appropriate treatment planning, a consultation is indicated. The consultant may be another physician, most frequently an internist or psychiatrist. The consultant may also be a clinical psychologist, a nurse, a social worker, or an alcoholism counselor whose credentials are not academic but result from the experience of his own recovery from alcoholism or work in alcoholism treatment. For such consultation, nonmedical people can be used very effectively.*

Such a consultant may be found on the staff of a community hospital, in an organized alcoholism treatment center in the surrounding community, or through a local voluntary alcoholism agency such as the various local affiliates of the National Council on Alcoholism. Not to be overlooked is the recovered alcoholic member of Alcoholics Anonymous (A.A) who may be a patient in the physician's office practice. This person may provide valuable assistance to the physician and the newly identified alcoholic in helping carry out a treatment plan. The consultation should confirm or rule out the preliminary diagnosis of alcoholism. Unless the physician has considerable experience in dealing with alcoholism, the consultant should be used to assist in the development of a treatment plan.

PRIMARY CARE (DETOXIFICATION)

Good primary care consists of detoxification that allows the patient to safely and comfortably go through the withdrawal process. The use of psychoactive drugs associated with detoxification should be discontinued, and the patient should no longer be using antianxiety drugs or minor tranquilizers. There should be a complete medical evaluation, including a drug screen, with special attention paid to potential cardiopulmonary, gastrointestinal, and hepatic problems. Appropriate medical treatment should be instituted, and there should be a plan for the future management of any unresolved medical problems. During this time, a complete psychosocial evaluation should be done. This psychosocial evaluation should include a history of early dynamics, and educational, vocational, social, and marital adjustment. There should be an in-depth history of alcohol and drug use. If indicated on the basis of preliminary assessment, psychiatric evaluation by someone skilled in dealing with alcoholism should be made. The period during primary care should be further used to help the patient begin to identify as having a problem with chemicals and to motivate him for treatment beyond primary care. Finally, the results of all of this activity should be put together in the form of a written treatment plan, always with the involvement of the patient (see Table 6–1).

*The majority of direct rehabilitation services for alcoholics in this country are provided by nondegreed people.

Table 6–1
Ancillary Uses of the Detoxification Period

Prove diagnosis to patient (e.g., both patient and physician witness withdrawal phenomena)
Establish a relationship between physician and patient (physician's concern with and efforts to relieve the patient's suffering fosters attachment)
Obtain a detailed history
Develop a short-term and possibly a definitive treatment plan
Introduce people with whom the patient can identify (e.g., A.A.)
Use all of the above to augment motivation for treatment and recovery

Certain facilities offer this type of care as part of a more comprehensive treatment program in which primary care* is one component and rehabilitation is another. The primary care component is seen as a part of an overall treatment program if followed by referral into the facility's own inpatient or outpatient components. On the other hand, there are specialized treatment centers that offer only primary care and referral. These facilities tend to use a broader spectrum of resources following initial treatment.

Although it is possible for the physician in office practice to accomplish some of the goals for primary care for the alcoholic, it is usually not feasible. For example, a primary care facility offers the alcoholic an opportunity to identify with other alcoholics. Optimally, primary care should be viewed as a multimodality process, leading to referral for rehabilitation, which will take place in a specialized environment organized specifically to deal with the problems of alcoholism. One very valid reason for referring to a primary care facility even when there are no other major medical problems is the patient's inability to stop drinking on his own.

It cannot be stressed too strongly that at the completion of primary care the patient still suffers from a chronic, progressive, debilitating disease that requires further treatment if the disease is to be arrested successfully and the patient stabilized. After those preliminary and basic steps have been taken, the next critical decision is the match between patient and the most appropriate type of further treatment available.

The matching process is very difficult for two reasons: the clinical spectrum of alcoholism varies greatly, and there is a great diversity of treatment approaches. Some are very appropriate for certain groups of patients, but none are appropriate for all.

First, a word about the diversity of the clinical pictures of alcoholism. It is quite apparent that the 55-year-old homeless, desocialized male alcoholic on skid row whose body is 10–15 years older than his chronologic age presents a very different clinical picture from the 40-year-old upper-middle-class housewife who has never drunk in a bar in her life, who has had extensive and unsuccessful psychotherapy for a variety of somewhat vague adjustment problems, and whose use of Valium

---

*The term *primary care* as used here refers to detoxification and treatment of complications or acute concurrent illness.

and Seconal could be characterized as regular and heavy. Yet another clinical picture is presented by the 18-year-old patient who comes to the attention of the physician for treatment of hepatitis and whose history indicates the patient's involvement in a life-style of drug abuse and addiction; although most of the drugs are acquired illicitly, alcohol is the drug of choice.

The diversity of treatment approaches reflects both the diversity in patient populations and differences in emphasis on the part of therapists. The remainder of this chapter will be an attempt to bring order to this diversity and confusion so that at the conclusion of primary care the physician can better answer the question "What's next?"

REHABILITATION OPTIONS

There are two major rehabilitation approaches for alcoholics—inpatient or outpatient treatment. Within these two broad categories, there are different levels of care as well as different settings. All of these have bearing on the patient-treatment match. Table 6–2 illustrates the different treatment approaches and the settings in which they are most commonly found. One or more settings/approaches may be used. When used in combination, the settings/approaches may be used consecutively or concurrently, as appropriate.

A more recent approach to alcoholism treatment gaining popularity is partial hospitalization (also referred to as intensive outpatient treatment, day treatment, or evening treatment). Partial hospitalization attempts to combine the advantages of the intensity of inpatient treatment with the lower cost and lesser life-style disruption of outpatient treatment. The current emphasis on cost containment has provided considerable impetus for the development of such programs.

Below we shall also discuss treatment for the family of the alcoholic, which includes residential care with or without the alcoholic, outpatient care, Al-Anon, and Alateen.

Table 6–2
Treatment Approaches and Options

Treatment Settings	Inpatient			Outpatient					
	Short-Term Intermediate	Long-Term Intermediate	Halfway House	Traditional Outpatient	Intensive Outpatient	A.A.	A.A. Clubhouse*	Al-Anon*	Alateen*
Acute care hospital	x			x	x	x	x	x	x
Psychiatric hospital	x	x		x	x	x	x	x	x
Freestanding facility**	x	x	x	x	x	x	x	x	x
Self-help						x	x	x	x

Note. Each facility may, but need not, possess each of the indicated (x) modalities.
* Although meetings may take place in hospital settings, they are otherwise unsupported by these environments.
** Defined as existing separately from a larger treatment facility.

Inpatient Rehabilitation

For the purpose of discussion, a few definitions are in order. Both short- and long-term residential treatments are sometimes referred to as intermediate care, because the intensity of treatment is less than that which is normally found in an acute care hospital; however, there is no doubt that care is being provided. Other terms sometimes applied to this sort of care are *psychosocial treatment* and, simply, *rehabilitation*.

We define as short-term that care ranging in duration from a minimum of 2 weeks to 6–12 weeks, the most common programs being approximately 4 weeks in length. Long-term programs are those that are usually no less than 3 months in duration and may extend up to 1–2 years. Some programs are time-limited, with a fixed time period that can be extended, whereas others are open-ended. Short-term programs usually provide more structure and a more intensive level of programming and therapy, and are more likely to view themselves as limited to initiating an ongoing recovery process. Long-term programs may or may not be structured but try to achieve more of the treatment goals within the duration of the treatment program itself rather than allowing these to be accomplished over a longer period of time after discharge. Longer programs tend to have a heavier emphasis on resocialization.*

Some treatment centers make a distinction in the expected duration of treatment between those patients whose primary addiction is to alcohol and those who may have a heavy involvement with other drugs in addition to the alcohol. This is particularly true if the other drugs are illicitly obtained. Current thinking is that it may take longer to effectively deal with other drug addiction problems, particularly if the drugs are acquired illicitly. In terms of duration of inpatient rehabilitation, use of alcohol alone requires the least amount of time, solid sedative addiction prolongs this period, and parenteral opiate use prolongs time to a multiple of this. On the whole, long-term programs tend to be separated from the traditional health care system, with less medical, psychiatric, and social service expertise. They also receive poorer third-party reimbursement than the short-term programs.

The alcoholism rehabilitation center, short- or long-term, is a specialized unit. Such treatment is provided through different treatment settings (see Table 6–2) and accordingly may vary in the style in which treatment is delivered. For example, an alcoholism unit in a psychiatric hospital tends to be more psychiatrically oriented, sometimes because of philosophic considerations but other times because of administrative and monetary considerations (e.g., financial support of psychiatric staff who may not be involved with the alcoholism unit). The same is

**Resocialization* is used to signify the process by which maladjusted persons attain those attitudes and skills that will facilitate their again becoming accepted members of the community. This is a particularly important aspect of treatment for addicts whose addiction has removed them from the general community (public inebriates and drug addicts who are totally integrated into a drug addiction subculture).

true in the acute care hospital setting. Alcoholism rehabilitation units found in psychiatric or acute care hospitals tend to be more expensive than freestanding facilities, but by the same token, they are usually able to generate better third-party reimbursement. One cannot assume from these facts, however, that units found within either the psychiatric or acute care hospital setting offer either better or worse care than the freestanding unit.

Often the setting can and does determine the nature of the treatment and therefore the appropriateness of the referral. There are three major treatment settings for intermediate care (frequently the differences among individual treatment programs in any one group of settings may be greater than the variance between treatment programs in different settings):

1. The psychiatric hospital, without a specialized alcoholism unit.
2. The alcoholism rehabilitation unit located in either a psychiatric or acute care hospital.
3. The freestanding alcoholism rehabilitation unit that is not part of another facility.

The psychiatric hospital without an alcoholism unit has traditionally treated alcoholism not as an addiction but as symptomatic of an underlying personality disorder. The focus is on cause and underlying problems. When this treatment is performed with full cognizance of the need to discontinue the addicting substance as a prerequisite to psychotherapy or any other intervention, one can appreciate that differing disciplines arrive at surprisingly similar therapeutic approaches. If the drinking continues unabated, there is little chance for successful resolution of the alcoholism.

Short-Term Residential Rehabilitation

The freestanding alcoholism rehabilitation program is the one that was developed about 20–25 years ago to fill a void for specialized alcoholism treatment. These programs range from highly sophisticated treatment facilities with considerable medical, psychiatric, and social services, to those with very little formal program. Depending on the facility, A.A. can play a minor or significant role in the treatment program. In the latter case, it is often interwoven into the psychosocial and therapeutic aspects of the program. These facilities may vary from "mom and pop" outfits run by charismatic and therapeutically effective individuals who have themselves recovered from alcoholism through A.A., to complex and sophisticated residences offering professional individual and group psychotherapy, vocational rehabilitation, and so forth. Turnover of personnel in the former may result in a disastrous change in therapeutic effectiveness, whereas the latter facilities tend toward greater reliability.

Although the program content in these inpatient treatment centers varies from facility to facility, there are components common to most. In many programs there will be an education component, which focuses on the program and steps of A.A., the problem of alcoholism, and cross-addiction, and which addresses living problems and so forth. Most facilities use some form of group therapy, usually as their major treatment modality. The nature of this therapy varies from discussion groups in which patients are simply seated in a circle, to psychodynamically oriented groups. Individual counseling is an essential part of these programs. There may also be work therapy, occupational therapy, or recreational therapy. This type of treatment setting will complete an in-depth psychosocial evaluation (in more depth than occurs in the primary care facility discussed earlier); from this overall evaluation the staff will develop a comprehensive medical and psychosocial treatment plan. Those treatment programs with heavy emphasis on A.A. may ask the patient to do a fourth step (a written personal inventory of "character defects") and a fifth step (sharing with another person the information that resulted from that inventory) after the patient has completed the first three steps (since they should be accomplished in order). They may provide A.A. meetings in-house or take patients to meetings away from the facility. Family counseling will be available, although the range of services provided for the family is very broad and will be discussed later in this chapter.

Short-term intermediate care programs of approximately 4 weeks' duration are effective for many alcoholic patients. Such programs not only keep patients from alcohol for 28 days but also give them sufficient time away from the potentially distracting home and job problems without creating a catastrophic disruption in lifestyle. Short-term inpatient rehabilitation programs should have relatively modest goals, and such treatment should be seen as the beginning of an ongoing recovery process rather than one that is a complete process. Reasonable goals to expect from such treatment include a beginning, meaningful identification with the problem of alcoholism, some realistic motivation for recovery, some insight into the addictive process and its effects, and most importantly, a concrete plan for continuing recovery (an aftercare plan). This plan should be developed jointly by the treatment staff and the patient and should be in the form of a written contract that details what the patient, possibly the patient's family, and the treatment center will do after discharge. There should be a follow-up system by the treatment center. The goal of the aftercare and follow-up part of the program is to consolidate the gains made during treatment. The treatment center staff must have a system that allows them to reach out to the patient who has difficulties with sobriety and/or living problems. This may be accomplished by representatives trained at the rehabilitation facility who are assigned by geographic coincidence to follow specific patients, private therapists (physicians or counselors) acquainted with the rehabilitation plan, or, when possible, local outpatient care supplied by the facility itself.

Long-Term Residential Rehabilitation

Long-term treatment, previously described as lasting from 3 months to 2 years, shares a number of program components with short-term programs. One feature that distinguishes it from short-term programs is a concentration on the resocialization of the patient. In short-term treatment there is usually an attempt to minimize disruption of life-style, whereas in long-term treatment such disruption is viewed as advantageous, if not necessary, to effect recovery.

Generally, the level of intensity of treatment is less than in the short-term programs, although there are exceptions. Some programs are modeled after the drug addiction therapeutic communities (TCs), which offer not only long-term treatment but also enforced separation from the outside world and the chemicals that accompany it. This separation is achieved by telephone blackouts (no phone calls—incoming or outgoing—permitted), confinement to facility grounds, and a restrictive visiting policy. At times, visitors are totally prohibited. This type of program is usually characterized by a rigid and authoritarian environment. Therapy is strongly confrontive and at times assaultive. Progress is measured by the degree of responsibility the patient exhibits. An example of such a program would be Synanon (as originally conceived).

Other long-term programs are essentially similar to the short-term programs but extend treatment over a longer time period. They lack the confrontive, authoritarian style of the previous type and are considerably less separated from the outside world.

Halfway Houses

A halfway house is basically a structured transitional living situation. It is commonly used following short-term rehabilitation care. It may follow primary care when the patient has previously had inpatient treatment and it is felt that return to short-term rehabilitation would not be as effective as a structured living situation. This type of program can be used for the patient who has a home but should not return to it. Examples of the latter would be the female patient who has been living with a drinking alcoholic spouse who physically abuses her. Another example would be the unmarried male alcoholic who lives alone in a room above a bar around which his entire social life revolves.

In halfway house programs there are 10–20 alcoholics living together, sharing the responsibilities for maintenance of the house but gainfully employed outside of it. The halfway house then represents their home, which provides a supportive living environment, a low level of treatment, and some A.A. meetings that are held within the house. The duration of halfway house care is usually 3–6 months, although there are programs that are open-ended, particularly for those alcoholics who suffer from chronic brain syndrome. For these people, the program may become a permanent home. Levels of program intensity in halfway houses vary, so that at one end of the spectrum there is a group living situation, while at the other end the program functions almost as an inpatient rehabilitation center.

OUTPATIENT REHABILITATION

Outpatient Alcoholism Services

Organized outpatient treatment is usually offered in the form of an outpatient alcoholism clinic or group practice and may directly follow primary care when judged sufficiently intensive to meet the patient's needs. It may also be used following residential rehabilitation when continued structured treatment is indicated. It is sometimes provided to a patient who is currently a resident of a halfway house. There are some specialists in alcoholism who provide this service in their office practice, but it is important to distinguish between outpatient treatment for the alcoholism and more traditional psychotherapy for the treatment of other problems. The latter is usually not effective unless begun 6–12 months after the cessation of drinking and after the patient has had some form of primary alcoholism treatment. In cases where traditional psychotherapy must begin earlier, some kind of alcoholism treatment, even if only supportive, should be taking place simultaneously.

Some outpatient alcoholism clinics are occasionally part of a larger mental health clinic or community mental health center, while others are alcoholism specific. These last may be located in general or psychiatric hospitals, may be part of a residential alcoholism treatment center, or may be freestanding. They specialize in providing treatment to both the alcoholic and the family members. They can be used by patients who need more structure than would be provided by A.A. alone, even after residential care, or those who are unable to "get away" for residential care. The latter problem should be checked out carefully because the real issue may well be one of resistance to treatment and not of time constraints.

While traditional outpatient treatment may involve 1–3 hours of care each week, intensive outpatient treatment may range from 5–25 or more hours of care each week. Programming may be offered during the day, evening, or weekends or in a combination of times.

Intensive outpatient treatment is a viable option when the patient is living in a relatively secure and stable environment, is moderately well motivated and does not have a history of previous treatment failure. Day treatment may be particularly appropriate for a single mother with school-age children. She can receive intensive treatment and still be home when her children arrive from school. It will enable someone working second shift to continue on the job. Evening treatment can be a most appropriate option for a patient whose days are otherwise occupied.

Alcoholics Anonymous

The oldest and most successful form of outpatient treatment for alcoholics is the program of Alcoholics Anonymous. Although informal, A.A. provides a worldwide recovery network for alcoholics. It is important to recognize that a significant number of alcoholics come to A.A., receive no other treatment, and recover; however, it appears that the combination of formal treatment in conjunction with A.A. increases the probability of recovery. In an employee alcoholism program, it was found that those patients who first went into short-term inpatient rehabilitation and then to A.A. maintained abstinence at twice the rate as those patients who went directly into A.A. Alcoholics Anonymous is effective and should be part of any treatment program, inpatient or outpatient. We would strongly urge any treatment person who will be working with alcoholics to attend some open A.A. meetings to learn more about the program of A.A.

One variation of the A.A. program is the A.A. clubhouse, a place that is open for long periods of time during the day and/or evening and that represents a place where the alcoholic can go, spend time, and chat with other recovering alcoholics. This setting will often provide a variety of benefits such as the replacement of the drinking environment, a new social group for the patient, and a supportive environment for a significant segment of the day.

It has been our experience that a number of professionals are ambivalent about use of and referral to A.A., particularly if their patients are resistant to A.A. What is not understood is that the patient's resistance to A.A. almost always represents resistance to sobriety because it poses a major threat to the alcoholic. The patient, and often the professional, may not recognize this, and therefore both may offer other reasons for not using A.A. The practice of good medicine, however, dictates that the physician use those approaches that have the greatest probability of creating positive change in the patient, even if the patient "doesn't like it." The attitudes of the referring physician about A.A. will have a major effect on whether or not the patient will accept the referral.

Aftercare

Although aftercare is not a separate treatment option, it is included here because it is offered in an outpatient format. Each treatment program, inpatient and outpatient alike, must have its own aftercare program. Aftercare is provided in a variety of ways, including: (1) aftercare groups conducted at a treatment center, (2) ongoing phone and letter contact between the treatment center and the patient, (3) aftercare groups located in the patient's home area if the patient lives some distance from the treatment center, and (4) "refresher courses" and postdischarge sessions. Most aftercare/follow-up programs continue from 3 months to 2 years after discharge. They may also include the family of the alcoholic patient. Aftercare, in the final stage of analysis, should be viewed not as another kind of treatment but as a component and therefore a continuation of the initial program. It is important to recognize that this differs from the usual alcoholism treatment offered in an outpatient clinic in that the goals are very limited and deal with the problems of reentry while simultaneously attempting to consolidate gains made during primary alcoholism treatment. Aftercare does not provide ongoing alcoholism treatment or psychotherapy, as is the case in an outpatient alcoholism clinic.

When patients are involved in aftercare groups, they may come back to the facility in which they received the original treatment for a period of 4–12 weeks, although some programs may extend from 1–2 years. The longer aftercare programs begin to blur the distinction between aftercare programs as previously defined (the purpose of which is to consolidate gains in treatment) and outpatient alcoholism treatment or psychotherapy. These shorter programs are time-limited and do not take the place of either more intensive treatment, when necessary, or A.A.

Because alcoholics now entering treatment are referred by increasingly different sources of referral, they represent a much more heterogenous group manifesting the entire range of emotional and psychological adjustment problems and psychopathology. Alcoholics on discharge are now being referred for specialized, intensive care (e.g., family therapy, sexual therapy, treatment of concurrent affective disorders, etc.) to deal with these other issues. When possible, a period of 6 months of sobriety may make this treatment most effective. In other cases (e.g., suicidal patients), such treatment may have to begin immediately. This treatment, no matter how necessary, should not be considered alcoholism treatment per se.

FAMILY TREATMENT

Appropriately, the family of the alcoholic is receiving growing attention. Almost all treatment programs currently have some kind of family program, which may range from a one-time evaluation and counseling session with the family to inpatient residential treatment for one or more of the family members. Residential treatment of the family member may coincide with the residential treatment of the alcoholic during all or part of the time the alcoholic is in primary treatment. Brief family residential treatment usually occurs in the last stages of the alcoholic's treatment and may range in time from 3 days to 1 week. Some inpatient treatment programs are beginning to mimic what outpatient alcoholism clinics have done for a long time, taking the family members of the alcoholic into treatment, even if the alcoholic himself or herself is not in treatment.

Family treatment is also being offered to adult children of alcoholics (COAs), to respond to the significant problems that result from being raised in an alcoholic home. Such treatment tends to focus more on "family of origin" issues than does usual family treatment in alcoholism. During the early months of treatment of the alcoholic, an Al-Anon approach to the care of the family is more appropriate.

A number of treatment centers are now providing an aftercare program for the family as well as for the alcoholic patient. Excellent outpatient resources for family members and/or significant others related to the alcoholic are Al-Anon, Alateen (for the teenage children of alcoholics), and Children of Alcoholics (COA groups) or Adult Children of Alcoholics (ACA) groups for COAs. All are very similar in philosophy to A.A. and oriented primarily to helping the family members/significant others with their own living problems (see Chapter 11).

THE CHOICE OF TREATMENT OPTION

Simply listing and describing treatment options does not answer the question "Why choose any of them?" At the risk of being repetitive, we reiterate that alcoholism is a chronic illness and that primary treatment or detoxification alone addresses only the physical and medical aspects of the disease process. Something now has to occur with reference to the psychosocial/behavioral aspects of illness if real recovery is to begin. Said another way, the problem for alcoholics is not stopping drinking. Many have stopped hundreds and thousands of times. The problem is staying stopped.

The physician has two responsibilities in this area. The first is to choose the appropriate type of treatment program, and the second is to choose the best treatment facility within that type for the patient. There are a number of parameters that can be used in making a decision about referral to postprimary care. Once again, for the physician who is uncertain about referral because of a lack of familiarity either with the treatment resources or with the specific needs of this patient, we strongly urge the use of consultation with people knowledgeable about diagnosis and treatment planning for alcoholics.

PATIENT VARIABLES AND CHOICE OF TREATMENT

In the past, the authors of this chapter had a definite bias for inpatient treatment, which appeared to be the most effective way to begin the treatment process. However, with more patients coming for treatment earlier in the progression of their illnesses and the increase in availability of intensive outpatient treatment, the formerly clear distinctions between inpatient and outpatient services have become blurred. What we would recommend is an intensity of treatment that results in an initial "push" that can carry the alcoholic over the rough spots in early recovery (Table 6–3). Given our bias, we would now like to describe some of the patient variables that can be used in selecting the most appropriate resource.

Coexisting Medical Problems

Obviously, the patient who has serious medical problems that will require ongoing medical treatment will need to be in a rehabilitative setting where such treatment is easily obtained. It is usually counterproductive to have an alcoholic patient continually interrupt alcoholism treatment in order to get medical treatment at another facility. Treatment settings providing such care include residential rehabilitation centers housed in acute care hospitals or freestanding treatment centers with associated medical care units.

Table 6–3
Advantages of Early Use of Intensive Rehabilitation

More probable period of abstinence during treatment
More rapid learning about illness and alternate coping mechanisms than likely to be achieved in traditional outpatient or in A.A. alone
Impresses patient with gravity of problem
More rapid opportunity to achieve identification with and relate to other patients with alcoholism
More integrated health care delivery

Coexisting Psychiatric Problems

The majority of alcoholics do not have such psychiatric problems as to require specialized psychiatric attention at that time. For those who do, the alcoholism treatment center may be faced with major management problems or other distractions from treatment. The most common problems are affective disorders or psychosis, which if adequately diagnosed can be managed by the use of an antidepressive or antipsychotic drug, a supportive environment, or both. Care must be exercised to ascertain that the psychiatric diagnosis is valid. Many alcoholics, when evaluated by professionals not experienced in alcoholism, are misdiagnosed because the symptoms of their alcoholism mimic a psychotic process, and they are mistakenly placed on antipsychotic drugs. It may require up to 6 weeks off psychotropic drugs in order to establish a nondrug-related psychiatric diagnosis.

If the patient does require an antipsychotic drug, care should be taken to avoid choosing a rigidly drug-free rehabilitation program. Some rehabilitation programs have recognized the dangers of prescribing psychoactive drugs to alcoholics, who frequently become dual- or cross-addicted. Unfortunately, some facilities have generalized from the dangers of specific drugs such as sedatives, barbiturates, and antianxiety medications, to antipsychotic and antidepressive drugs. They sometimes go so far as to prohibit such things as vitamins, hormones, and so forth. Obviously, such a program will be inappropriate for the patient requiring antipsychotic drugs. There are treatment facilities that, while recognizing the potential that psychoactive drugs have in reinforcing the addiction, will evaluate each situation individually, often permitting the use of other than antianxiety drugs when indicated. If ongoing psychiatric treatment is required and/or management problems are in evidence, the obvious choice would be an alcoholism unit within or attached to a psychiatric hospital.

A word of caution about psychological depression in alcoholics: depression, particularly reactive depression, is a very common symptom of addiction and does not necessarily indicate a separate affective disorder or indicate a need for antidepressant drugs. Although there are some alcoholics with affective disorders, it is difficult to make that kind of diagnosis within a few months of the cessation of drinking. Frequently, when this diagnosis is made too early it is in error. When possible, it is better to offer the alcoholic emotional support and reassurance than to immediately prescribe antidepressant drugs. The period of depression will frequently end of its own accord after a period of recovery from alcoholism. On the other hand, if the depression is profound and associated with significant sleep disturbances, high levels of agitation, serious suicidal ideation or threats, history of previous manic episodes, family history of serious affective disturbances, and somatic and other delusions, prompt intervention is obviously required.

The patient who manifests a character disorder along with the alcoholism will require a long-term, highly structured, and highly confrontative (although not necessarily psychiatrically oriented) program. Alcoholics who are particularly immature and/or dependent may also require a long-term program that is highly structured but not confrontative. On the other hand, these patients may best respond to a program wherein they are confronted gently at first and to a greater degree as the transference allows. Problems such as chronic brain syndrome may require a very supportive program with a high degree of structure and of substantial duration. (See Chapters 9 and 10 for further discussion of these problems.)

Degree of Structure Required

Patients with poor impulse control, those who have suffered at least a moderate degree of organic impairment, those who are younger and require major help in socialization or resocialization, those who are very immature and dependent, and those with a previous history of unsuccessful treatment generally can benefit from a more structured environment. Although this is not always true, usually the more highly structured programs are also of longer term. Obviously, a process such as resocialization will not take place in a 4-week period. On the other hand, there are some very good short-term treatment programs that are highly structured, so that the variables of both time and structure should be considered.

Current Living Arrangements

The patient who is living with an intact family that can provide emotional support, who has shown a gradual decline into an addiction over a period of years, who is employed, and who can generally function in a responsible manner can benefit from either a short-term inpatient program or an outpatient program. On the other hand, the alcoholic who lives alone, or who lives with a drinking alcoholic spouse, is best separated from that living situation and should, at least temporarily, be removed from that environment. The probability of an alcoholic maintaining abstinence in early recovery while living with a drinking alcoholic family member is not very good. The family member may have been the alcoholic's drinking partner. Abstinence by the patient will represent a threat to the family member, which may result in an unconscious attempt to sabotage the abstinence of the newly sober person. In this situation the patient may be a candidate not only for inpatient residential treatment but possibly for a halfway house after residential treatment.

The alcoholic who is also a drug addict and who has supported the addiction by dealing in drugs obviously cannot go back to his old "vocation" and expect to stay straight. A return to the "old neighborhood" usually means a return to drugs.

It is important to recognize that merely separating the alcoholic from the drinking environment will not bring about recovery. In A.A., this known as a "geographical cure." The problem is that alcoholics bring the alcoholism with them wherever they go. Sometimes the presence of the drinking or drug-using environment is either a distraction or so destructive a force that it impedes the delivery of effective treatment, particularly on an outpatient basis.

Family Relationships

The level of psychologic health and supportiveness of the significant others is very important. Family members, because of their own psychodynamics, can at times be tremendously destructive forces in the alcoholic's attempts to recover. Their attitudes can mitigate the gains that occur in treatment. Even those who are not themselves drinking alcoholics may unconsciously attempt to sabotage the sobriety of the patient. The family, including the alcoholic, should be viewed as a dynamic system in which the family members adapt to the alcoholism in various pathologic ways. No matter how vigorously family members complain about "their alcoholic," they often receive some sort of gratification from the situation. Some members may adopt the role of a martyr, suffering long and loudly but unwilling to do anything that might change the situation; they may attempt to control the alcoholic, the alcoholism, and even treatment; they may become rescuers who continue to help the alcoholic avoid the consequences of the alcoholism. If the alcoholic recovers, thereby changing roles in the system, the system changes. This interferes with the ability of the family members to continue receiving gratification from their respective roles, which results in a considerable threat and creates stress on the system. It is for these reasons that the situation must be evaluated to help not only the alcoholic but the family.

Depending on the extent of the family pathology, a referral to family treatment (alcoholism-specific), Al-Anon, or Alateen may be sufficient. If the problems are severe enough, formal family therapy in an outpatient setting is indicated. There are times when the extent of the pathology is so drastic that the only solution, if the alcoholic is to stay sober, is at least a temporary, if not permanent, separation from the family. This is especially indicated in cases where the family members refuse to accept referral for treatment themselves.

Employment Situation

Another issue that must be examined is the employment situation. Close proximity to drinking environments may be a factor leading to a referral to treatment that removes the patient from the job: that is, residential treatment. For example, although there are recovered alcoholics who are employed as bartenders, returning to bartending early in recovery may place additional stress on the patient. Other job-related indications for residential treatment are the shifts worked and the amount of work-related travel. The patient who works varying shifts may not be able to receive consistent or intense enough treatment in an outpatient setting. Extensive travel may produce the same problem. In general, freelance as opposed to more structured employment tends to greater isolation and is therefore less desirable.

Attempts at Previous Rehabilitation

The treatment history of the patient has to be examined very closely. When the history indicates that a particular type of treatment program has been used without success, the physician should think in terms of a different kind (e.g., replacing outpatient with inpatient or short-term with long-term treatment). The recurrent use of the same inpatient treatment center, in light of repeated relapses, is usually unwise. There are some long-term treatment centers (extended care) that view themselves as offering treatment primarily to alcoholics who have been unsuccessful in previous treatment attempts. It is not unusual for such programs to require a history of numerous treatment failures as a criterion for admission.

In taking the treatment history, it is helpful to distinguish between an admission to a general hospital for the medical treatment of the sequelae of the alcoholism and one characterized by direct treatment of the alcoholism itself. Although a previous history of treatment for the medical complications of alcoholism can be used to confront the alcoholic with the extent of the problem, it should not be considered as an "unsuccessful" rehabilitative experience.

Time Availability

Although this concern is obviously important, it cannot be considered the major factor. For example, the patient who has been unsuccessfully involved in outpatient treatment over an extended period of time may simply have to find the time for residential care. On the other hand, it is appropriate to consider outpatient treatment if the patient can accomplish the objectives effectively in this setting. This is especially true if residential treatment creates a major hardship. One example would be a divorced or separated woman with young children and no one to care for them while she is in residential treatment.

Be prepared for the fact that many alcoholics will "not have the time" (as they perceive it) to do anything about their drinking. Perhaps an agreement can be made that if the patient can remain abstinent by means of outpatient care for a significant period of time, he does not have to go to a facility. Thus, the need to go away (possibly threatening a job) becomes the patient's own responsibility, not the doctor's. The patient who slips must blame the illness, not the physician's philosophy. On the other hand, when your assessment of this situation indicates that you are dealing with resistance to treatment rather than a real problem, the role of the physician is to be supportive but firm in his or her recommendation.

Consequences of Relapse

Certain conditions create a greater than usual risk to patients should they relapse and resume drinking. In certain instances the consequences of relapse may be disastrous. For example, the patient who has had extensive medical problems, such as esophageal varices and a subsequent portal caval shunt, must be regarded as a "last chance." This patient will not likely have the opportunity to fail more than once in a treatment experience, and all pressures should be brought to bear on such a patient to follow the most appropriate treatment program. Another situation with potentially dire consequences is the patient who may have been placed on probation; and if the patient drinks again, the probation will be revoked and the patient jailed. The situation makes the choice of appropriate treatment most critical. The same choice is critical also in situations where another drinking episode will result in termination of employment or the break-up of the family.

Pattern of Substance Abuse

When alcoholism is complicated by a history of secondary drug use, the problem is somewhat more difficult to treat and therefore may require additional time in treatment. Dually addicted or cross-addicted patients generally respond better to intensive treatment. The method of acquisition of the drug is another issue. The patient who has acquired drugs illegally (on the street) must be separated from that drug-using subculture. In this situation, outpatient treatment is almost always a failure, since the entire subculture consists primarily of users and suppliers of the drugs. A comparable situation would be the use of a legal drug (alcohol) in which the alcoholic is a member of "taproom society." Here all of the significant others in the life of this alcoholic are drinking companions, and home is the bar. This pattern will definitely require separation from that subculture.

Age

Age is a very significant factor. In the past, many alcoholism treatment people believed that there were significant differences between those patients who were addicted to alcohol and those who were addicted primarily to opiate drugs. What has become apparent is that the differences are based not only on the drug of choice but also on age. The majority of opiate or polydrug addicts seen by the physician are young people who have been involved in an addictive life-style for most of their adolescent and later years. They will require longer-term, more structured treatment with emphasis on resocialization. Many alcoholics, on the other hand, particularly those whose problem drinking began later in life, are people who have accomplished something in their lives and possibly lost it as a result of the drinking. For them, recovery is returning to an earlier level of successful functioning rather than learning a drug-free coping style for the first time.

Some treatment programs have a relatively narrow range of patient ages, while others are much broader. Adolescents, unless they are quite mature, usually do better in a program geared to the specific needs of their age group. Young addicts also have difficulty identifying with the "older" patients in treatment. Parental consent and continued schooling are also considerations when treatment is going to be of long duration.

Older patients may need greater structure and/or longer-term programs. Experience indicates that they require more time to recover from the physical effects of the drinking, and many times in short-term treatment program they begin to "clear" only at about the time the other patients are being discharged. When there is disruption in affective or cognitive functioning due to early arteriosclerotic or senile or Alzheimer's changes, a high degree of structure is helpful.

Sociocultural and Economic Factors

Socioeconomic level is another variable to be considered in choosing a program. It is inappropriate to refer someone into a program when the patient will experience cultural shock, as might be the case in which a young alcoholic/drug abuser from a rural community is sent to an inner-city drug program. Also, patients should not be referred to programs too far above their socioeconomic level; the patients will feel chronically uncomfortable and out of place and will not be able to identify with the other patients. The converse is also true. Some treatment programs provide a broad socioeconomic cross-section, which prevents this kind of problem. The physician must also be alert to a potential language problem (a Hispanic who speaks very poor English cannot be sent to a treatment center where there are no Spanish-speaking members of the treatment staff).

Intellectual/Educational Factors

If intellectual ability and educational level present problems, care should be taken to assure that a good patient/program match is made. When intellectual functioning is significantly impaired because of chronic brain syndrome or when the patient is borderline mentally retarded, a long-term, highly structured, relatively simple program with heavy use of reality therapy is a good choice. Analytically oriented programs that require a good deal of introspection and insight are wasted on such patients. In cases where the patient is of average intelligence but illiterate, care should be taken that the treatment center to which the patient will be referred has the capability for handling the situation.

Physical Handicaps

The presence of a physical handicap, such as significant hearing loss, speech impairment, blindness, or learning disability, may severely restrict the number of treatment opportunities available. A sometimes overlooked problem is the patient who lacks ease of mobility because of a handicap. If the patient is being referred to a residential treatment program, it should be determined beforehand that the handicap will not impede treatment. When considering referral to outpatient treatment, keep in mind that the major obstacle to receiving such care may be associated with travel. The necessity of using public transportation may further compound the problem.

CHOICE OF THE SPECIFIC TREATMENT FACILITY

Whatever type of treatment is chosen for the patient, you should be familiar with the treatment center itself. Begin by determining if it is licensed and by what agency and whether or not it is accredited by the Joint Commission on Accreditation of Hospitals (this is more appropriate to inpatient rehabilitation centers than halfway houses or outpatient clinics). Try to ascertain its general reputation by checking with people who are involved in the alcoholism treatment field (A.A., National Council on Alcoholism, or their affiliates). Much can be determined by a request for literature from the treatment center as well as by talking with the staff or representatives directly by phone. Do not hesitate to ask very pointed questions about costs, program duration, treatment philosophy, aftercare, or whatever else will assist you in making the most appropriate referral for your patient. The ideal arrangement, whenever possible, is a personal visit to the facility. Again, when trying to choose the specific treatment facility that best suits your patient, don't hesitate to use the consultants you may have used previously to confirm the diagnosis or help with treatment planning.

THE ROLE OF THE PHYSICIAN VIS-A-VIS THE TREATMENT CENTER

It is important that the referring physician supply the treatment agency with as much information about the patient as possible. Valuable information includes a medical history, particularly as it relates to the alcoholism, drug history (if any), and the symptoms (vocational, familial, social, etc.) that have led the physician to a diagnosis of alcoholism. Of special importance is the physician's assessment of patient identification with the alcoholism, motivation for recovery, and level of credibility when patients discuss their use of chemicals and resultant problems. There are times when the treatment program will call the physician for additional information. Be open and available to them. In return, the physician should expect to receive a history and physical examination report and a summary letter from the facility about the patient's progress, prognosis, and aftercare plans, including the specifics of the aftercare contract to which the patient is committed. (The physician may also be asked to participate in the development of the aftercare plan.) Any existing medical management problems should also be brought to the physician's attention.

Depending on the duration of treatment and on the arrangements made between the physician and treatment centers, progress reports may be sent to the physician on a regular basis. In any case, the physician should expect a verbal progress report about a patient in response to a phone call.

Expectations of Successful Outcome

Since alcoholism is a chronic, progressive illness characterized by exacerbation and remission of symptoms, the goal of treatment is to achieve permanent remission. No responsible treatment person would recommend any course other than abstinence. Abstinence, however, although a necessary beginning step in recovery, is not necessarily synonymous with recovery. Patients who function as irresponsibly when abstinent as they did when drinking represent something less than recovery. We are reminded of a patient who was a "hit man" for organized crime. After completing our treatment program, he did not drink again. As we were congratulating ourselves on the fine job we had done with him, we recognized that what we had really accomplished was to help improve his aim.

Recovery is best defined in terms of improved psychological adjustment, satisfaction with self, job performance, and interpersonal relationships. All of these things take place with greater likelihood with abstinence.

Early indications of successful treatment are reduction of the patient's denial or minimization of the problem of alcoholism and a general positive change in attitude, including a reduction of the anger originally felt toward the physician for the diagnosis and referral into treatment. Patients should exhibit greater awareness of the relationship between their other problems and the use of chemicals and should have firm commitments to follow through with aftercare plans.

Continued Role of the Physician with the Patient

If, in fact, the physician has been responsible for getting the patient into successful rehabilitation, then the major part of the physician's role has been completed; however, this does not and should not terminate the relationship involving the patient's alcoholism. The physician may be required to continue the treatment of the sequelae of the alcoholism. He can remain an ongoing supportive resource to the alcoholic and his family, recognizing that alcoholism is a chronic illness and that there may be a relapse. The doctor's continued involvement with the patient around other medical problems can be helpful because there is now an awareness of and sensitivity to such things as the danger of prescribing elixir of terpin hydrate with codeine for a cough. The physician has now played an extremely valuable role by recognizing and communicating to the patient that primary care alone is insufficient, and by referring the patient to appropriate rehabilitation. Ongoing emotional support can be an invaluable aid to the now recovering patient. Follow-up contact will help prevent relapse or help constructive referral if a relapse occurs.

7

Long-Term Management

Joseph J. Zuska
Joseph A. Pursch

The long-term treatment of the alcoholic requires rethinking of the "medical model" and the usual definitions of alcoholism that place the site and cause of the disease within the individual.[1] A more appropriate working definition for the long-term management concept is as follows: Alcoholism is an illness that is a reciprocal relationship between the individual and the social environment. It is characterized in the individual by the developing dependency on alcohol resulting in alienation, dependency, loss of self-esteem, role dysfunction, and an apparent irreversible inability to safely ingest alcohol. The illness is characterized in the community by responses and practices that actively create social pressure to drink and that reinforce individual alienation and dependency. The illness is further characterized by denial of the problem by the individual and/or the community, unless and until visible dysfunction results in recognition.[2]

Long-term recovery has no time limit—it is a lifetime program dealing with a chronic, relapsing illness, and although less and less professional aid will be necessary after the first year or two, the physician interested in the long view may well maintain contact with patients indefinitely. Indeed, many of them may become the physician's close friends—a phenomenon that is often discouraged in other fields of medicine.

ALCOHOLISM:
A Practical Treatment Guide

ISBN 0-8089-1912-1

The physician then must be prepared to enter into a lifetime relationship with recovering alcoholics and their families. This means accepting them as equals and being willing to attend signficant happenings in the course of patients' progress, such as an Alcoholics Anonymous birthday celebrating each year of sobriety. The physician must be willing to share his feelings and, yes, even shortcomings when counseling alcoholics or participating with them in group settings. Above all, the physician must be aware of the limitation of the one-to-one relationship in a disease that has medical, social, and spiritual facets. Not only other physicians but also other agencies, recovery homes, paraprofessionals, volunteers, and especially a peer group of recovered alcoholics will be needed from time to time. A thorough working knowledge of appropriate community resources is essential. By enmeshing alcoholics and their families in a continuum of services that includes Alcoholics Anonymous and maintaining a close personal interest as a physician-friend, one can play a pivotal role in guiding alcoholics and their families into recovery.

As the physician's interest and knowledge grows, he will often participate in community education on matters of early diagnosis and prevention and stimulate the development of appropriate curricula in medical schools and schools of nursing. Such outreach accomplishment increases physician credibility and convinces patients of his genuine and abiding interest in their problems. A fringe benefit to the physician will often be a lessening of his own drinking.

The essence of this concept is that one cannot adopt a classical psychoanalytic model in the treatment of the alcoholic. Patients seeking psychological treatment implicitly request that the therapist play a role in their life patterned on figures from their pasts (the magical father, nurturant mother, etc.). In classical analysis the therapist rejects this role and instead analyzes (i.e., destroys) it. In psychotherapy, on the other hand, the therapist utilizes this role. For the alcoholic, such a relationship can lead the patient to, and help maintain, sobriety; however, it is critical that the therapist avoid excessive involvement such as to facilitate the very behavior he is attempting to treat. An example of this may be observed with the overly dependent patient who uses alcohol (i.e. slips) as a means of controlling the therapist—exactly as the patient had previously done, for example, with a spouse. Thus a balance must be established between participation in the patient's life experiences and excessive dependence.

GOALS OF LONG-TERM TREATMENT

A case of alcoholism cannot be closed in a few weeks or months of treatment; solid recovery requires at least 2 years in most instances.

The self-medication of anxiety and depression with alcohol over a span of years has resulted in exacerbation of these symptoms partly because of the drug and partly because of the failure to learn healthy means of dealing with moods that are common in normal existence. Recovery from alcoholism is a long, slow relearning process with continued wide mood swings even after many months of sobriety[3] (Fig. 7-1).

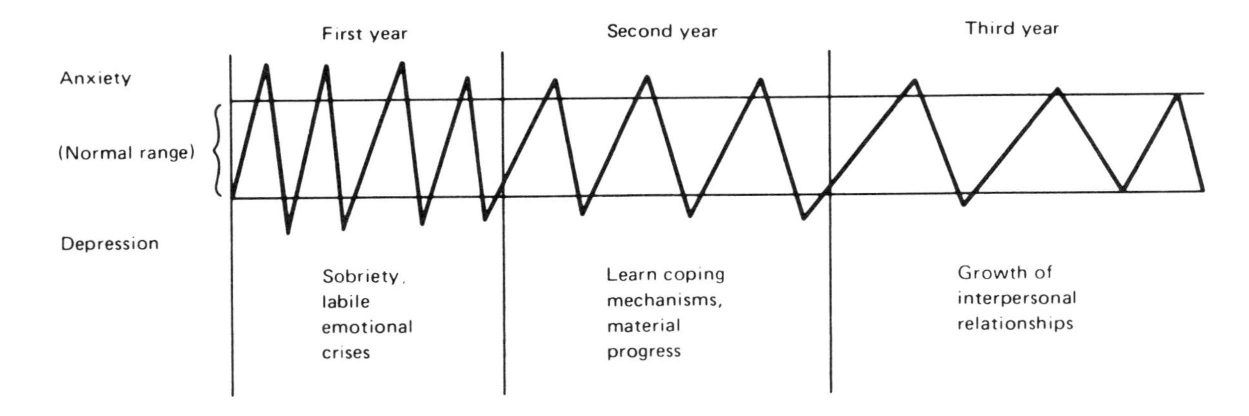

Fig. 7–1. Dynamics of mood swings.

The question often arises as to when the alcoholic can return to work after a course of treatment. Although it is important to consider the type of work, degree of responsibility, the supervisor's cooperation, the severity and duration of the illness, and the progress made in early recovery, it is usually felt that the sober alcoholic who is participating in a sound program at least twice weekly can return to work 4–6 weeks after the onset of treatment. In some cases it may be necessary to assign recovered alcoholics to less stressful jobs temporarily or to part-time work or in unusual cases to advise them to change jobs if present employment is too productive of anxiety.

From a physical standpoint, recovery proceeds rapidly in the first few months and is fairly complete at the end of the first year. By the end of the second year, physical and emotional health are leveling off and often reach above the level of most of the drinking years.

Figure 7–2 indicates a feeling expressed by most recovered alcoholics that sometime between the first and second year of recovery they rise above their pretreatment levels in feelings of well-being and ability to work. Statistics reported by industry corroborate this impression (Fig. 7-3).

Many alcoholics in telling their stories state that they are glad they became alcoholic because their recovery carried them in growth of emotional and spiritual maturity beyond the level of their predrinking period. Certainly, many alcoholics with long sobriety are stable, dependable, and concerned over the welfare of their fellow humans to the point that their earned sobriety must be viewed as a strong plus factor.

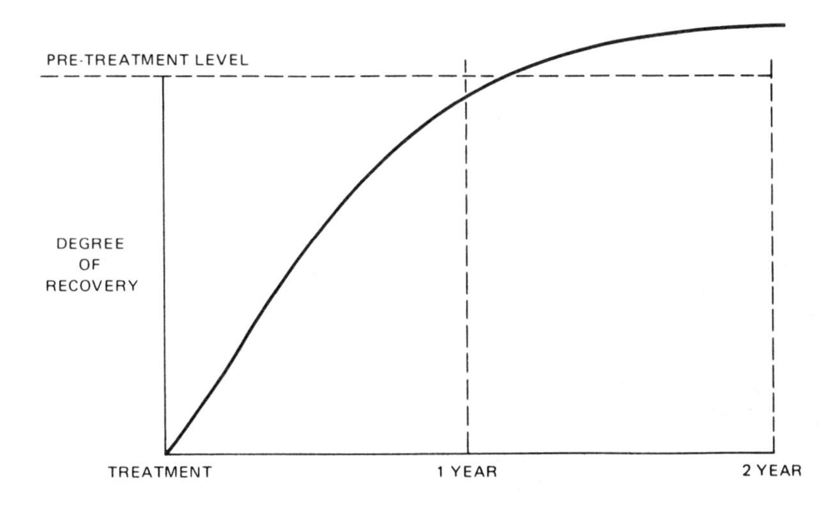

Fig. 7–2. Physical and emotional health levels.

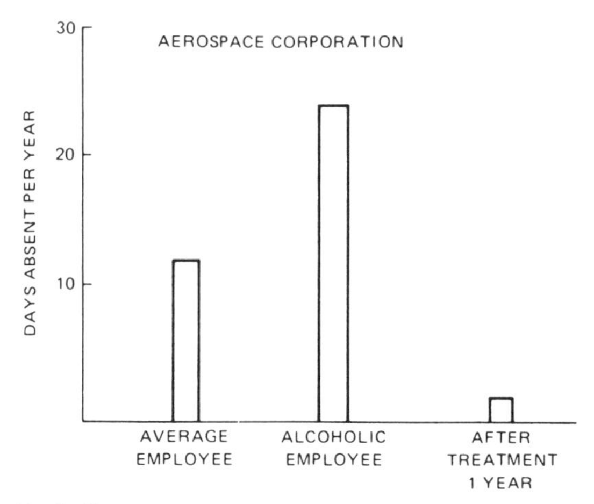

Fig. 7–3. Alcoholism recovery statistics reported by an aerospace corporation.

Many crises, including relapse, will occur, especially during the first 2 years after treatment. By developing and maintaining a warm, open relationship with the alcoholic and the alcoholic's family, the physician will be more apt to be consulted when such crises occur.

In response to the emotional turmoil that these crises often produce, the physician might be tempted to refer the patient for psychiatric care. This should be avoided if at all possible until the patient has had at least 1 year of sobriety in the A.A. program. An exception to this underscores the specific need of a small number, perhaps 2–5 percent, of these patients who require early psychiatric consultation for possible use of specific therapy for schizophrenia, manic depression, or other severe psychiatric disturbance. When psychiatric opinion is finally sought, this consultant should be a psychotherapist who is thoroughly familiar with the principles of A.A. and who understands the priorities involved in abstinence.

Enhancing motivation for remaining in treatment is one of the most important building blocks in nourishing the recovery process. Clearly pointing out the alternatives, giving positive feedback to the patient of improvements noted, and, above all, allowing the patient to have a choice in selecting treatment modalities are strong motivating factors.

DISULFIRAM AS AN ADJUNCT TO TREATMENT

Total abstinence is still the single most important criterion for day-by-day progress, and resumption of drinking must be viewed as a symptom of relapsing into active alcoholism. The main reason for abstinence being so necessary to recovery is that no reliable therapy has yet been found that would enable alcoholics to recover from their illness while still drinking. As a matter of a fact, society has a curious contradiction in its thinking that alcohol is an addicting drug that would probably not be approved by the Food and Drug Administration if it were a new discovery but that alcoholics must be defective in some way because they cannot control the use of alcohol as a social pleasure. We are reluctant to come forth as we do in tobacco, opiate, and other drug dependencies and point to the drug in question as being high in addiction potential and dangerous when repeated use occurs; with alcohol, we say that the normal state is to master the drug and be able to use it at will without harm. This attitude has begun to be questioned.[4]

Total permanent abstinence is the goal of therapy because the histories of thousands of alcoholic individuals who returned to drinking after a period of sobriety have revealed a progressive downward course with resumption of the active illness of alcoholism. One might summarize the reasons for abstinence thus:

—Alcohol causes alcoholism in the alcoholic individual (the drinking is the disease)
—Meaningful participation in a growth program cannot be obtained under sedation (alcohol or pills)
—The alcoholic is addicted to alcohol and needs a great deal of it to feel comfortable (more than is safe to drink)
—The required spiritual changes necessary for recovery cannot be made while drinking

Disulfiram (Antabuse) is a useful chemical barrier to impulsive drinking, especially the first year or two of sobriety. Instead of having to make many decisions not to drink during a particular day, the patient on disulfiram need make only one—the taking of a single pill.

Disulfiram is advised in the following circumstances:

—For patients who are willing to take it
—To test motivation when it is in doubt
—During periods of stress (examinations, spouse ill, etc.), particularly after the stress is over
—For the impulsive drinker
—For the repeated failure in rehabilitation
—For the drunk driver or parolee who is sentenced to enforced administration and rehabilitation

Disulfiram is a safe medication with relatively few side effects, which can generally be controlled by temporary reduction of dosage. Disulfiram, by interfering with the action of aldehyde dehydrogenase, results after ethanol ingestion in the rapid accumulation of its catabolite, acetaldehyde. Within minutes after alcohol is consumed the face turns beet red, and sweating, palpitation, dyspnea, tachycardia, hypotension, nausea, and vomiting occur. The intensity and duration of the symptoms depend on the dose of Antabuse and time interval since last dose, the amount of alcohol taken, and individual variation of response.

Disulfiram must always be prescribed with the full knowledge and consent of the patient. Although any alcoholic substance, including mouthwashes, aftershave lotion, food sauces, and cough medicine, can produce a reaction, the likelihood has been exaggerated anecdotally, and when it occurs it usually means that alcohol has deliberately been consumed; however, the patient should be given a list of common products containing alcohol and be thoroughly briefed on the symptoms of the reaction. Ayerst Laboratories issues an identification card that patients should carry at all times in order to alert medical personnel that they are taking Antabuse. Initiation of the alcohol-Antabuse reaction as a part of treatment is no longer considered necessary.

Treatment of the alcohol-Antabuse reaction is mainly supportive to restore blood pressure and to control shock when present. Most reactions are mild and last 30 minutes to several hours. Intravenous antihistamine (benadryl 50-100 mg) or ascorbic acid (1000 mg) will usually suffice.

Antabuse is slowly excreted; therefore reactions to alcohol usually occur for up to 5 days (more rarely as long as 2 weeks) after cessation of its administration. The drug is usually given as a 500 mg tablet daily for 5 days followed by 250 mg daily thereafter. No alcohol must have been consumed during the 12 hours prior to starting Antabuse.

Side effects are generally mild and consist of fatigue, somnolence, headache, dizziness, skin rash, gastrointestinal distress, and a peculiar taste and odor (garlic-like) to the breath. The last is due to the presence of carbon disulfide in the breath and can be controlled by reducing the dosage.[5] Side effects generally disappear in a week or two or may be controlled by lowering the dosage for 2 weeks and then returning to previous levels.

There are few contraindications to Antabuse. Ruth Fox, after experience with several thousands of cases, withholds it only in overt psychosis or a decompensated heart.[5] The drug may be given with practically any condition as long as the risk of treatment is weighed against the risks of continued drinking. It has been taken for many years without ill effect. Antabuse should be used with caution with isoniazid, coumadin, and dilantin administration. Rare instances of psychosis have been observed following administration of Antabuse.

Certain judges and traffic courts have sentenced drunk drivers to enforced Antabuse administration. The drug is given three times weekly for 1 year after a physical examination. Pharmacists and alcoholism treatment centers have been authorized to supervise the administration of Antabuse in these programs, which have shown some promise particularly when coupled with A.A. counseling, education, and peer group sessions.

Antabuse administration may be continued indefinitely but is usually needed only in the early months or years of sobriety. The patient's willingness to take it is a sign of commitment to sobriety and that denial is lessening. Decision to terminate the drug is best made jointly by the physician, spouse (or significant other), and Alcoholics Anonymous sponsor acting in consultation with the alcoholic on the strength of sobriety as evidenced by the alcoholic's progress. Important guidelines in this decision are as follows:

—Active participation in A.A. (no longer needs to drink)
—Coping with crises without recourse to drinking
—Improved family relationships
—Dissolution of denial
—Social ease (diminution in social anxiety)
—Growth in self-esteem
—In excess of 12–24 months of sobriety

The use of disulfiram while patients attend Alcoholics Anonymous meetings causes them at times to be criticized by some members who reject all drugs as "crutches." They need to be counseled that crutches are necessary to tide one over a period of disability and that willingness to "go to any length" to achieve sobriety can be a source of quiet pride. Fortunately, Antabuse is more acceptable today by most A.A. groups, and such criticism is on the wane (see Appendix D).

As a part of the goal of abstinence one must teach alcoholics how to become social deviants in a culture that not only encourages drinking but tolerates heavy drinking and intoxication. A key point in this endeavor is to advise them to be open with their friends and relatives about recovery programs (most of them know only too well about the drinking problem) and refuse alcoholic beverages when offered by saying frankly, "No thanks, I am an alcoholic." This action will usually stop all pushing and offering of drinks except by those who are involved in the alcoholic's illness and in need of treatment themselves or who are practicing alcoholics and feel uncomfortable when a drinking friend is abstinent. As a general rule it is well to counsel alcoholics who have just been discharged from inpatient treatment programs to avoid cocktail parties and bars until they have developed a solid base of sobriety—this usually requires at least a year.

Gentle coercion is often necessary to accelerate the motivation process.[6] The physician is in a favored position to point out worsening health problems in a nonjudgmental, supportive manner—not as a scare tactic. On the other hand, health improvement is a strong positive motivating factor and should be shared adequately with the patient. Other coercive levers are the possible loss of a spouse and children, loss of a driver's license, job loss, revocation or suspension of a professional license, and loss of any skill or talent that the patient values.

ALCOHOLICS ANONYMOUS

There is no longer any doubt that Alcoholics Anonymous is responsible for the sobriety of more alcoholics than any other single treatment modality.[7,8] It is available in 92 countries and offers long-term continuity to a program with "contented sobriety" as its goal. Alcoholics Anonymous emphasizes action and places the responsibility for recovery squarely on the shoulders of the alcoholic. Participation in Alcoholics Anonymous does not damage the therapeutic alliance with a counselor or physician. Physicians desiring to become better acquainted with alcoholism as an illness and its continued management should attend various Alcoholics Anonymous meetings in their communities. Much can be learned and observed, and striking changes can be noted in individuals who are "surrendering" to the process and who are genuinely participating. Not the least of what is learned will be that alcoholism is generally misdiagnosed and mismanaged by physicians.

Attendance at Alcoholics Anonymous meetings should be prescribed with the same degree of seriousness as a cardiac consultation, and patients should feel that the doctor respects Alcoholics Anonymous as a potent and valuable step in recovery.[9] Having their physician attend an occasional meeting is refreshing to alcoholics, convinces them of a genuine human interest, and allows for sharing the recovery process. Physicians who cannot enter into the ways suggested above are advised to refer their alcoholic patients to someone who can for long-term care and follow-up.

Much can be said about the advantages of Alcoholics Anonymous,[7] but suffice it to say for our purpose that alcoholics can find warmth, friendship, firm guidance, appropriate and supportive confrontation, resocialization, no need to drink, and growing confidence in their own recoveries by a regular working attendance. As a matter of fact, one of us[10] first became interested in alcoholism through feelings of envy when he noted the striking changes that were occurring in naval patients who were coerced into Alcoholics Anonymous attendance for 10–20 meetings and could not at first understand what was causing those changes. He was at a loss to explain a healing phenomenon that he, a physician, could not bring about.

Early in his Alcoholics Anonymous affiliation the alcoholic should select a sponsor from the community network of alcoholics recovered through Alcoholics Anonymous. The sponsor will guide the alcoholic's progress and advise in crises. The problems of recovery are so many and varied that a sponsor is a welcome member of the interdisciplinary team, and conflict with the physician or any other therapist need not arise. As a matter of fact, conferences can be held when a crisis such as relapse occurs and a course of management decided upon as the result of discussion between physician, sponsor, "significant other," marriage counselor, Al-Anon member, etc. Care should be taken to shift dependency of the patient to the program rather than to any particular individual, however.

Alcoholics Anonymous is a worldwide fellowship of men and women who are banded together to solve their common problems of alcoholism and to help fellow sufferers to recover.[11] The only requirement for membership is a desire to stop drinking. By sharing their experience, strength, and hope as recovered alcoholics and guided by a philosophy embodied in the "Twelve Suggested Steps" the members are able to maintain sobriety.

The Twelve Suggested Steps*

1. *We admitted we were powerless over alcohol—that our lives had become unmanageable.* (Taking this step implies giving up and surrendering to the program and admitting one is whipped as far as control over drinking is concerned.)
2. *We came to believe that a power greater than ourselves could restore us to sanity.* (Giving up one's ego control and throwing oneself on the power of the group, God, or whatever we believe to be our higher power.)
3. *We made a decision to turn our will and our lives over to the care of God* ***as we understood Him***. (Surrender to a spiritual program—*not a religion.*)
4. *We made a searching and fearless moral inventory of ourselves.* (Must be written in order to thoroughly examine all the material that one has been rationalizing, minimizing, denying, or distorting in various ways.)
5. *We admitted to God, to ourselves, and to another human being the exact nature of our wrongs.* (Reading and discussing step four inventory with another person of our choice.)

   The vast majority of people who fail in A.A. have not taken the fourth and fifth steps.
6. *We were entirely ready to have God remove all these defects of character.*
7. *We humbly asked Him to remove our shortcomings.*
8. *We made a list of all persons we had harmed, and became willing to make amends to them all.*
9. *We made direct amends to such people whenever possible, except when to do so would injure them or others.*
10. *We continued to take personal inventory and when we were wrong promptly admitted it.*
11. *We sought through prayer and meditation to improve our conscious contact with God* ***as we understood Him,*** *praying only for knowledge of His will and the power to carry that out.*
12. *Having had a spiritual awakening as the result of these steps, we tried to carry this message to alcoholics, and to practice these principles in all our affairs.*

It is important in using A.A. as a referral source to realize that A.A. gives no concern to the reason for drinking and considers all such reasons merely as excuses. A.A. feels that alcoholics drink because of a compulsion to do so and that they have lost the power of choice as to whether or not to drink even when they are not aware of such loss. It is believed that alcoholics are unable to help themselves in this situation in spite of any amount of willpower, intelligence, or moral integrity. Relief comes from accepting powerlessness and then accepting help from an outside source. *Alcoholics cannot keep themselves sober but end up sober by trying to help other alcoholics stay sober even when the latter do not find sobriety.*

---

*Reprinted with permission of A.A. World Services, Inc.

The A.A. program is a spiritual way of life; this fact must be understood by physicians who are managing an alcoholic in A.A. The physician's tendency to prescribe mind- and mood-altering medications is the greatest cause of conflict with A.A., and patients would be better served by being informed that their symptoms were of emotional origin. Turning to their 12-step program would be preferable to medication in the average case. The physician should not accept the responsibility for relief of distress in these individuals unless it is disabling. Very often the anxiety symptoms are a manifestation of an unconscious desire to drink or a resentment, and it is safer for such patients to work the A.A. program without sedation.

"A.A. doesn't work for me" is a commonly heard statement that need not force the physician to quickly assume the responsibility for producing an alternative for such a patient. The A.A. program will work for anyone who "thoroughly follows our path"[16]; however, not all patients are willing to make the necessary surrender immediately, and it may be necessary to try other methods of treatment until patients become ready for A.A. In their attempts to avoid A.A., patients may complain about the "religious" approach, the cigarette smoke, the coarse language of the repetitive "drunkalogues." We feel that these are all excuses and can be avoided if the patient is sincere by merely shopping around in the community for a satisfactory meeting.

In general, it is surprising how many meetings of all types and sizes one can find not only in one's own locale but throughout the world. There are speaker meetings, discussions, participation or question-and-answer meetings, and special meetings for beginners, men only, women only, or people under 30 or 40 years old. Some meetings concentrate on a study of the "Big Book," others on the Twelve Steps and Twelve Traditions or on just certain steps such as the 4th or 11th. Some meetings are "open" to the public; others are "closed" and admit alcoholics only or those who are trying to decide whether or not they are alcoholic. In addition to the more than 12,000 meetings listed with the A.A. General Service Office in New York City, there are a great many unlisted meetings of A.A. members who get together just for the pleasure of holding a meeting. Such groups may be composed only of priests, physicians, attorneys, movie stars, politicians, military personnel, homosexuals, nonsmokers, agnostics, or others who wish to share common problems. Members of "special interest" groups are far more likely to stay sober if they also attend regular membership meetings where all are considered to be equal and suffering from the same disease.

Beginners' meetings are smaller, more intimate, and have question-and-answer sessions to aid newcomers. New members usually are not asked to speak about their own experience with drinking until they feel ready to do so and may pass if called upon. They are asked to read a chapter from the Big Book from time to time as a means of developing comfort in appearing at the podium in front of a group. When newcomers feel ready to do so they may volunteer or respond when called upon to tell their stories in front of the group. This type of ventilation helps to develop honesty and remove guilt. Within a few weeks a spiritual transformation begins to take place as the result of not drinking "one day at a time." The emphasis is on "today," and the desire to drink is put off for 24 hours by following the successful experience of those who have achieved significant sobriety.

It is important that the physician realize that neither alcoholism nor A.A. is restricted to skid row derelicts or "hopeless" drunks. Just as the majority of alcoholics in the U.S. are not bums and not on skid row, so also are the members of A.A. successful business and professional men and women of social stature and financial means. The physician, then, should be willing to recommend A.A. knowing that *it can work and is working for all classes of society.*

Anonymity is at the very heart of the program and is best expressed in the Twelve Traditions.[11]

Tradition Eleven states: "Our public relations policy is based on attraction rather than promotion; we need always maintain personal anonymity at the level of press, radio, and films."*

Tradition Twelve: "Anonymity is the spiritual foundation of our traditions, ever reminding us to place principles before personalities."*

For newcomers, anonymity serves to allay their fears of being labeled as alcoholics by everyone they know. The larger significance of anonymity, however, is the key to understanding the strength of A.A. It is a symbol of personal sacrifice without the dangerous rewards of fame and fortune that might be reached for by an individual seeking publicity as an A.A. member doing great work for alcoholics. The latter behavior would most probably reinflate vanity and might very likely result in a relapse that would tend to destroy the unity and credibility of the A.A. fellowship and imperil its very survival. Breaking anonymity at the private level is desirable whenever the alcoholic is ready for extending a hand to another.

A.A. World Services publishes five books. The first is *Alcoholics Anonymous* (also known as "The Big Book"), which comprises the personal stories of recovered alcoholics. The initial 164 pages outline the A.A. recovery program as written by the original members, who stated in the preface to the first edition:

> We of A.A. are more than 100 men and women who have recovered from a seemingly hopeless state of mind and body. To show other alcoholics *precisely how we have recovered* is the main purpose of the book.
>
> For them, we hope these pages will prove so convincing that no further authentication will be necessary. We trust this account of our experiences will help everyone to better understand the alcoholic. Many do not comprehend that the alcoholic is a very sick person. And besides, we are sure that our way of living has its advantages for all.*

This book deserves serious study as a part of any rehabilitation program and is an excellent vehicle for discussion and readings. It should be read by the physician just as any other book dealing with clinical medicine.

The only authority of the A.A. program is the book *Alcoholics Anonymous*. Of further relevance may be the *Twelve Steps and Twelve Traditions*, which is an

*Reprinted with permission of A.A. World Services, Inc.

elaboration of the meaning of the steps and traditions, *A.A. Comes of Age*, a history of A.A., and *As Bill Sees It*, which features brief excerpts of the writing of the cofounders of A.A. selected for daily reading. A new paperback entitled *Living Sober* has an excellent selection of A.A. approaches to the problem of what to do when the desire or compulsion to drink returns. In general, an A.A. member who is actively engaged in the A.A. program is not troubled by the desire that previously had been an obsession or irresistable compulsion. Members are often so impressed with this change that they consider it miraculous.

The ease with which members stay sober is often a trap in that they may feel they no longer need the meetings or other A.A. activities. Drinking almost invariably follows, which sooner or later results in a progressive downhill course that is as bad as or worse than that which had originally brought them into treatment. In this sense the alcoholic is not considered as "recovered" but only as "recovering" even after many years of sobriety.

As progress is made in Alcoholics Anonymous alcoholics are encouraged to begin "twelfth-step work"—the helping of other sick alcoholics. This reinforces their own progress, makes them feel needed, and is one of the strong factors behind the success of Alcoholics Anonymous. There is hazard when the neophyte fails, and one must caution novice twelfth-steppers not to get too emotionally involved. Helping another alcoholic in efforts to remain sober can be of the greatest importance to the progress of patients in their own recoveries.

As patients grow in confidence and ability to cope with stress, they can often assist the physician as volunteers by helping new patients into Alcoholics Anonymous and participating in community educational work with the physician. An advantage is that the physician can hand-pick a particular recovering alcoholic to indoctrinate a new patient. Many recovering alcoholic patients, and their spouses, will seek further training in alcoholic rehabilitation as a step toward becoming qualified counselors. This should be encouraged only after 1 year or more of sobriety has been attained.

INDIVIDUAL AND GROUP COUNSELING

As an adjunct to patients in Alcoholics Anonymous or for those who initially refuse to attend, it is valuable to arrange for or refer them to an ongoing series of group or individual counseling sessions conducted by a professional or paraprofessional familiar with the complex disease of alcoholism. The group should be open-ended and consist mostly or entirely of other alcoholics who are in various stages of recovery. The peer group identity is a necessary ingredient of long-term management and is valuable in dealing with anxiety, isolation, loneliness, and anger, and especially with the inconsistent messages that alcoholics receive from the community.

The individual counseling sessions should involve support, confrontation, ventilation, and clarification of current living problems. The primary focus should be on total abstinence and a "here and now" approach, coupled with a firmly stated *avoidance* of a search for "why the patient drinks." A constant theme of all sessions should be that patients are being prepared for group counseling and A.A. because they have a disease that is best healed by group counseling and peer-group support.

PSYCHOTHERAPY

Psychoanalytically oriented psychotherapy of the recovering alcoholic, be it individual or group therapy, is doomed to failure if the patient is using alcohol or any other sedative drug. Even supportive psychotherapy of the alcoholic is ineffective if the patient is still drinking. Because of the alcoholic patient's manipulativeness and because of the therapist's tendency to search for the "underlying cause" of the drinking, the patient will gradually get sicker.

Only a relatively small number of recovering alcoholics will actively seek out or need intensive psychotherapy. This kind of therapy should not be undertaken until the patient has 1 or preferably 2 years of uninterrupted sobriety and a thorough grounding in Alcoholics Anonymous or another support system. If drinking or use of some other medication is resumed, the psychotherapy should be temporarily or permanently stopped because it indicates that the patient still needs to use sedatives to control anxiety or depression. Peer-group support should continue.

PASTORAL COUNSELING

Spiritual counseling by a minister trained in alcoholism is an important addition to the interdisciplinary team for patients that express a need for this type of support. Renewed faith in a higher power represents a recovery from the effects of excessive narcissism and offers hope and meaning in the growth out of alienation and isolation from family, friends, and the church of one's belief.

EDUCATION OF THE ALCOHOLIC PATIENT

During the initial few weeks of treatment the alcoholic is usually exposed to lectures by physicians, recovered alcoholics, and others, along with films and discussions on the nature of the disease of alcoholism. This should be continued and should include the changes that must be made in the patient's life if recovery is to be achieved and maintained. Such education is an important part of the growth process. Physicians willing to undertake the long-term management could well arrange for a monthly evening discussion group on subjects pertinent to their patients' needs. Spouses or significant others should be included.

THE FAMILY OF THE ALCOHOLIC

It is assumed that the family and significant others become involved in treatment during the initial phase. Al-Anon for the spouse, Alateen for the children over 10 years old, and even Alatot for the younger children are helpful group meetings for family members as continuations of the learning process in dealing with their anxieties not only over the past but especially over the changes now occurring in the alcoholic as the result of treatment. Should a relapse occur, these self-help groups can be very supporting to the family.

When indicated, family counselling, couples groups, and conjoint therapy can be very useful providing that the therapist understands alcoholism and its recovery process.

THE PROBLEM OF THE "ENABLER"

An "enabler" is anyone who has enabled or perhaps even encouraged the alcoholic to continue destructive drinking. Although the enabler can be a spouse, friend, child, roommate, homosexual partner, physician, corporation, the military, or society itself, the enabler is usually the spouse or an adult son or daughter. The enabler will initially be quite concerned and forceful about the need for the alcoholic to stop drinking, but the enabler's enthusiasm for cooperating with the therapy tends to diminish when it becomes evident that the enabler will need to undergo some psychological changes if he plans to have a satisfying relationship with the abstinent alcoholic. The physician should get enablers to attend Al-Anon meetings as soon as possible. In these meetings enablers will learn to manage their own lives and to live comfortably with the idea that alcoholics will gradually have to accept responsibility for themselves and for the consequences of their drinking. The enabler may need the physician's support when it comes to "letting go" of some of the controls that alcoholics are trying to accept back as they gain sobriety (these are the same controls—e.g., family finances and child rearing—that the enabler had taken over, sometimes eagerly, as the alcoholic was getting sicker).

All the problems of "normal" families, such as sexual difficulties and role struggles, will present themselves in the recovering alcoholic's family and will require skillful management by use of A.A., Al-Anon, the alcoholic's sponsor, and (rarely) appropriate consultation by medical specialists.

A special problem is the marriage that was never meant to be or that began when one spouse was already drinking alcoholically. The enabler may prefer divorcing and marrying another drinking alcoholic to undergoing the necessary emotional growth. Another problem is that of the enabler who is also drinking alcoholically. Immediate introduction into Al-Anon will often lead to the enabler switching over to attending A.A. meetings in a few weeks or months. Another frequent problem is that of the enabler presenting to the physician to seek help for the allegedly alcoholically drinking mate. After getting a fair idea from the enabler that the mate is in fact drinking alcoholically, the physician will have to assess the emotional maturity and economic self-sufficiency (actual or potential) of the enabler. Dynamically, the underlying problem often is that the enabler fears loss of the alcoholic if confronted. A skillful therapist can often convince the enabler of the necessity for confrontation by showing that alcoholism is a progressive, relapsing disease, and that it results in loss of the lover gradually but steadily. The only way to prevent this loss is to confront and bring about rehabilitation. Otherwise the loss of the alcoholic is only a question of time—and will occur later, when the enabler has become more cynical, older, and therefore less flexible for undergoing such changes as proper mourning, getting a job, and establishing new relationships. Not infrequently, emotionally crippled, widowed, middle-aged enablers will, in the face of the above life problems, begin to drink alcoholically themselves and eventually find help in A.A.

After a brief explanation of alcoholism as a disease, they need to be persuaded to (1) immediately begin attending Al-Anon meetings, (2) tell their spouses that they have discussed their problems with the doctor, and (3) suggest that the spouses see the physician. They will learn at Al-Anon how their spouses' illness trapped them into anger, defensiveness, protection, and controlling, blaming, and finally enabling them to avoid the consequences of their drinking because they unconsciously assumed responsibility for their actions. Actually, proper management of the spouse has often resulted in a previously uncooperative alcoholic seeking treatment.

Society as a whole or a large subculture can also be viewed as an enabler because, like an individual, it will encourage or discourage the alcoholic's tendency to drink excessively. Normal American drinking customs suggest that we use alcohol when we feel good, when we feel bad, as a "pick-me-up," to calm down, as an "eye-opener," and as a "nightcap." At cocktail parties we use it to say hello, to "get in step," to "unwind," as an ice-breaker, courage-maker, socializer, or friendship-maker, and, finally, as "one for the road." At a dinner party we use it as an appetizer, as a main beverage (beer or wine), as an after-dinner drink, and as "more of the same" during later evening socializing until we drive home with "one for the road" toward the nightcap before bedtime.

Executives discuss business while having cocktails, and salesmen buy another round when they land contracts. If a sales pitch falls through and the customers leave, the salesman is apt to buy a double to control frustration.

In sports, we drink at the clubhouse, at the golf shack, on the beach, during the hunt, at the races. We drink cold beer at baseball games because it is hot in those bleachers, and Irish coffee at football games because it is cold in those bleachers. The winners of the World Series shower in champagne before cameras and the press, and the losers drink heavily, silently, resentfully, and alone at the hotel.

We drink when we hear good news, when we get bad news, go off to war, celebrate peace, commemorate a birth, or mourn a death. We drink at birthdays, reunions, Christmas, Halloween, and the New Year. Drinking goes with courting ("Candy is dandy but liquor is quicker," said Odgen Nash), with engagements, marriages, anniversaries, and, nowadays, even with divorces.[27]

An example of a subculture as an enabler is the world from which the alcoholic Navy pilot comes.

> In naval aviation we drink at happy hours, after a good flight, and after a near midair collision to calm our nerves. To celebrate our first solo flight, we traditionally present our instructor with a bottle of his favorite liquor. We drink when we get our wings, when we get promoted (wetting-down party), when we get passed over (to alleviate our depression), at formal dining-in, at change of command ceremonies, chief's initiation, and free wine at "beef and burgundy night." At birthday balls we drink our door prize if we had the lucky ticket.
>
> When a diver inspects the hull of the ship we give him "medicinal" brandy and we "prescribe" the same "treatment" (for equally questionable medical indications) for the man who fell overboard and was fished out of the Caribbean Sea on a hot day in July.
>
> Night carrier landings from sunset to sunrise rate medicinal brandy dispensed by the well-meaning flight surgeon. We "hail and farewell" frequently, and the first liquid that wets the bow of a newborn ship at its christening is champagne. We drink from enlistment to retirement and from teenhood to old age. For those who have predisposition to alcoholism there seems almost no escape. And those who want to abstain because they are trying to recover from alcoholism find it difficult to live with such national myths as the hard-drinking, two-fisted pioneering frontiersman, the hard-charging tiger of an aviator who can drink with the best of them, the ruggedness of the guy who can hold his liquor like a man, and the notion that "you can't trust a man who doesn't drink."*

The extent to which it is embedded in our culture may be reflected in our use of alcohol in those very religious rituals in which the higher power, i.e., God, is praised or communed with.

The alcohol-orientation of the enabler plays an important role in the life of the recovering alcoholic. An individual enabler can change and grow—through Al-Anon or other support systems—as recovering alcoholics can grow away from the

---

*Reprinted by permission from Pursch JA: Alcoholism in aviation: A problem of attitudes. *Aerospace Med* 45:318-321, 1974.

enabler who refuses to change a relationship toward them. In the case of a subculture as an enabler, recovering alcoholics need to be enlightened about the "enabling" nature of the drinking practices of their society because the desired change in that society is going to take place very slowly and will continue to present stresses and pitfalls for alcoholics who continue to try and find peer acceptance and approval by living up to peer drinking expectation. A clear, forthright explanation of these conditions from the therapist will increase the alcoholic's chances for continued growth.

THE PHYSICIAN'S OFFICE

Recovering alcoholics should be seen at least weekly to monthly during the first year, especially when they are well—that is, when they tend to drop the program. The family is requested to accompany the patient at every other visit. (Occasionally it is wise, however, to maintain separation of treatment personnel in dealing with the patient and the spouse.) Evidences of emotional growth and physical improvement are shared with patients and their continuance in the program reinforced.

The physician should try to involve at least one other person in the patient's life in the treatment of his alcoholism. This is usually the spouse, but it could also be a parent, adult son or daughter, brother or sister, friend, employer, etc. Care is needed here to reassure the alcoholic that the significant other requires education about the disease of alcoholism as much as the alcoholic does and that the other's presence does not necessarily imply a plot to defeat the alcoholic (although at times it could literally be true). The main purpose is to educate, introduce to A.A. and Al-Anon, and encourage relatives or friends to work alongside the alcoholic for their own welfare as well as to understand the disease process and its effect on relationships. The alcoholic may become angry and object to any other person being brought into the treatment. This resistance must be viewed as a part of the denial process and needs working through before progress can be made.

Attendance at Al-Anon for spouses or significant others is preferable to "advice" or "therapy" by the physician, since it puts them in touch rapidly with people who have been healed after similar experiences and offers them hope as well as a uniquely sustaining fellowship.

Secretarial and nursing staff need to develop positive attitudes toward the alcoholic and learn to accept the fact that alcohol on the breath is no more a cause for rejection than acetone on the breath of a diabetic. Comment on the breath should be made in the same manner that one comments on the presence of a rash.

IATROGENIC SABOTAGE VERSUS PROPER USE OF PSYCHOACTIVE MEDICATION

The prescription blank is one of the major stumbling blocks for the alcoholic on the way to recovery.[12] Many a "dry" alcoholic was returned to active sedativism by the sincere but unaware physician who did not know about the relationship between alcohol and other drugs and who therefore responded to the dry alcoholic's problem of pain, depression, anxiety, or apathy with a prescription for drugs instead of prescribing ongoing rehabilitation, A.A., and counseling. All sedatives, analgesics, minor tranquilizers, opiates, psychedelics, and stimulants should be avoided by the recovering alcoholic because their "high" or "downer" effects can easily become a substitute for the effects previously obtained from alcohol. If the alcoholic patient's anxiety is such that a minor tranquilizer would control it, then it is best that the patient learn to live with that anxiety and cope by participating in A.A. and other support programs rather than risk developing dependence or addiction to a new substance.

Since alcoholics already have cross-tolerance for sedatives (e.g., barbiturates) and minor tranquilizers (Librium, Valium, Meprobamate, Serax), they will, usually in a relatively short time, begin to take these substances in increasingly larger doses, at first for stressful situations, then for daytime sedation, and finally for sleep. Eventually in combination with a return to drinking they will probably be hospitalized because of overdosage. This will complicate detoxification procedures because of the cumulative effect and longer half-lives of these drugs, which may lead to patients having grand mal seizures a few days to a few weeks after detoxification for alcohol withdrawal has begun.

Also, the recovering alcoholic must be made aware of the need for being honest with the physician and the anesthesiologist prior to surgery so that the doctors will be aware of the patient's high tolerance for sedative-hypnotics.

Drugs in the amphetamine family present chemical traps for recovering alcoholics who are primarily troubled by depression and apathy. These patients will tend to increase their use of stimulants, try to titrate them with alcohol or other sedatives, and frequently end up being hospitalized with symptomatology that is initially indistinguishable from paranoid schizophrenia and that then requires a prolonged period of detoxification. A similar problem often stems from the use of amphetaminelike drugs by the (usually female) alcoholic desirous of dieting. More recently, cocaine has resulted in these complications most frequently.

The recovering alcoholic who presents with pain (psychosomatic or posttraumatic) often becomes addicted to Darvon, Talwin, or opiates if these drugs are prescribed and if counseling and A.A. are allowed to diminish in importance.

Phenothiazines, because they do not produce euphoria, may be carefully prescribed for recovering alcoholics if in the opinion of a physician who understands alcoholism the patient's mental functioning will be improved by phenothiazine maintenance therapy. The same can be said for the use of tricyclic antidepressants in the case of retarded depressions and lithium for recovering alcoholics with manic-depressive disorders.

Recovering alcoholics who are being maintained for necessary brief intervals on some of the above medications may find that in some Alcoholics Anonymous groups[13] the feeling against drugs of any kind (including disulfiram) is strong and expressed frequently enough so that it could jeopardize their sobriety. The psychiatrist or other physician who treats alcoholics should be familiar with the Alcoholics Anonymous resources in his community so that he can help the patient understand the basis of the position taken by the antidrug A.A. groups. The physician should be willing and able to describe a rationale for short-term use of such drugs so that the patient is reassured by the awareness that the physician is as concerned with misuse of drugs as are these antidrug groups.

A major concern of the long-term manager must be the prevention of the unnecessary, harmful, mood-changing, and mind-changing brought about by physicians who are unaware of the alcoholic's susceptibility to the abuse of these drugs and of the fact that the prescription pad can sabotage the recovery process by renewing the dependence on sedative medication. Until all physicians have learned about the addiction susceptibility of the alcoholic, it will be necessary to educate recovering alcoholics about their disease so that they have the confidence to speak up when medication is being "pushed" on them by unaware physicians.

CONTROLLED DRINKING

The recent literature on alcoholism treatment reveals a growing number of papers on attempts at teaching "controlled" or "social" drinking and claims that abstinence may have been overemphasized as the sole criterion of recovery from the disease.[14] The very word "controlled" implies that rigid and structured limits must be placed upon the drinking or trouble will ensue. A curious fact is that in no other drug addiction do we attempt to teach controlled use of the drug. (The exception is methadone treatment for heroin addiction, where the rationale is not really controlled social use but rather substitution of a prescribed drug in order to block the desired effect of an illegal one that fosters criminal behavior. Even in this instance, gradual tapering off and withdrawal of the methadone is a prelude to abstinence whenever possible, and control of the drug remains in the physician's hands.) In alcoholism those who recommend controlled drinking are attempting to train the alcohol addict to self-prescribe.

Society by its "pious pushing" is constantly reminding alcoholics that they are not "normal" unless they can drink "socially" without harm. Most alcoholics try innumerable times with great suffering and loss to live up to this image but eventually learn that they cannot drink in moderation. Warnings have been issued by the American Medical Association, the American Medical Society on Alcoholism (now A.M.S.A.O.D.D.), and the National Council on Alcoholism that continued drinking is dangerous to the alcoholic (see below).

We do not deny that an occasional alcoholic may recover the ability to drink in moderation—what we question is the frequency of this phenomenon and our present ability to make it happen.[15] The very attitude on our part that drinking may be "necessary" for some alcoholics is an invitation for too many of them to try it. The experience of the authors indicates that this goal is unwise, fraught with failure, and an admission of defeat. Let careful research continue; when proof is available that a significant number of alcoholics can achieve controlled drinking *after reentry into society* and that we can select and predict which ones will make it, then we shall reconsider our opinion. In the meantime, the combined statement of the National Council on Alcoholism and the American Medical Society on Alcoholism is a safe guide:[28]

1. Abstinence from alcohol is necessary for recovery from the disease of alcoholism.
2. Although abstinence is a means of achieving recovery, other factors by which a person's life is enriched are important: improved physical and emotional health, better work performance, more rewarding relationships with the family and society, and increased economic efficiency.
3. As in many other diseases, relapses may take place but must never be thought to indicate that recovery is beyond reach. Any improvement is positive and should be recognized and encouraged as a prelude to recovery.
4. There is a need for responsible research into alternate approaches, carried out with proper controls as well as the judicious publication of results when pertinent. However, in the present state of our knowledge, we firmly believe and emphasize that there can be no relaxation from the stated position that no alcoholic may return with safety to any use of alcohol.*

The "Big Book" of Alcoholics Anonymous recommends in Chapter 3 a technique of self-diagnosis—to try a period of controlled drinking as a test to determine whether or not one is alcoholic.[16] Failure to maintain control *over an extended period* is considered indicative of an alcohol problem. Perhaps this is one of the fringe benefits of a controlled drinking program—convincing alcoholics that they are unable to drink even in a controlled program and helping them decide that sobriety is the best course. Indeed, controlled drinking experiments have yielded reports that some subjects were found to be abstinent on follow-up studies.[17] In accordance with the medical concept of the disease of alcoholism, "The only generally accepted and time-tested technique for treatment of this highly recidivistic illness entails the achievement of abstinence."[18]

MANAGEMENT OF THE RELAPSE

Relapse is common and seems to occur especially during the early weeks or months of sobriety and again between the 11th and 13th months. Resumption of drinking will not always necessarily proceed immediately to serious alcoholic drinking, although it certainly may and often will do so eventually. In some individuals, however, there will be a period of weeks, months, or even a year or more of "controlled" drinking without the onset of the signs and symptoms of alcoholism. Sooner or later drinking will proceed to the alcoholic variety, with a recurrence of serious medical and social problems. Without treatment alcoholism commonly becomes progressively worse.

*Position statement on abstinence reprinted by permission of the National Council on Alcoholism and the American Medical Society on Alcoholism.

On obtaining a history from the patient in relapse one often finds that a characteristic chain of events occurred after the ground was laid by one or more of the following:

—Disappointment in sobriety
—Emotional conflicts
—Peer pressure of social drinking by persons significant to the alcoholic
—Excessive mood swings
—Various life crises
—Psychoactive drug prescription after an illness or injury
—Excessive zeal as a "twelfth-stepper"—too soon
—Investing too much of oneself in the rescue of a new member of the program (i.e., a "baby" or "pigeon")

A phenomenon referred to as "building up to a drink"[19] begins with a change in mood, anxiety, and psychosomatic complaints and culminates in a state of emotional irritability and confusion referred to by sober alcoholics as a "dry drunk." This state may precede the onset of drinking by several days or weeks and can often be recognized by family, friends, or A.A. members. Treatment consists in the acceptance of the vulnerable state by the alcoholic, verbalizing feelings with a sponsor in A.A. meetings, and taking action along the lines of the recovery program. Medication is almost never advisable, although counseling by the physician can be supportive. Hospitalization or attendance at a daycare facility for a few days may occasionally be necessary.

If drinking has occurred and trouble becomes evident, the physician should confront the patient, making use of the present crisis to motivate, pointing out the alternatives, and employing whatever coercive levers are appropriate to reinstitute the previous program of sobriety. Hospitalization may be necessary to interrupt or prevent the drinking cycle. The physician, spouse, friend, industrial alcoholism counselor, A.A. sponsor, Department of Motor Vehicles, county and state professional societies, state professional licensing bureaus, police, and others can exert pressures that may be useful to help convince the relapsing alcoholic that serious loss can occur if drinking continues.[6] Although confidentiality is a sacred cow in the physician-patient contract, it must not be rigidly adhered to in the face of recurring disability and deterioration, particularly when a little pressure on an area valued by the patient can effect a resumption of the recovery process. Here, the physician as a kindly "SOB"* can play a major role in not only saving the alcoholic's life but protecting the general public as well. Permission in writing, authorizing the physician to contact any person or agency having a possible bearing on the patient's course, can be crucial.

THE CHAIN REACTION OF HEALTH

As alcoholics progress in their own sobriety and growth they often reach out more and more to help other alcoholics in their circles of friends and neighbors.

*"Specialist on booze"—a personal communication from Max A. Schneider, M.D.

This phenomenon has been called the chain reaction of health[10] and represents real hope of a breakthrough in enhancing a greater rate of recovery from the serious epidemic disease of alcoholism. When the number of recovered alcoholics begins to approach a critical mass sufficient to create a herd immunity, an "epidemic of health"[20] could be initiated in our communities—a distinctly possible outcome from the partnership of Alcoholics Anonymous and the health sciences. A good example is that of the Navy rehabilitation experience, which has resulted in 85 "Dry Dock" A.A. groups located worldwide that were started by recovering men and women who had completed the treatment program.[26] This type of seeding of our communities with a growing referral network of recovered alcoholics unashamed of their illness and willing to assist health professionals and paraprofessionals, such as counselors, social workers, A.A. sponsors, etc., is an exciting prospect.

EVALUATION OF LONG-TERM MANAGEMENT

Criteria for the evaluation of the effectiveness of long-term care would emphasize the number of patients and their families that remain in treatment versus those that drop out. Sobriety, employment, and ability to relate would be basic. An additional factor of great significance is the number of "alumni" or recovered alcoholics managed by the physician or program who remain in touch and volunteer their services when called upon to help guide a neophyte into recovery. How many of them are willing educators of the community? Case-finders? How many have sought additional training and have entered the field of alcoholism?

An additional indicator is the comparison of the frequency of use of medical facilities before and after alcoholic rehabilitation. In a study of 161 alcoholic patients, the Naval Health Research Center reported that for subjects in the 2 years before treatment 4251 days were spent on the sick list as contrasted with 1985 days in the 2 years following treatment.[21]

OTHER MODES OF THERAPY

Aversion therapy, systemic desensitization, behavior modification, hypnotherapy, acupuncture, transcendental meditation, megavitamin therapy, and therapy with lysergic acid diethylamide (LSD) all have their advocates.

The very fact that so many modes of therapy are available for alcoholism, and have their apparent successes, indicates that there is no specific technique of treatment. In fact, technique may not be as important as the therapists' warmth, understanding, and acceptance of the alcoholic as an equal with optimism about the recovery process.[22]

At the present time it is generally agreed that the only recovery method that has proven widely successful is Alcoholics Anonymous. Research on effective therapists suggests that an important characteristic is the commitment to the client.[23] "The inmost growth of self grows only in relation to another" (Martin Buber). Certainly this characteristic and principle is what A.A. is all about.

THE PHYSICIAN'S ROLE

The physician, in the long-term management of alcoholics and their families, should be an intelligent shoehorn for the introduction into A.A., Al-Anon, Alateen, and other community helping agencies. The physician is also a friend, educator, counselor, and crisis interventionist in addition to being an important initial contact for the necessary development of growth in interpersonal relationships. To do this, the physician must have his own house in order as far as attitudes and personal use of alcoholic beverages are concerned.

A few simple rules:[12]

1. Don't assume responsibility for keeping the patient sober—that is the *patient's* problem.
2. Be careful with your prescription pad—it is one of the greatest hazards to sobriety.
3. Don't try to treat the patient alone.

SUMMARY

Long-term recovery involves abstinence and restructuring and reshaping the alcoholic's life not in terms of "cure" but in terms of helping him find new friends that value sobriety instead of a social group that just tolerates it.[24] The physician as an important member of the interdisciplinary team will be more successful in matching patient needs with the community services if he understands and respects those services as at least equal in value to his own effort.

Long-term recovery of the alcoholic therefore is an ongoing growth process without an endpoint, implying that the case can never be closed.

REFERENCES

1. Beauchamp DE: Alcoholism as blaming the alcoholic. *Int Addict* 11(1):41-52, 1976
2. Dodd MH: Alcoholic recovery homes; A community model at work in the home and community. Presented to the Alcohol and Drug Problems Association Conference, Recovery Home Section, San Francisco, December 1974
3. Fox V: Dynamics of substance abuse management. Eleventh Annual Distinguished Lecture Series in Special Education and Rehabilitation, University of Southern California, 1973
4. Hayman M: The Myth of social drinking. *Am J Psychiatry* 124:585-594, 1967

5. Fox R (ed): *Alcoholism: Behavioral Research, Therapeutic Approaches*, New York, Springer, 1967
6. Knott DH, Beard JD, Fink RD: Alcoholism: The physician's role in diagnosis and treatment. Presented as a scientific exhibit at the American Academy of Family Practice, 23rd Annual Scientific Assembly, Miami Beach, October 1971
7. Hayman M: Current attitudes to alcoholism of psychiatrists in Southern California. *Am J Psychiatry* 127:7, 1971
8. Trice HM, Roman PM: *Spirits and Demons at Work: Alcohol and Other Drugs on the Job*, Ithaca, N.Y. State School of Industrial and Labor Relations at Cornell University, 1972
9. Rogawski AS, Emundson B: Factors affecting the outcome of psychiatric interagency referral. *Am J Psychiatry* 27:7, 1971
10. Zuska JJ: Beginnings of the navy program. *Alcoholism Clin Exper Res* 2(4):352-357, 1978
11. *Twelve Steps and Twelve Traditions*, New York, A.A. World Services 1965
12. Ohliger P: No pills to alcoholics. Orange County, Calif. *Med Assoc Bull*, February 1974
13. Bissell L: The treatment of alcoholism: What do we do about long-term sedatives? *Ann NY Acad Sci* 252, 1973, pp. 396-399
14. Ewing JA, Rouse BA: Outpatient group treatment to initiate controlled drinking behavior in alcoholics. *Alcoholism* (Zagreb) 9:64-75, 1973
15. Hirsch J (ed): *Opportunities and Limitations in the Treatment of Alcoholics*, Charles C. Thomas, Springfield, IL, 1967
16. *Alcoholics Anonymous: The Story of How Many Thousands of Men and Women Have Recovered from Alcoholism.* New York, Alcoholics Anonymous Publishing, 1955
17. Chalmers DK: Controlled drinking as an alcoholism treatment goal: A methodological critique. Paper presented at Proceedings of the North American Congress on Alcohol and Drug Problems, San Francisco, December 1974
18. Gitlow SE: Alcoholism: A disease, in Bourne PG, Fox R (eds): *Alcoholism: Progress in Research and Treatment.* New York, Academic Press, 1973, p 5
19. Valles J: From Social Drinking to Alcoholism. Dallas, Tane Press, 1972, pp 89-115
20. Seixas FA: A possible effect of major efforts to treatment of established alcoholism: Initiating an epidemic of health. *Prevent Med* 3:83-96, 1974
21. Bucky SF, Edwards D, Berry NH: A note on hospitalization and discharge rates of men treated at the Navy's alcohol centers. Report No. 75-41, Naval Health Research Center, San Diego, May 1975
22. Emrick CD: A review of psychologically oriented treatment of alcoholism. II. The relative effectiveness of different treatment approaches and the effectiveness of treatment versus no treatment. *J Stud Alcohol* 36:1, 1975
23. Swensen CH: Commitment and the personality of the successful therapist. *Psychol Bull* 77:400-404, 1972

24. O'Briant RG, Lennard HL, Allen SD, et al: *Recovery from Alcoholism: A Social Treatment Model.* Springfield, Ill, Charles C. Thomas, 1973
25. Paulson S, Kraus S, Iber F: Development and evaluation of a compliance test for patients taking disulfiram. *Johns Hopkins Med J* 141(3):119-125, 1977
26. Pursch JP: What do you do with a drunken sailor? Address at the 40th International Convention of A.A., Denver, July 1975
27. Pursch JA: Alcoholism in aviation: A problem of attitudes. *Aerospace Med* 45:318-321, 1974
28. Position Statement Regarding Abstinence, National Council on Alcoholism/American Medical Society on Alcoholism, Sept. 16, 1974

8

The Medical Complications of Alcoholism

Stanley E. Gitlow
Frank A. Seixas

In recent years, an accumulating body of research has led to the identification of a large group of diseases specifically engendered by alcohol addiction. Some of these pathologies arise directly from the toxic effect of ethanol upon the tissues and others from the malnutrition that at times accompanies alcoholism.

Alcohol generates a large caloric yield (7 cal/g) without supplying any essential nutrients. Alcoholics may therefore suffer from severe malnutrition without feeling hungry or suffering substantive weight loss. While this dietary deficiency is extremely important in itself, it has become increasingly clear that direct toxic effects of alcohol on tissues responsible for absorption, modification, and storage of essential nutrients augments such malnutrition. For instance, high-dose ethanol produces histologic abnormalities of the intestinal mucosa, decreased absorptive capacity, and alterations in the intestinal permeability, as well as motility. In addition, it interferes with the cellular metabolism of vitamin B_6, folate, and iron, and impairs absorption of vitamin B_{12}. It is therefore common to find interference with processing of nutrients to their absorbable state, inadequate absorption, in-

ALCOHOLISM:
A Practical Treatment Guide
ISBN 0-8089-1912-1

creased loss through the affected intestinal mucous membrane (backflux), decreased intestinal transit time, as well as deficient intracellular conversion to their active congeners and decreased storage. What with a disruption in the quantity and quality of foodstuffs common to active alcoholism and its resultant acute and chronic gastritis, there is little wonder that malnutrition results. To aggravate these circumstances, there is strong evidence that chronic ethanol ingestion results in elevation of splanchnic oxygen consumption and overall basal metabolic rate. The huge energy load associated with the oxidation of large quantities of ethanol (via alcohol dehydrogenase and aldehyde dehydrogenase to form acetaldehyde and acetyl-CoA, respectively) results in a marked decrease in the ratio of NAD to $NADH_2$ and interference with the citric acid (Krebs) cycle. The redox change associated with the lowered NAD:NADH ratio results in shifts of lactate:pyruvate and α-glycero phosphate:dihydroxyacetone phosphate toward their reduced forms rather than permitting adequate regeneration of ATP with its associated mitochondrial function. This metabolic derangement results in changes in the manner in which the body handles innumerable vital substances, including but not limited to acetate, lactate, pyruvate, urate, indolealkylamines, catecholamines, sex hormones and other steroids, lipids, lipoproteins, cholesterol, fatty acids, carbohydrates, and amino acids. As an example, the metabolic shift from pyruvate to lactate not only results in an elevation of urate (thereby explaining in part the occasional acute gouty attack following an episode of drinking), but also deprives the pyruvate carboxylase and phosphoenol-pyruvate carboxykinase catalyzed reactions essential to gluconeogenesis. In conjunction with the inadequate hepatic glycogen storage associated with malnutrition (starvation) or diabetes, such impaired gluconeogenesis may result in life-threatening episodes of hypoglycemia after ethanol ingestion. Major chronic illnesses, such as arteriosclerosis and hypertension, are also affected by these ethanol-induced metabolic/physiologic changes. Acute ethanol administration favors mobilization of fat stores with an elevation of fatty acids, but more chronic ethanol use elicits an increase in the synthesis of neutral fats (triglycerides), especially in the liver. A concomitant increase in the synthesis of high-density lipoprotein (HDL) cholesterol has been suggested as a possible mechanism for a reduction in coronary heart disease amongst modest drinkers (although the increase is of the HDL_3 rather than the more critical HDL_2 subtype). Alternatively, a substantial hyperadrenergia results from ethanol ingestion, norepinephrine synthesis increasing during continous drinking and epinephrine rising acutely immediately thereafter (drinking withdrawal). That portion of the population hypersensitive to pressor substances (primary hypertensives) might well be expected to respond to even modest doses of ethanol with elevation of blood pressure.

It should not be entertained that ethanol modifies metabolism only through inhibition of the malate-aspartate and/or glycerol-3-phosphate shuttles. The shifts in catabolism of the indolealkylamines and catecholamines from the oxidized (acidic) forms to their reduced congeners after ethanol administration (i.e.,vanillylmandelic acid to 3-methoxy, 4-hydroxyphenylethylene glycol) might more likely result from competitive inhibition of aldehyde dehydrogenase, the enzyme used commonly during the catabolism of ethanol as well as these neurohumors. The very multiplicity of these effects may lead to critical interactions that, over time, result in certain of the pathologic entities commonly considered to be sequelae of alcoholism.

Whereas a compromised diet appears to explain the riboflavin (B_2), ascorbic acid (C), and calciferol (D) deficiencies occasionally associated with alcoholism, thiamine (B_1) and pyridoxine (B_6) are inadequately converted to their active congeners thiamine pyrophosphate and pyridoxal-5′-phosphate during periods of substantive ethanol ingestion. Unfortunately, and perhaps as a result of these circumstances, the administration of thiamine fails to elevate transketolase (for which it is the coenzyme) without considerable delay. Slow and possibly incomplete recovery of such enzyme systems essential for carbohydrate metabolism might be related to the inordinately long time required for recovery from peripheral neuropathy and the relatively poor prognosis of the organic mental syndromes characterizing long-term recalcitrant alcoholism.

Retinol (vitamin A) levels may be compromised in the alcoholic by elevated hepatic catabolism and or steatorrhea. Interference with the other fat-soluble vitamins appears to follow only cholestasis or chronic pancreatitis.

Cobalamin (B_{12}) malabsorption may accompany alcoholism but this cannot be rectified by correcting the abnormally low gastric intrinsic factor. Apparently it results from the failure of pancreatic digestion of R protein, the latter competitively inhibiting the binding of intrinsic factor to cobalamin. Folate absorption, on the other hand, does not appear to suffer from ethanol ingestion except in the presence of malnutrition. Rather, there is evidence that further compromise of serum folate may result from abnormalities in hepatic storage and (elevated) renal excretion.

Anomalous mineral metabolism has long been accused of playing major roles in the pathophysiology of alcoholism. Despite such claims, serum iron levels are usually unaffected, calcium levels are unchanged in the absence of steatorrhea, and abnormal magnesium and zinc levels are probably largely the result of muscle wasting with elevated urinary excretion. Thus far, the data concerning these minerals fail to warrant enthusiasm in their therapeutic use.

THE LIVER

The most conspicuous physical effect of taking high quantities of alcohol is fatty infiltration of the liver. This results largely from increased hepatic lipogenesis. The fatty liver appears clinically as hepatomegaly accompanied by minimally disturbed liver functions and, rarely, mild jaundice. There have been a number of unexplained sudden deaths among alcoholics in which the only postmortem finding was a fatty liver (hepatic steatosis, lacy liver). These have been attributed to many factors including sudden and severe hypoglycemia; cerebral fat emboli have also been postulated but not demonstrated. Paroxysmal arrhythmias independently related to drinking are more likely the cause of these sudden deaths.

Alcoholic hepatitis is considerably less common than fatty liver. The condition is characterized by jaundice, fever, leukocytosis, and, sometimes, liver tenderness. Hepatic functions are disturbed, with greater elevation of SGOT than SGPT, and a rather typical histologic picture with the presence of inclusions called Mallory bodies and centrilobular hepatocyte swelling with accumulation of polymorphonuclear leukocytes has been described. Unfortunately the prognosis with this illness must be very guarded. There is not only a 30 percent mortality rate early in its course, but the notable propensity for later conversion to hepatic cirrhosis.

There is evidence that alcoholic hepatitis is one of the major pathways from fatty liver to hepatic cirrhosis. It is now accepted that the pathology of alcoholic cirrhosis varies in the amount and distribution of fibrous tissue, and can include both the small nodular "classically Laennec" type and the large nodules once associated with the "postnecrotic" variety. Studies in France and Germany have shown that prolonged high levels of ethanol ingestion were more conclusively related to the incidence and occurrence of cirrhosis than were dietary deficiencies.

The observation that there are correlations between the incidence of cirrhosis and both the quantity as well as the duration of alcohol ingestion has led some observers to conclude that ethanol per se (with the fatty liver) is "the cause" of cirrhosis. That the majority of heavy drinkers fail to develop cirrhosis despite untold numbers of debauches, each with its episode of fatty liver, suggests that the latter lesion represents no more than exposure to some secondary and determinative event (viral, genetic, or alternate chemical injury). Outdoor high-wire walking does not in and of itself cause fractures, but the more frequently it is practiced the more likely that a sudden and unexpected wind will occur concurrently and result in just such morbidity. The coincidence of such unhappy events appears to be the key etiologic circumstance leading to a number of the medical complications of alcoholism. From a pathologic standpoint, considerable suspicion of an early conversion to cirrhosis is warranted upon the observation of not only fat but more importantly centrilobular fibrosis in a liver biopsy. Only somewhat later does the development of fibrous and necrotic bridges (bridging) and regenerative nodules clearly establish the diagnosis of cirrhosis.

From a clinical standpoint, the diagnosis of cirrhosis should be suspected in any alcoholic suffering from chronic or recurrent anorexia, nausea, weight loss, asthenia, change in bowel habits, upper abdominal pain, or low-grade fever in conjunction with a tender enlarged liver. More rarely, the diagnostic suspicion may be greatly assisted by the appearance of mild jaundice, bleeding, pruritis, or dependent edema. Splenomegaly leads to palpation of a spleen (tip, usually) in no more than one half of the cases, whereas hepatomegaly is clinically absent in one third. Spider telangiectasia, palmar erythema, Dupuytren's contracture, testicular atrophy, gynecomastia, loss of masculine hair distribution, parotid enlargement, evidence of collateral circulation, and findings of organic mental dysfunction can individually or collectively offer the clinician a greatly increased likelihood of diagnostic accuracy, but abnormal liver function tests persisting beyond the 3- to 5-day withdrawal period of inpatient abstinence and ultimately the results of a liver biopsy are desirable for clinical certainty. Hepatic failure, gastrointestinal hemorrhage, sepsis, and an elevated incidence of hepatoma all serve as paths to the often fatal outlook of this illness.

Management of cirrhosis consists of abstinence, prolonged rest, and carefully balanced nutritional therapy. The reader is referred to more detailed texts for methods to control portal hypertension, gastrointestinal bleeding, ascites, hepatic insufficiency, and coma. Although there are some cases (approximately 15 percent) of cirrhosis unassociated with alcoholism, i.e., those secondary to schistosomiasis, chronic infectious hepatitis, or kwashiorkor, and separate cirrhotic disease such as Wilson's disease and biliary cirrhosis, the failure to make and formally list the diagnosis of alcoholism when applicable along with cirrhosis on the hospital record may account in part for the frequent failure to advise appropriate treatment of the alcoholism. Advice to cut down on ethanol ingestion is a useless shibboleth under such circumstances. Active and aggressive treatment for alcoholism is required in order to attain effective therapeutic results for the cirrhosis.

THE PANCREAS

About 75 percent of cases of pancreatitis stem from alcohol ingestion. The precise etiology is still under investigation, but more and more emphasis is being placed on the direct effect of large doses of ethanol over long periods of time. Ethanol influences pancreatic function both directly and indirectly through gastric acid and secretogogue release as well as through neural control. The response of each of the physiologic mechanisms varies with dose and chronicity of ethanol administration. Unfortunately, major species differences make interpretation of animal research difficult or impossible. In general, ethanol inhibits markedly both volume and bicarbonate secretion by the pancreas but protein content remains relatively unaffected. It has been presumed that these effects might relate, as a result of increased viscosity, to the obstruction of pancreatic ducts with protein plugs early in the course of pancreatitis. There is also evidence that ethanol injures pancreatic exocrine cells in much the same manner as hepatocytes, since lipid accumulation, swelling of mitochondria, and cytoplasmic degradation results from such exposure. It is a noteworthy coincidence that ethanol-induced cellular lipid accumulation increases with elevated levels of food ingestion, that acute pancreatitis commonly follows the combination of an ethanol binge with a food binge, and that recurrent episodes of pancreatitis are also associated with a genetic form of hyperlipidemia.

Although chronic alcoholic pancreatitis can rarely appear without a history of recurrent abdominal pain, such pain remains the cardinal symptom of acute pancreatitis. It is usually epigastric, severe, transmitted through to the midback and relieved in part by sitting and leaning forward. The addition of nausea, vomiting, fever and shock in conjunction with a "surgical abdomen" often yields a clinical picture at once nonspecific and urgent. Assay of amylase in blood and urine and studies of the abdomen with sonography or CT scanning may be rewarded with a presumptive diagnosis. Treatment remains nonspecific but total body and alimentary rest (intravenous feeding with continuous nasogastric suction) with meperidine, anticholinergics, and histamine-2 blockade are commonly used. Recovery may be complicated by pseudocyst formation, mild obstructive jaundice, and mild diabetes mellitus. Recurrent episodes commonly result in pancreatic calcification (visible on a plain abdominal radiograph), and evidence of inadequate endocrine function (glucose intolerance) and exocrine function (steatorrhea). On rare occasions, a mixed system syndrome with involvement of skin, joints, kidneys, and a migratory thrombophlebitis has been noted. One can survive many acute attacks but progressively, pancreatic tissue becomes destroyed. Failure to abstain from ethanol increases the rate of recurrence threefold. In some patients not responding to treatment, surgical interventions such as cholecystostomy, enterostomy, drainage of the peritoneal sacs, and total or partial pancreatectomy have been used with limited success.

GASTROINTESTINAL TRACT

As an astringent, alcohol has a direct irritating effect upon mucous membranes. Anomalous esophageal motility and decreased sphincter pressure following an ethanol meal may well explain the increased frequency of reflux and heartburn. In the stomach it may produce acute gastritis characterized by nausea, vomiting, pain, and other signs of indigestion. Superficial gastric erosions, petechial hemorrhages, and an occasional acute duodenitis have also been observed. Chronic atrophic gastritis is less common and characterized by loss of the glandular portions of the mucosa with some irregularity of the epithelial cells and inflammatory infiltration of the stroma. At times, persistent vomiting may lead to a tear or rupture of the esophagus at the esophagogastric junction, the Mallory-Weiss syndrome.

At the turn of the century ethanol was used as a test meal in order to evaluate patients for achlorhydria. More recently it has been found that rather than increase gastric acid secretion, ethanol alters the integrity of the gastric mucosal barrier. Salicylates duplicate this lesion but the literature is indecisive as to whether the adverse effects of these substances (gastric erosions and hemorrhage) are additive or synergistic.

Although the incidence of peptic ulceration is increased fourfold amongst patients with alcoholic cirrhosis, there remains some doubt concerning the clinical teaching relating peptic ulcer disease to ethanol ingestion etiologically. Nonetheless, discontinuation of ethanol in association with a bland diet will likely result in prompt recovery from the usual peptic problems incumbent upon excessive ethanol ingestion.

Ethanol is largely, if not completely, absorbed in the stomach and jejunum, thereby explaining the startling rapidity with which this substance finds its way into the bloodstream. Its concentration in the ileum is likely related to backflux (bloodstream to intestinal lumen). Whether related to a direct toxic effect of ethanol upon the mucous membrane of the small bowel or to the biochemical defects remaining from the oxidation of ethanol by mucosal cells, the ultimate result is that of an anomalous membrane permeability. Backflux becomes significant and the activities of those enzymes that are membrane-bound or energy-dependent diminish. These include the disaccharidases and ATPase. The former circumstance leads to lactose intolerance, and the latter to deficient absorption of D-glucose, amino acids, salt, and water. Thus, at least three (backflux, disaccharide intolerance, and defective function of the Na^+, K^+ ATPase energy pump) mechanisms may explain the colic and diarrhea that is commonly associated with drinking. To complicate matters, either malnutrition or chronic ethanol ingestion can lead to shortened villi and other morphologic changes in the small bowel mucosa. Nonetheless, well-nourished periodic binge drinkers regularly suffer the enterocolitis associated with ethanol. Fortunately, this syndrome disappears without specific treatment within a few days after becoming abstinent.

THE CARDIOVASCULAR SYSTEM

For many years, heart disease in alcoholics was thought to be rooted solely in malnutrition. Researchers working during the last 20 years have determined that chronic alcohol intake has a direct toxic effect on the myocardium. Alcoholic heart disease has been conveniently divided into toxic, conductive, and nutritional.

The nutritional variant, largely the result of thiamine deficiency and historically referred to as the wet type of beri-beri, is rarely seen in western countries any longer. It is characterized, however, by high-output congestive heart failure in conjunction with a peripheral neuropathy. Administration of thiamine may yield a prompt cardiac response, though the neuropathy usually requires many months to improve. Occasionally, treatment fails to reverse the cardiac lesion, a circumstance that leaves the patient with no more than the less effective general supportive cardiotonic regimen on which to rely.

The other two cardiac problems appear to stem from the direct toxicologic effects of ethanol upon the myocardium. Even modest and short-term ethanol administration results in a deleterious effect in cardiac performance. Ethanol is a direct depressant of inotropic activity of the myocardium, a circumstance that can be measured in normal men within a few hours of achieving blood alcohol levels no higher than that with which it is legal to drive in many states (0.1%). Similar blood levels in the dog result in depressed dp/dt^2 and elevated left ventricular filling pressures and dimensions. Such effects from rather common degrees of social drinking only achieve immediate clinical import when coupled with an enormous volume overload, a circumstance described in 1884 as the "Munich beer heart," but little is known concerning the long-term repetitive subclinical effects of such ethanol use upon the heart. It also remains unclear why one person appears to suffer progressive cardiac impairment after a level and duration of drinking that fails to substantively affect another. As with cirrhosis, such a circumstance suggests the presence of some concomitant factor or factors. Along this line of reasoning, it is of special interest to note that women seem unusually prone to the complication of cirrhosis but resistant to that of alcoholic primary cardiomyopathy, despite the fact that both illnesses are otherwise related to prodigious ethanol ingestion of long duration.

Although cardiac biopsies from patients with this illness reveal mitochondrial, myofibrillar, and sarcoplasmic changes, along with an increased ratio of triglycerides to fatty acids, reduced calcium uptake ability, and a marked alteration in mitochondrial enzymes, contrasting studies of other types of cardiac disease raise serious questions regarding the specificity of such findings. Thus, the precise mechanism whereby ethanol produces cardiac injury is unknown.

Acute intoxication as well as the early withdrawal period have been observed clinically to be associated with abnormalities in cardiac rhythm. Although no more than palpitations may be noted by the patient, the electrocardiogram may reveal a prolonged QT interval, spinous or cloven T waves, abnormal P waves, premature contractions, bundle branch or intraventricular block patterns, supraventricular tachycardias (usually atrial flutter or fibrillation), or heart block. As little as a few ounces of whiskey exert a negative chronatropism in patients with previous cardiac disease, and there is adequate evidence to confirm that even small amounts of ethanol exert adverse effects upon the cardiac function of such individuals. Sudden death during or immediately following weekend "benders" (the holiday heart syndrome) are believed to be related to ethanol-induced ventricular arrhythmias (despite the fact that no more than a fatty liver appears on the routine postmortem examination).

Even moderate drinking appears to be associated with increased levels of systemic blood pressure and likelihood of cerebrovascular accidents. Hypertension, with its attendant elevated morbidity and mortality, therefore represents another cardiovascular contraindication to ethanol use. The failure to appreciate these untoward effects of ethanol may have stemmed from age-old observations that its direct and immediate action was as a vasodilator and that the patient with angina pectoris occasionally felt less discomfort after its use. Unfortunately, the latter is unassociated with electrocardiographic or physiologic improvement, and perhaps due to ethanol-induced hyperadrenergia, the dominant and overall effect upon the vasculature is one of vasoconstriction.

Ecologic and angiographic studies have revealed a negative correlation between ethanol consumption and coronary artery disease (atherosclerosis). This might stem from the ability of ethanol to elevate HDL-cholesterol (although subtype 3 rather than the more critical subtype 2), to increase the antiatherogenic neutral lipid metabolites of ethanol in the vascular wall, or simply be related to subtle differences in the diets of drinkers and abstainers. On the other hand, a panel of experts at the first ARUS conference in Washington, DC in 1985 concluded that "it is impossible on scientific grounds to recommend any alcohol consumption pattern as being protective against coronary heart disease." Unfortunately, an American Heart Association public pronouncement in 1986 failed to concur with the caution inherent in such an approach.

The first observable clinical manifestations of primary myocardiopathy tend to be fatigue and dyspnea, usually exertional, but the latter sometimes presenting as a nocturnal paroxysm. Arrhythmias are prominent in the clinical course and an isolated paroxysm of atrial fibrillation may even announce the illness. Shortly thereafter, multiple-chamber (not restricted to the left ventricular outflow tract) cardiomegaly appears on chest x-ray examination and echocardiography may reveal chamber enlargement with depressed fractional shortening. At that time a careful history will usually reveal "fifth a day" drinking for at least 10 years. If immediate abstinence is not achieved, more pronounced congestive heart failure intervenes, the heart becomes massively enlarged, and peripheral edema with hepatomegaly appears. Intracardiac thrombosis and recurrent embolization may occur.

Such an event or an arrhythmia often concludes the course of the illness within a few years of the onset of congestive heart failure. Late-stage treatment response occasionally follows abstinence, long-term bed rest, a low-sodium high-nutrient diet, diuretics, and cardiotonics with or without afterload reduction.

Physical examination reveals the usual manifestations of left and right heart failure in conjunction with other complications stemming from the use of excessive ethanol. On the other hand, the ultimate diagnosis tends to await demonstration of a hypokinetic heart without coronary artery disease by cardiac catheterization.

About 20 years ago there was a short flurry of a severe perimyocardiopathy related to the simultaneous administration of ethanol and cobalt by a beer industry too eager for a long-lasting "head" on their product. After a number of deaths they ceased adding cobalt to their brews.

THE NERVOUS SYSTEM

The thiamine depletion that causes nutritional alcoholic heart disease is also responsible for a number of debilitating neurologic conditions frequently encountered in the alcoholic. It must be stressed that those nutrients required for coenzyme production often develop patterns of depletion at times of metabolic load rather than during periods of starvation. Thus, evidence of thiamine deficiency may not appear until the dietary improvement coincident with treatment for the withdrawal syndrome. What with the time required for conversion of such vitamins to their biologically active congeners, prompt administration would seem to be more critical than size of dose.

Peripheral neuropathy is one of the most striking and widespread of these syndromes. It appears clinically as progressive numbness, pain and paresthesias in the legs and/or arms, as well as motor weakness, usually bilateral and symmetric, of the peripheral parts of the limbs (feet more commonly involved than hands). The sensory deficit is of a glove and stocking type. As a rule, the lower extremities are affected first; walking becomes difficult or impossible.

The disease is reversible with thiamine, but recovery may take as long as 24 months. Treatment consists of a diet rich in calories and vitamins, polyvitamin supplements, bed rest, and unfailing abstinence. To prevent contractures, the affected limbs may require splinting, and physical therapy should be instituted as soon as possible.

Toxic or "tobacco-alcohol" amblyopia is a neuritis of the optic nerve leading to progressive failure of central vision and difficulty in distinguishing red from green. Clinical testing reveals impaired visual acuity and bilateral central scotomata. The condition is reversible with thiamine and abstinence.

Wernicke's encephalopathy, often accompanied by Korsakoff's syndrome and more rarely by peripheral neuropathy, is a brain disorder in which severe thiamine depletion results in acute hemorrhagic lesions primarily in the gray matter about the third and fourth ventricles and aqueduct, especially the mammillary bodies. When found in conjunction with Korsakoff's psychosis, there is uniform involvement of the medial dorsal nuclei of the thalamus as well. In the latter circumstance one also sees more diffuse neuronal injury, greater chronicity, and lesser likelihood of a complete therapeutic response. It results from prolonged alcoholism, but as with so many of the organic complications of this disease there is confusion as to the relative roles of nutritional deficiency, direct ethanol toxicity, and concomitant but apparently unrelated factors such as genetics and sex. Since Wernicke's syndrome coincident with starvation without ethanol use rarely if ever results in the amnesic residua common to alcoholic patients with Wernicke-Korsakoff's syndrome, it appears that Wernicke's more likely results from thiamine deficiency whereas Korsakoff's probably stems from a direct toxic effect of ethanol. However, one cannot rule out the possibility that such chronicity might result from repetitive subclinical vitamin deficiency in the alcoholic.

Patients suffering from Wernicke's encephalopathy are unable to move their eyes conjugately either horizontally or vertically (ophthalmoplegia). They exhibit nystagmus, ataxia, disorientation, and confusion. In the syndrome's earliest stages, thiamine rapidly reverses the ophthalmoplegia and should be combined with intensive oral or parenteral polyvitamin therapy as well as abstinence.

Korsakoff's disease is clinically characterized by both retrograde (memory) and anterograde (learning) amnesia. Patients are often verbal and affable but confabulate readily, apparently unaware of their amnesic defects. They are usually disoriented in time and space and do not benefit from being taught mnemonic strategies for new learning. It seems likely that this illness represents but a severe and perhaps complicated (by malnutrition) form of the toxic neurologic deficit produced directly by ethanol and referred to below as alcoholic dementia (alternatively as chronic brain syndrome or organic mental syndrome secondary to ethanol). Again, as though to stress etiologic factors concomitant with long-term and high-dosage ethanol ingestion, the incidence of this illness is less in women than in men (as in cardiomyopathy) and no correlation with cirrhosis can be demonstrated. Treatment parallels that for Wernicke's encephalopathy, but mental recovery may take 12 or more months and in half of the patients may not take place adequately to permit outpatient function. Even with the more satisfactory outcomes there is usually residual memory impairment.

Alcoholic cerebellar degeneration is a syndrome in which atrophic cerebellar changes produce progressive unsteadiness of gait and stance and, in some cases, mild to moderate nystagmus, hypertonia, and deep tendon hyporeflexia. The disease has a rapid course, reaching maximum severity and then stabilizing within days or weeks of onset. Abstinence and nutritional therapy may produce some limited abatement of symptoms.

Central pontine myelinolysis and Marchiafava-Bignami disease are rare neurologic conditions found almost exclusively in malnourished chronic alcoholics. Both diseases are difficult to diagnose clinically; they are normally discovered on autopsy.

In central pontine myelinolysis, a dense concentration of demyelinized lesions in the pons produces rapidly progressing weakness of the bulbar innovated musculature, which first manifests as dysphagia and dysarthria. Within days, there is aphonia and total inability to swallow, as well as complete ophthalmoplegia, fixed or dilated pupils, and lack of corneal response. Initial quadriparesis is usually succeeded by hyporeflexic or areflexic quadriplegia, which may be rigid or flaccid. In the terminal stage, death is preceded by a sequence of drowsiness, stupor, lethargy, and coma.

Marchiafava-Bignami disease involves severe atrophy of the corpus callosum, the lesions resembling those of central pontine myelinolysis and multiple sclerosis. Progressive psychologic deterioration occurs within days or months of onset. Patients exhibit agitation, confusion, hallucinations, negativism, impaired judgment, and disorientation. The neurologic damage is evidenced physiologically by dysphagia, echolalia, disturbance of gait and motor skills, incontinence, grasping, sucking, perseveration, and delayed initiation of action.

Although generating considerable disagreement, the notion that ethanol alone could produce a chronic brain syndrome distinct from those CNS disorders resulting from nutritional deficiencies has achieved broad acceptance. In its most extreme form, cerebral degeneration is an irreversible progressive dementia characterized by confusion and memory loss and complicated by spacticity of the lower extremities, and "astasia-abasia" type of gait disturbance, retropulsion, fine picking movements, digital and labial tremulousness, and dysarthria.

In its earlier phases, the syndrome of alcoholic dementia may be ubiquitous among those patients ingesting large quantities of ethanol for protracted periods. Subtle interference with mentation and memory such as to lead to difficulties with job or school performance and failure to appreciate the logical consequences of specific behavior are common. One may judge change in mental status of a patient not previously known to you by reference to a standard such as previously accomplished schooling or job performance.

On the other hand, excellent psychometric tests can readily illustrate the common organic mental deficits following ethanol ingestion, especially in areas of visual-spatial, memory, and rapid psychomotor skills. Although diffuse CNS injury resulting in cognitive deficits were apparent to experienced clinicians many decades ago, neuropathologic confirmation did not appear in patients without the Wernicke-Korsakoff syndrome until pneumoencephalographic evidence of brain atrophy in alcoholics was first published 30 years ago. This evidence has been confirmed and extended more recently by CT scan data. There are encouraging data suggesting that CT scan lesions may remit after many months of abstinence. These findings are in concurrence with those psychometric data that depict early improvement (within 1-3 weeks of abstinence) followed by a slower phase of cognitive recovery requiring many months. Clinical experience supports these observations, but serves to caution that some patients never achieve full recovery and others require a few years to do so despite continuous abstinence. Addictive use of benzodiezapines or other psychotropic agents apparently complicates, aggravates, and prolongs such a recovery. Moreover, persistence of memory deficits is related to age: ethanol either accelerates the aging process, or tolerance to the toxic CNS effect of this agent is diminished after 50 years of age. At this time it appears that initial and periodic psychometric evaluation of problem-solving ability, memory, abstract reasoning, visual-spatial function, and timed psychomotor ability has a potential role in motivation, choice of therapy, and prognostic evaluation for the alcoholic patient.

Severe hepatic insufficiency also induces a cerebral dysfunction known as portalsystemic encephalopathy. It may be accompanied by elevated blood ammonia levels, a common result of hepatic failure, especially after a portocaval shunt. It is associated with astrocyte hyperplasia and neuronal degeneration. It may be induced by elevated protein ingestion, administration of a diuretic, a gastrointestinal hemorrhage, or sepsis. It may start with behavioral, intellectual, or neuromuscular symptoms including asterixis (flapping tremor of the extended hand), dementia, dysarthria, ataxia, and athetosis but rapidly progresses to stupor and coma. The prognosis is poor but temporary responses may follow treatment of the initiating event along with administration of lactulose, neomycin, metronidazole, a low protein diet, and/or branch chain amino acids.

THE MUSCULOSKELETAL SYSTEM

Over the last three decades, clinicians and researchers have defined an alcohol-induced muscle disease affecting the muscles of the thoracic cage and the proximal muscles of the extremities, characterized by acute muscle tenderness, pain, muscle weakness, frank rhabdomyolysis, and sometimes myoglobinuria. This syndrome, which may cause death by acute tubular necrosis with renal failure, is fortunately quite rare.

More commonly one sees muscle pain, tenderness, and weakness involving the proximal limb girdles especially, and occurring in conjunction with and for up to a week following the acute alcohol debauch. Careful study has revealed a leakage of muscle enzymes with transient elevations of SGOT and CPK. Return to full function within 5-7 days is the rule, but a chronic myopathy may intervene should ethanol ingestion persist. Occasionally the chronic myopathy appears in the absence of a preceding acute episode. Wasting and weakness of the proximal limb girdles is the rule, and diminished response of blood lactic acid elevation to ischemic exercise may be observed. Distal limb findings of a similar nature should always make one suspect dysfunction of the peripheral nerves rather than a myopathy. Myopathy improves with abstinence and adequate nourishment.

Inebriation is connected with a high incidence of traumatic fractures due to falls, brawls, and automobile accidents. In some alcoholics, the risk of fracture is increased by osteoporosis. The normal homeostatic cycle of bone formation and bone resorption is disturbed by a combination of calcium depletion, poor diet, and decreased activity. The resulting "metabolic" fractures (i.e., those superimposed upon osteoporosis) most commonly observed are in the hip, wrists, humerus, and spine, whereas the usual locations of the "traumatic" fractures of the alcoholic are ribs, legs, and skull.

Osteonecrosis of the hip is a rare syndrome seen mainly in patients with alcoholism. Limping and severe hip pain, usually bilateral, progress to femoral dislocation as the head of the femur necroses. It has been suggested that the bone tissue dies as a result of hyperlipemia, fat emboli obstructing the blood supply of the femoral head. Previous treatment with cortisone, possibly for an unrelated illness, may also play an etiologic role in this condition.

When osteonecrosis is suspected, usually from hip pain seen in alcoholics with no other signs of arthritis, the patient should be taken off weight bearing immediately. Needless to say, drinking should cease at once. Hip reconstructive surgery is often needed.

BLOOD

Ethanol interferes with hematopoiesis at multiple levels, producing various anemias and clotting disorders.

At the nutritional level, the restricted diet may be deficient in B-complex vitamins, especially B_6, B_{12}, and folate. Although an iron deficiency anemia is not uncommon among alcoholics, this does not usually result from a nutritional deficiency but rather from excessive iron loss (via gastritis, hemorrhoids, or varices). In fact, consumption of alcoholic beverages high in iron (occasionally due to manufacture) may result in hemosiderosis. Alcohol may even speed the development and manifestations of hemochromatosis where the genetic predisposition is present.

It must be understood that blood levels of such essential substances as iron and vitamin B_{12} may not solely reflect total body storage levels but may be elevated by a maturation block of the marrow or a release of hepatic stores due to injury. Their true metabolic status may therefore require studies of tissue levels or turnover (excretion relative to absorption). The manifold problems of absorbing the various nutrients following ethanol were pointed out earlier in this chapter. A block of intestinal folate absorption was accepted as the major hemopoietic problem for alcoholics after the observation that indigent alcoholics (derelicts), especially those with cirrhosis, revealed low serum folate levels. More recent studies have labeled that as too simplistic. The dietary content of folate and the general nutritional adequacy of the diet are more determinative of folate absorption during drinking. Even urinary folate excretion and hepatic storage and enzyme induction appear to play roles in the development of this deficiency. In normal volunteers, ethanol elicits a fall in reticulocytes and platelet counts along with an increase in serum iron. These observations are quite compatible with the major recognized ethanol effect on the marrow, that of producing a maturation arrest. The fall in serum folate, which also occurs, fails to explain this phenomenon since folate administration will not reverse the block until the ethanol is discontinued. The marrow reflects these phenomena with vacuolated proerythroblasts and promyelocytes. When malnutrition and/or chronic drinking are added to these circumstances, one may also see megaloblasts and ringed sideroblasts. The failure of conversion of pyridoxine to its active form, backflux of nutrients across the ethanol-injured intestinal membrane, and interference with cobalamin-intrinsic factor binding may each further complicate this picture.

The maturation arrest affects all marrow cellular elements: red cells, white cells, and platelets. Fortunately the resultant abnormalities in the circulation are not of clinical import unless complicated by other factors, such as liver disease. Since a significant number of narcotic addicts are also ethanol dependent and this community has suffered from the recent onslaught of the acquired immune deficiency syndrome (AIDS), the relationship of ethanol to immunologic mechanisms has been carefully scrutinized. Despite the leukopenia and diminished leukocyte mobilization and chemotactic properties associated with ethanol, this drug appears to exert minimal influence upon tissue resistance to infection in the absence of liver disease. Similarly, only in the presence of cirrhosis is there a significant reduction in RBC lifespan (hemolytic amemia).

Discontinuation of ethanol ingestion in conjunction with an adequate diet is followed by a rapid return of hematopoiesis, often with the appearance of reticulocytes, which should not delude the observer into the mistaken impression of hemolytic syndrome.

As we have seen, the maturation arrest and nutritional problems associated with ethanol ingestion often result in anomalous RBC production characterized by an increase in cell size (MCV). Measurement of MCV and various liver function tests have been used as a screening technique for the presence of alcoholism in various populations.

The maturation arrest of thrombocytes is complicated by a decreased platelet lifespan, abnormal platelet function, and the possibility of diminished clotting factors resulting from a damaged liver.

INFECTIOUS DISEASES

As noted above, ethanol administration has been long known to result in WBC dysfunction. Decreased serum bactericidal activity against *Escherichia coli* and *Haemophilus influenzae*, as well as an elevated mortality in rodents given both sepsis and ethanol, have also been observed. An enormous amount of recent literature evaluating more subtle aspects of immunologic function has failed to reveal a significant effect of ethanol unless hepatic injury has been produced.

Pulmonary tuberculosis is an infectious disease frequently associated with alcoholism; the population of tuberculosis hospitals shows a disproportionately elevated percentage of alcoholics. The tuberculosis is often complicated by peripheral neuropathy and liver disease. Although ethanol is not a primary cause of tuberculosis, its effect on leukocytes may lower resistance to the infection and undoubtedly compromises any long-term therapeutic plan. V. Hudolin has found a definite correlation between improved cure rates and abstinence.

The heavy smoking that almost universally accompanies alcoholism (even heavier during withdrawal) is a complicating factor in bronchopulmonary disease. Poor bronchial toilet associated with excessive sedation may account in part for the high incidence of suppurative bronchopulmonary disease in patients with alcoholism. There is clinical validity to the teaching that in the absence of an immunocompromised patient, the presence of a pulmonary abscess without bronchial obstruction strongly suggests the diagnosis of alcoholism. The same lesson may be applied to the presence of exceptionally slow clearing of a bacterial pneumonia. A Danish study of brewery workers, however, failed to demonstrate elevation of mortality rates due to infection among those with high ethanol ingestion.

CANCER

There is little doubt but that ethanol ingestion can be dose-correlated with elevated incidence of cancer of the mouth (tongue and palate), pharynx, larynx, esophagus, and liver. There is a strong likelihood that this may be true of cancer of the lungs and possibly of the pancreas as well. Cigarette smoking can be shown to represent a further, separate, untoward factor. The type of alcoholic beverage apparently influences carcinogenesis, since certain specific regions of wine-producing countries reveal disproportionate elevations of esophageal cancer.

Although the incidence of alcoholism varies widely among the European wine-drinking nations, Spain and Italy, as well as France, share the same onerous burden of elevated levels of these malignancies. The Danish study of brewery workers demonstrated elevated overall mortality rates as well as higher incidence of the aforementioned neoplasms among those supplied with free daily six-packs of beer. Other malignancies, such as colonic, occurred in normal numbers. Other studies, however, show increased incidence of cancer of both the cardia of the stomach and the colon. The increased incidence of cancer seen among alcoholics may be due at least in part to the enhanced capacity of these individuals to activate procarcinogens in the intestine, according to C. S. Lieber.

SURGERY

Because of alcohol's cross-tolerance with other members of the hypnotic-sedative group of drugs, one may expect an abnormal response to preoperative and general anesthetic medications. In addition, the sudden cessation of sedative ingestion coincident with surgery and/or injury-illness frequently results in an acute withdrawal syndrome, often DTs, in the immediate postoperative period (within 3 days for ethanol and 5-14 days for solid sedative withdrawal).

The anesthesiologist must also bear in mind that ethanol interferes with pulmonary function by decreasing ciliary activity, diffusion capacity, and surfactant production while increasing shunting. Obviously, the elevated incidence of hepatic dysfunction, poor wound healing, and metabolic abnormalities must also be considered in preoperative decision-making as well as during and after surgical care.

ENDOCRINE

Ethanol has its major effects upon the hypothalamus-pituitary-gonadal axis. It can cause pseudo-Cushing's syndrome, which may be indistinguishable from Cushing's syndrome in every way except that it disappears within a few weeks of abstinence. It is possible that this endocrine effect of ethanol might explain the elevated incidence of aseptic hip necrosis with alcoholism. This same endocrine axis may demonstrate insufficiency upon challenge with hypoglycemia or other stress. It is possible that this system may respond to ethanol administration with the development of tolerance. The major gonadal response to this drug appears to be that of a fall in plasma testosterone, apparently stemming from inhibition of Leydig cell function. Gonadotropic defects have been noted. Feminization of males may also be related to increased estrogens, a circumstance that apparently does not require the presence of liver damage. FSH secretion in the female has also been shown to be inadequate.

Ethanol is one of the few substances capable of depressing the secretion of ADH. This effect is reversed as the blood ethanol level falls.

In the absence of liver disease, there is little clinical evidence of other major endocrine abnormalities following ethanol administration.

PERINATAL AND PEDIATRIC

During the 20 years following the repeal of prohibition, it was almost heresy to suggest that ethanol was directly responsible for any of the circumstances noted in this chapter. Bad nutrition was the usual scapegoat for DTs and cirrhosis, while a host of other problems recognized since antiquity as the direct toxicologic result of ethanol ingestion were simply forgotten. One of these happened to be the leading preventable birth defect and the third most common such lesion overall in the United States, fetal alcohol syndrome (FAS). Jellinek was one of the earliest to refer to this syndrome in this century and even he thought it was related to nutrition rather than the teratogenicity of ethanol. It remained for Rouquette, Lemoine, Jones and Smith, and Streissguth since 1957 to rediscover and scientifically authenticate the observations of biblical times.*

*Dr. John Wallace found recently a text entitled *Handbook of Modern Facts about Alcohol* by C. F. Stoddard, which listed the major findings of FAS in 1914.

Ethanol is able to pass the placental barrier, and in that sense, when a mother partakes of this drug so does her fetus. Animal experimentation suggests that such passage of ethanol is critical at about the third week of human pregnancy, a time period when many women may still be unaware of their pregnancy. Apparently for each child that suffers the complete teratogenic injury FAS, four develop incomplete forms of the illness, alcohol-related birth defects (ARBD). Since many of the latter children lack a complete enough syndrome to achieve etiologic specificity, some researchers have been slow to accept the responsibility of ethanol for their anomalies. Nonetheless, even moderate drinking during pregnancy has been observed to lead to increased risks for spontaneous abortion, stillbirths, and low birth weight children.

The full FAS picture includes three sets of problems:

1. Growth deficiency, both pre- and postnatal with hypotonia and poor sucking.
2. CNS injury, characterized by microcephaly, an irritable tremulous infant, mental retardation, and an abnormal EEG.
3. Facial injury, characterized by hypoplastic philtrum, thin upper lip, small pug nose, short palpebral fissures, epicanthal folds, ptosis, strabismus, and retrognathia. Other anomalies involve the heart (atrial septal defect), joints, genitalia, and skin (altered palmar crease).

Although there is little doubt that the severe lesions are reserved for the children of those mothers who drink severely throughout their pregnancies, the cutoff points for both degree and duration of drinking below which full safety resides are simply unknown at present. It is alarming to realize that 13 percent of children enrolled in learning disorder units are believed to have had alcoholic mothers.

"No ethanol with pregnancy" would appear to represent the only responsible course at present.

On rare occasions infants are born so intoxicated with their mothers' choice of drugs that they must experience withdrawal phenomena. Among alcoholic women this has become especially dangerous when their drugs have included not only ethanol, but other longer-acting sedatives and cocaine as well. The infants then suffer not only withdrawal (from the sedatives) but experience direct toxicity from the stimulant as well (CNS and cardiovascular, especially).

Among the pediatric complications of alcoholism, one must not ignore two that are equally tragic to that already noted: child abuse and the tendency to hand the illness of ethanol and other drug dependency down to the next generation.

PSYCHIATRIC

One often hears of the danger of abstinence for patients who treat their own premorbid psychopathology with ethanol and/or other sedatives. If one fails to observe such patients for a long enough period of sedative abstinence, the presumption may be reached that the acute toxic mental disorder during withdrawal represents the patient's true underlying mental state. If the physicians then act in haste, the issue becomes a self-fulfilling prophecy and they confirm for themselves that they had best always hesitate to recommend the course of sobriety for their alcoholic patients. The critical issue becomes the manner and duration of observing the abstinent patient.

CONCLUSIONS

It appears from this brief survey that alcohol can generate multisystem problems of extreme gravity, any number of which may be present in an individual patient. It must be emphasized that the drug produces this damage primarily when consumed in large quantities over extended periods of time.

The thousands of these patients who die from suicide, malnutrition, accidents, withdrawal complications, and the myriad pathologic processes noted previously are all victims of a single disease: alcoholism.

While the countless symptoms may range all the way from indigestion, anxiety, and broken bones to cirrhosis, dementia, and unbearable family tragedies, they all require continued ingestion of ethanol for their ultimate expression. In that sense abstinence becomes the single most critical therapeutic achievement. Only in this manner may the medical complications of alcoholism achieve maximal rates of regression. In fact without abstinence most therapeutic efforts are ultimately doomed to failure.

BIBLIOGRAPHY

Bayliss RIS: Medical disorders associated with alcoholism, In Dawson AM (ed): *Third Symposium on Advanced Medicine*. Baltimore, Williams & Wilkins, 1968, pp 328-339

Fifth Special Report to the US Congress on Alcohol and Health. Washington, DC, US Department of Health and Human Services, NIAAA, 1983

Gitlow S, Dziedzic LB, Dziedzic SW: Alcohol and hypertension: Implications from research for clinical practice. *J Subst Abuse Treat* 3:121-129, 1986

Kissin B, Begleiter H (eds): *The Biology of Alcoholism: Clinical Pathology*, Vol 3. New York, Plenum, 1974, pp 291-586

Lieber CS: Alcohol and alimentary tract. *Adv Alcohol* 1, 1979

Petrakis, PL (ed): *The Effects of Alcohol on the Immune System*. Summary of a workshop held Nov 4-5, 1985. NIAAA, Rockville, MD

Seixas FA, Eggleston S (eds): Work in progress on alcoholism. *Ann NY Acad Sci* 273:146-302, 1976

Seixas FA, Williams K, Eggleston S (eds): Medical consequences of alcoholism. *Ann NY Acad Sci* 252:10-377, 1975

Sherlock, S (ed): Alcohol and disease. *Br Med Bull* 38, 1982

Streissguth AP, Landesman-Dwyer S, Martin JC, et al: Teratogenic effects of alcohol in humans and laboratory animals. *Science* 209:353-361, 1980

Tarter RE, Van Thiel DH (eds): *Alcohol and the Brain: Chronic Effects*. New York, Plenum, 1985

Tuyns AJ: Alcohol and cancer. *Alcohol Health Res World*, summer 1978, pp 20-31

Wilkinson DA (ed): *Cerebral Deficits in Alcoholism*. Addiction Research Foundation, Toronto, 1984

World MJ, Ryle PR, Thomson AD: Alcoholic malnutrition and the small intestine. *Alcohol Alcoholism* 20:89-124, 1985

9

Alcoholism and Clinical Psychiatry

Herbert S. Peyser

Alcoholism and the other substance abuse and dependency disorders are recognized as diseases in all the important medical classifications (e.g., ICD-9 and DSMIII-R). They are included within the category of psychiatric disorders, but the differentiation of the addictive disorders from the other psychiatric illnesses, crucial as it is for prognosis, management, and treatment, is not always clear. Alcoholism and other drug dependencies can mimic many psychiatric illnesses such as schizophrenia, the affective disorders, and the character and personality disorders, with the psychiatric picture clearing up on sobriety alone. They can coexist with such disorders and they can aggravate them. They can even cause illnesses such as borderline or schizophreniform disorders to appear as affective disorders or as true schizophrenia, thus distorting the picture, the course, and the treatment of patients with these diseases. Finally, where they do coexist with other psychiatric illnesses they markedly complicate the diagnosis, prognosis, management, treatment, and course of each of the combined disorders.[1]

This problem of combined psychiatric and addictive diseases is not as uncommon as one would think if one's experience were derived primarily from an office practice or from an association with a freestanding rehabilitation center. In the first case, that of the office practice, one is dealing with a relatively healthy population from a psychiatric point of view. In the second instance, the rehabilitation center, the population of more seriously ill alcoholics and drug abusers will

ALCOHOLISM:
A Practical Treatment Guide
ISBN 0-8089-1912-1

tend to include more people with psychiatric disturbances, but the number will still be relatively low. In the former situation the number of significantly psychiatrically ill people may be under 2 or 3 percent: in the latter perhaps up to 10 or 15 percent.

In the state psychiatric centers, however, the incidence of the coexistence of these disorders rises greatly. Here we are dealing not with the existence of psychiatric illness in an alcohol and/or other drug dependent population but with the reverse: the existence of alcoholism and other drug dependence in a population with significant and severe psychiatric illness.[2] Despite the literature, which reports anywhere from 25 to 40 percent of psychiatric inpatients to be dependent on alcohol or other drugs, informal estimates from such state hospitals as Manhattan State, Rockland State, and Nassau County Psychiatric Centers in New York estimate that 50 to 80 percent of their psychiatric patients have a history of serious alcohol and/or other drug use. (Rockland State Psychiatric Center is an unusual hospital in that it has a great awareness of drug dependency disorders and has had for over 10 years a special unit for the treatment of psychiatric patients with combined psychiatric and addictive disorders. Most other psychiatric hospitals do not have such a special unit; they do not report such statistics, but then again they do not look for them.) Studies show how infrequently questions about or objective evidence of alcohol and other drugs enter into the examination of patients by medical and psychiatric professionals.[3] Other studies note how infrequently the staff will report or record alcohol and, even more so, other drug use incidents.[4] One study, interestingly enough, using urine screens, discovered that over 60 percent of the patients in that psychiatric center were secretly using drugs.[5]

The converse is true as well. In the nonpsychiatrist's office, in the self-help group meetings, in lay groups and the freestanding rehabs, in the longer-term halfway houses, and in the therapeutic communities and recovery homes, all staffed by lay people in great part, these psychiatric illnesses are not looked for and hence are not found and reported. The staff is just not trained to diagnose nor are they oriented toward discovery of psychiatric pathology. The question of the diagnosis of a psychiatric illness and/or drug disorder is related, therefore, to the proportion of psychiatric professionals as opposed to lay people on the staff as well as the specific institution's program, orientation, and philosophy.

The conclusion is that there are no good statistics as to the coexistence of alcohol and other drug disorders with the other psychiatric disturbances. Everything depends upon the population studied and the background and orientation of those doing the studies. Nevertheless the incidence of combined disorders is not small and it increases rapidly as one enters more and more into populations of increasingly serious psychiatric disturbances. This may be true as well for the converse: psychiatric illness in alcoholics and other drug dependent patients. Here, however, the objective surveys and scientific reports are even more scarce and the issues and diagnostic criteria even more poorly defined and reported. Here the caretakers and therapists in the freestanding rehabs and so on tend to be more therapeutically and less scientifically and diagnostically oriented. Therefore, we are left more with impressions than with facts but it is best to review here what we do know: the reports from psychiatric sources in regard to the coexistence of alcohol and drug disorders with (1) schizophrenia, (2) affective disorders, (3) sociopathy, (4) borderline and other personality and anxiety disturbances, and (5) organic disturbances.

ALCOHOLISM AND SCHIZOPHRENIA

As to schizophrenia, there seems to be no established relationship between the two illnesses. Except for one epidemiologic study,[6] all the others found that alcoholism and schizophrenia were unrelated from a familial perspective and were hence unrelated biologic entities.[7-10] However, there is definitely an increased incidence of schizophrenia in patients with addictive disorders and vice versa. How much of an incidence is undetermined and reports vary. Studies report anywhere from 1 to 45 percent of groups of alcoholics to be schizophrenic, most of them reporting over 8 to 10 percent. Studies of addictive disorders in schizophrenia vary from 3 to 63 percent but here, too, most of the studies report the incidence to be above 10 percent.[11-13] Many factors influence these statistics: outpatient versus inpatient, diagnostic criteria of DSM-II versus DSM-III, and the sociologic and cultural nature of the groups studied. There is, for example, a "natural incidence" of alcoholism and other addictive disorders in different cultural groups and this must affect the incidence of such disorders in the psychiatrically ill members of these groups. Therefore, various studies show addiction to be absent in Chinese schizophrenics[14] and very low in Italian as opposed to Irish schizophrenics.[15] Other problems in determining the incidence such as underreporting, failing to look for or question on examination, and so forth, have been previously noted. All in all, the frequency of the combined disorders has most likely been underestimated in the general population.

There are some similarities in the course of each of the illnesses, at least in large groups of patients with either schizophrenia or the addictive disorders. With many of these patients there is a tendency in both illnesses toward onset in adolescence or early adulthood; toward chronicity, for the most part, with a relapsing, progressive course; toward physical, interpersonal, and occupational deterioration; and toward an earlier death. In addition, the course of each of the illnesses will certainly modify the other. The patients with coexisting schizophrenia and alcoholism tend more to resemble the pure alcoholics than the schizophrenics in terms of the course of the disorder, and are more apt to use other addicting drugs as well, even more than the nonpsychotic alcoholics. (One study showed a history of excessive use of alcohol and other drugs in the premorbid functioning of the schizophrenics prior to their first hospitalization; the use of alcohol was heavier in the chronic cases and was connected with readmissions as, even more so, were hallucinogens and stimulants.)[16]

The onset of combined illness tends to be a bit later than the onset in the usual schizophrenics. The former tend to be older, are more suicidal, and have a shorter hospital course (probably related to the significant degree of improvement on merely attaining improvement in the alcoholic part of the picture). As noted, they tend to continue using drugs secretly in the hospital and present many more behavior and management problems on the ward.

In regard to diagnosis and management, it is probably best to pay initial and primary attention to the addictive aspects than to the schizophrenia, except, of course, for the necessary emergency concerns where self-destructive or dangerous behavior is present in the form of suicide or violence, inability to take care of oneself, or other medical or psychiatric emergencies. Often enough, an acutely and flagrantly psychotic picture is not schizophrenia but is due to intoxication with alcohol, a stimulant (such as an amphetamine or cocaine), or a hallucinogen, and will clear within hours. Or it may be due to withdrawal, most unlikely from narcotics but rather from sedatives, including alcohol; here the use of phenothiazines will tend to lower the threshold for central nervous system (CNS) excitation and make matters worse. Giving a benzodiazepine may remarkably relieve the acute picture.

Urine screen by thin-layer chromatography is probably inadequate except for emergency rooms; it is the least specific, accurate, and sensitive of the tests and therefore tends to produce both false positives and false negatives. Testing by high-performance liquid or gas chromatography with mass spectroscopy to back up enzyme or radio immunoassay, although more expensive, is far more accurate, sensitive, and specific and can even be used for legal purposes. In certain situations the determination of blood levels is often preferable. It goes without saying that the blood alcohol level is the useful laboratory determination where that is the drug in question. As the blood level drops the picture should clear in the case of alcoholic intoxication, which fact can aid greatly in a differential diagnosis. Here, too, certain clinical findings are of diagnostic help in differentiating the picture from CNS trauma, other neurologic disorders (e.g., multiple sclerosis or cerebellar dysfunction), other sedative intoxications or withdrawal pictures, and various metabolic disturbances (such as hypoglycemia): spider nevi, palmer erythema, hepatomegaly, and so forth.

It should also be noted that abuse of antiparkinsonian drugs such as trihexyphenidyl or benztropine can produce acute atropine-like toxic metabolic psychotic states with agitation, delusions, and hallucinations, primarily visual, and with a warm, dry skin, diminished secretions, and tachycardia.

THE PROLONGED WITHDRAWAL SYNDROME

Thus, to make an adequate diagnosis of schizophrenia one may have to wait for the picture to clear. One may find oneself dealing with a pure toxic metabolic psychosis due to intoxication or withdrawal, or perhaps a drug- or alcohol-precipitated transient psychosis in a borderline, schizophreniform, or schizoaffectiuve disorder, rather than a true schizophrenia. The height of the withdrawal reaction from alcohol is 1–3 days after cessation of drinking and is largely completed from a physiologic standpoint after 5 days. It may go on, however, to the so-called prolonged withdrawal syndrome, lasting several weeks to a few months, occasionally even longer, with anxiety, depression, physiologic symptoms (involving respiration, blood pressure, and pulse), tremors, cognitive difficulties, irritability and emotional lability, and, perhaps, but rarely, transient psychotic states. The solid sedatives take longer with the height of withdrawal for many being about 5–10 days following stopping the drugs. The benzodiazepines take even longer and withdrawal psychoses have been reported as late as 14 days after the cessation of those drugs. Even abrupt discontinuing of "therapeutic" doses of benzodiazepines taken over several years can produce withdrawal phenomena, and other reports indicate that short active benzodiazepines can produce withdrawal symptoms after only a few weeks of continuous therapy.[17]

It may be helpful in dealing with the prolonged withdrawal syndrome or a similar state following cessation of stimulant or hallucinogenic drugs to give, if the anxiety is high, one of the more sedative neuroleptics: chlorpromazine or thioridazine in small doses, starting with 25 mg and increasing as necessary. One must be careful, for the effect of these psychotropic agents can be to "space out" the individual and frighten him or her, causing more trouble with fears of loss of control, vivid dreams, and increased suicidal ideation (this is particularly true in paranoid or obsessional people). Other nonaddicting sedatives that can be used are: hydroxyzine 25–100 mg, or better, diphenhydramine 25–50 mg. It is best, however, not to use any such medication, if possible, for it diverts the patient from a program of abstinence and the necessity of avoiding any medication to solve his or her problems.

For the depression of the prolonged withdrawal syndrome or that following cessation of stimulant or hallucinogenic drugs, one can give imipramine 25–50 mg up to full therapeutic dosage, or desipramine in similar doses. The latter is less apt to cause orthostatic hypotension and dizziness. Other tricyclic antidepressants can be used as well (e.g., nortriptyline). Amitriptyline has a sedative effect and can be abused; it is probably better to avoid that drug unless one really needs the sedative effect. There is some evidence that disulfiram can decrease the metabolism of tricyclic antidepressants, just as with phenytoin and benzodiazepines, and can therefore potentiate and prolong the effects of these drugs. Care must be therefore be exercised here.

The major problem is that the addictive disorder can, as noted, mimic schizophrenia (as well as the other disorders) and it is important to wait until the picture clears to make a good diagnosis. It is easier to differentiate between acute schizophrenia and DTs or even acute hallucinosis (considered a withdrawal syndrome but with a clear sensorium and unclouded consciousness). These clear in a matter of a few days to a week. Alcoholic hallucinosis may rarely go on and become chronic, in which case it is indistinguishable from schizophrenia save for the lack of family history, premorbid history, and so forth. But hallucinosis, DTs, and the amphetamine- or cocaine-induced psychoses should in general clear in a matter of days or weeks, a few months at the outside. They usually can be easily differentiated from schizophrenia in a few days to a week.

PROBLEMS IN TREATMENT

Treatment regimens for combined schizophrenia and addictive disorder can present problems, for the therapeutic programs for each can find the programs for the other somewhat contraindicated. Disulfiram, for example, can present problems. The literature tends to oppose its use in schizophrenia, even in situations where there is only a past history of psychosis.[12] Individual practitioners, however, state that in their experience, especially with the use of 125- to 250-mg dosage (instead of the 500-mg dosage used in the past), that they have had no such trouble with the drug. Institutionally based psychiatrists in state hospitals often feel, in addition, that the dangers of alcohol intake in their schizophrenic patients greatly outweigh the dangers of disulfiram as to exacerbation of the psychosis. Their only problem, they report, is outpatient compliance with the disulfiram regimen, which they can attempt to enforce by monitoring with carbon disulfide breathalyzer tests. Many people believe that disulfiram should not be a treatment in itself, but must be part of a total program and its use should be dependent on the patient's degree of participation in such a program; monitoring then would be with the patient's consent.[18,19] Implants of disulfiram present strong legal as well as medical problems, and do not have a good history of success. The office practitioner, not covered by a government or institutional professional liability insurance, must remember the malpractice implications of giving disulfiram in the presence of the existing literature.

There are other problems in treatment programs for the combined disorders. Schizophrenics often do best with a more "medically" oriented, supportive, gently directive approach without too much in the way of intense emotional expression and interpersonal interaction. Alcoholics and those with other addictive disorders in pure form, on the other hand, often require intervention and confrontation (and sometimes strong confrontation) to overcome denial and resistance to involvement in the therapeutic program. Such denial and resistance constitute the initial and usually the major problem in dealing with these disorders. The therapist desperately needs the very active participation of the patient in the recovery process, just as in the cases of diabetic or cardiac patients. This is unlike the situation of the schizophrenic, of whom (by necessity) much less is required in the way of active participation, often merely cooperation with the therapist-directed program. Emotional expression and interpersonal sharing, as in the 12-step self-help groups, are aspects of the therapeutic regimen as the alcoholic or chemically dependent patients move in the direction of substituting a reliable relationship or, better, a network of such relationships as a replacement for the addiction ("People—not pills.") It is necessary, therefore, to have adequately trained therapists, staff personnel, and lay coworkers and counsellors trained in, sensitive to, and deeply aware of both illnesses to deal with the situation and to titrate, so to speak, the amounts of the opposing and contradictory approaches.

Indeed, the giving of medication itself constitutes a problem. Sedatives, including benzodiazepines, may be useful at times in schizophrenics but are cross-addicting with alcohol and with each other and thus present severe problems in the postdetoxification period of treatment of addictive disorders. After all, it is ideal to be able to be as simple, as direct, and as clear as possible to the addicted patient in the early period of recovery from the use of alcohol or other drugs, and to oppose the drive to drink or use drugs as rigidly, as compulsively, and with as much force as the drive itself was forceful and peremptory. It is much clearer to the recovering patient if he or she can avoid all mood-changing psychotropic drugs, but, of course, the schizophrenic patient often cannot and may well have to take some antipsychotic medication. Then again, the caretakers, lay and professional, may espouse the principle of no psychotropic medication and may interfere with such needed psychopharmacology in the case of patients with the combined disorders.

Therefore, it may well be best not to treat such patients with dual diagnoses in a general unit, but rather in a special unit designed for that purpose with specially trained personnel, both professional and lay, as described previously. (Such personnel will be skilled as well in detecting illicit alcohol or drug abuse on the ward.) The unit will be under the direction of a specially trained primary therapist and the 12-step self-help groups involved will also be appropriately trained and experienced. There must be available continuing outpatient resources to prevent fragmentation of care and to funnel the patients into compatible 12-step groups—A.A., N.A., and so forth—on the outside where their programs, in conjunction with properly trained psychiatric clinics, will continue the care. The supportive, widespread network of the fellowship, as described elsewhere in the book, and the adjunct groups for the significant others—Al-Anon, and other such organizations—will aid in the environmental support of the recovering patient.

One lesser step if the above is not practical is to have a liaison psychiatrist-addictionist on the staff, full-time or part-time, to do both liaison and consultative work, to make rounds, to look for neglected or overlooked combined disorders, to recommend treatment procedures, to do education and training, and to work in the direction of the development of such a special unit. Such a psychiatrist-addictionist program is modeled on the former career teachers program set up by the National Institutes of Drug Abuse and of Alcohol Abuse and Alcoholism.

The last point is the question of the relationship between schizophrenia and alcoholism (and the other addictive disorders). It is erroneous to conceive of the latter disorder as a "defense" against the former, for alcoholism itself has been demonstrated, as noted, by family studies and twin studies as a separate biologic entity. It is true that schizophrenics may use alcohol and other drugs initially in an attempt to ameliorate the schizophrenia (thus tending to develop a latent addictive predisposition into a full-fledged disorder) but the development of the addictive disorder is a separate process leading to its own set of symptoms and its own course, and it will, sooner or later, usually aggravate the psychosis and produce the picture of the combined disorder. It is also true that the alcoholism or other drug disturbance may dominate the clinical picture and "mask" the schizophrenia for a while. In these instances we see the schizophrenia emerge more clearly after the recovery process has taken place. In such instances, one may on occasion discover, after sobriety has been well established, that there has been a long history of covert hallucinations, delusions, and schizophrenic behavior in interpersonal situations with withdrawal, excessive self-consciousness, perfectionism, and so forth extending back in childhood.

ALCOHOLISM AND MAJOR AFFECTIVE DISORDERS

In the case of the major affective illnesses and alcohol and other drug disorders, the relationship, although still not clear, is much closer with much more overlapping than that of schizophrenia and those latter disorders. However, here there are more problems in terminology and nosology that render the relationship less than clear. There is no doubt that alcoholism and other chronic narcotic and sedative use are associated with depression, both clinically and on rating scales, but there is the difficulty that the term depression describes not only an affect or ubiquitous mood state, but also describes a clinical condition in which the mood may not be the predominant characteristic. Instead, in the latter, the psychiatric condition, one might see apathy, anhedonia, fatigue, anorexia with weight loss, terminal insomnia, loss of sexual desire and other interests, withdrawal, somatic complaints, and a diurnal mood variation with either retardation or agitation. The problem here is that many such symptoms of discomfort with sleep disturbance and suicidal tendencies exist in both affective and addictive disorders and therefore both primary and secondary (to the addiction) depressions resemble each other. (The only exception is that one may tend not to find true psychomotor retardation in alcoholism or secondary depression; indeed, the rebound hyperexcitable phase of the drug's effects tends to turn retarded depressions into agitated ones.) Also to be noted here are the atypical depressions with hypersomnia, hyperphagia, and so forth, which also show an increased tendency towards alcohol or drugs, thus complicating the picture of such depressions.

A second problem is that of differentiating which came first, which is primary, the addiction or the depression. On the one hand, symptoms of depression are very common during heavy drinking. Primary depressions are in themselves often self-limited and can remit over time, unrelated to and regardless of whether one is drinking or not. Other depressions can, when secondary to the alcohol or drug, remit with sobriety after a matter of several days to a week or two for alcohol or somewhat longer for sedatives and narcotics. On the other hand, depression may appear for the first time after cessation of alcohol, sedatives, narcotics, or stimulants, sometimes a very severe depression. There has been much discussion of primary versus secondary depression in alcoholism, but it tends to come down to the practical issue of whether to use psychiatric medication or not. But such medication is symptomatic, not etiologic. As with schizophrenia it is best to wait—if one can and if the picture is not too severe, the depression not psychotic (delusional), and the patient not noticeably suicidal—before instituting medication. If necessary, however, medication can be given as described earlier in the section on depression in the prolonged withdrawal syndrome under the discussion of schizophrenia. If this is of no avail, one may have to resort to other antidepressant medication or even electroconvulsive therapy, should the depression be severe, for it can be life-threatening at times. Many of the factors and concerns discussed previously regarding the treatment of combined schizophrenic and alcohol/drug disorders apply here as well.

Alcoholism and sedative or narcotic dependence is significantly associated with suicide, it should be noted, both during active alcohol and drug taking and after withdrawal, particularly from narcotics. Suicide is a serious danger as well during the depression that may follow cessation of stimulants, especially cocaine. Hence serious depression is a true psychiatric emergency and calls for an appropriate referral.

The dysphoric state produced by the chronic intake of alcohol and other drugs is partly physiologic and partly due to the interpersonal, occupational, and financial difficulties caused by the addiction. As such it will improve with sobriety and involvement in a treatment program, but it may take weeks and even at times as long as months to have the full depression and sleep patterns improve.

Physiologically, alcohol is a weak elevator of mood and, despite the general feeling, there is no good evidence that depression causes alcoholism. Small amounts may lift the mood in alcoholics and in depressed people (predominantly when the blood alcohol level is rising) but large amounts increase depression in both (especially as the blood alcohol level drops). Indeed, in bipolar disorders there are many reports that there is increased alcohol intake in the manic rather than the depressed phases, and bipolar alcoholics tend to show aggravation of their addictive disorder when "high."[20,21] (Alcohol seems, at times, to work to decrease the unpleasant effects of the manic phase, but in any event there are tendencies in both conditions to loss of control and, therefore, increased alcohol or drug intake.) In these instances, of course, lithium (or other such medication) may be essential for the control of the bipolar aspect of the illness and hence for the control of the alcoholism. Some people have even tried lithium and other medications, as a result of this, in the pure alcoholic, especially the "periodic" (episodic) alcoholic, but the results are not clearly beneficial. [18]

Family studies are variable (as to genetic influence). Some show increase of depressive illnesses in alcoholic families and increased alcoholism in families of bipolar patients, but others fail to show this.[20,21] One concept to be mentioned is the notion of a subgrouping of a genetically based "depressive spectrum disorder" with alcoholism or antisocial personality disorder in the men and depression in the women;[22] this is not well established either. The women's depression may possibly be environmental, and the population studied, it has been pointed out, is too heterogeneous for clear and solid conclusions.[21] In short, there is no definite correlation between bipolar disorders and alcoholism, nor is there good evidence that recurrent unipolar depressives drink more when they are depressed, although it must be stated that many psychiatric clinicians still feel that excessive alcohol or sedative intake can mask or initially ameliorate a primary depressive disorder, at least for a while.

One other note: what appears to be an acute manic state, with or without delusions, can be the result of the toxic effect of stimulants such as amphetamines or cocaine, can be the result of hallucinogens or antiparkinsonism drugs, or can even be seen in acute withdrawal states. It is useful then to do urine or blood screens as discussed in the section on schizophrenia. Finally: alcoholics with primary affective disorders tend to show a picture and a course more like pure alcoholism than pure affective disorders.

ALCOHOLISM AND SOCIOPATHY

Sociopathy, according to the literature, shows a close relationship to alcoholism and drug abuse and there is marked overlapping between these disorders as found in family and epidemiologic studies in the clinical pictures of the personality disturbances, and in the incidence of antisocial and violent acts.[23] Nevertheless, they are not the same disorder for it is not the rule for alcoholics and sedative addicts to show such behavior and not all injectible narcotic patients commit criminal or other antisocial acts or exhibit sociopathic personality traits. On the other hand, not all patients exhibiting such personality traits develop dependency on alcohol or other drugs. Indeed, the usual middle-class alcoholic is not commonly antisocial. It may be more the parameters of social class, of socioeconomic conditions, and of cultural and personality factors existing prior to the emergence of the addictive disorder that determine the behavior.

Antisocial and sociopathic behavioral manifestations when present markedly complicate the treatment of alcoholism and other addictions, and vice versa. Indeed, one can almost say that the alcoholics and other drug users are treatable and true sociopaths are not. When both disorders coexist the prognosis, therefore, is very poor; one sees markedly greater use of drugs with overdosing, death, aggressive behavior, violence, and criminal acts. Here one sees most clearly the effects of the disinhibition produced by alcohol and sedatives, or the cocaine or injectible narcotic-dependent patient's loss of judgment and need to support his or her habit. It should be added that antisocial behavior is in general greater among the young and among the younger-onset alcoholics.

However, just as in schizophrenia and the affective disorders, it is crucial not to make the diagnosis too early but to give treatment a chance. Alcoholism and other drug dependencies can mimic sociopathy as well as the other disorders. It is best not to write off such patients too quickly for, regardless of the primary diagnosis, as in the other psychiatric disorders, controlling the alcohol and other drug dependency is the primary goal of therapy. Nowhere does one see this more clearly than with the impaired physician—be it alcohol, sedative, injectible narcotic, or cocaine use—whose behavior has been most antisocial and dangerous to his patients and the community. Upon entering a treatment program and achieving sobriety, perhaps over a matter of months, perhaps less, he or she becomes a solid citizen, an honorable and valuable physician, and a credit to the profession. It may seem like a miracle but it is not. It is merely the recovery from the disease and the reemergence of the basic person who had been imprisoned within his or her disorder.

One last caveat: Benzodiazepines and other sedatives, and probably all psychotropic medication, must be strictly avoided among this group of patients for there is no good indication for any such medication in sociopathy. It will only be abused. Even amitriptyline and trihexyphenidyl are abused.

ALCOHOLISM AND OTHER PSYCHIATRIC DISTURBANCES

As to *borderline, other personality disturbances, and certain anxiety and somatization disorders*, there are no hard facts as to frequency or epidemiology as regards alcoholism and other drug disorders. The concept of the borderline personality disturbance is a relatively more recent diagnosis and, although included in DSM-III, is not always strictly defined in general use. Indeed, the various personality disturbances tend to grade into one another and are often not clearly distinguished. Most psychiatric clinicians report an increased incidence of alcohol and drug use in borderline disturbances but it is often difficult to say which is primary and which is secondary. Just as with the other psychiatric disorders, alcohol and drug dependencies can mimic these illnesses and on just sobriety alone one can see marked improvement. Often enough the therapist pays too much attention to the dynamics and too little to the altered ego states, the weakened defenses, the loss of impulse control, and the emergence of regressive mental mechanisms and regressive "acting out" behavior, all secondary to the drugs. The withdrawal of drugs alone can suddenly remove the management and behavior problems and change the entire picture. It must be the first thing the therapist thinks of when confronted with such a patient, and one must not, here too, make the psychiatric diagnosis too early. In addition, one must not give benzodiazepines or sedatives to the borderline or masochistic character with depression or anxiety to allay his or her chronic suffering, for one is apt to contribute to an addiction, which only makes matters worse. Where the patient can turn to drugs for relief, he or she will be less inclined to turn to the therapist and the therapy. The therapist has nothing in his or her arsenal as magically powerful, as quickly effective, or as potentially dangerous as a drug or a drink.

The therapist must also be alert to the possibility that the patient, suffering and not given immediate relief by the therapist, will turn to other physicians, to the street, the liquor store, or to the bar for relief, and then guilty, will hide this from the therapist. Sudden changes in the transference relationship, negativism, hostility, evasiveness, missed sessions, and other changes in behavior may be due to the patient taking drugs or alcohol secretly and hiding it from the therapist.

Some medications can be given cautiously if absolutely necessary, such as antidepressants or even sedative neuroleptics (e.g., chlorpromazine or thioridazine) as in the situation noted in the discussion of the prolonged withdrawal syndrome in the section on schizophrenia. It is probably better, however, if one can avoid even this type of medication. It too easily turns the patient in psychotherapy away from concentrating on the etiology and dealing with his or her symptoms, and toward paying too much attention to the effects of the symptoms and complaining about them instead of analyzing or at least handling them. It also turns the patient away from the therapeutic (or other interpersonal) relationship as the solution to problems, and toward the direction of autistic, magical solutions through chemical substances. This is further discussed in Chapter 10 on Implications of the Disease Model for Psychotherapy and Counselling. It must be recognized, however, that should the anxiety or panic be too high, psychotherapy is not possible, and some form of pharmacologic intervention, as noted, is in order.

One must remember that it may take several weeks to several months after detoxification for the patient to recover fully. The physician is cautioned not to make a primary psychiatric diagnosis here too quickly.

Patients reporting panic attacks may be using amphetamines and/or cocaine but not admitting to those drugs. Those patients and others with dysthymic or generalized and other anxiety and somatization disorders may seek to ameliorate their difficulties with alcohol or other drugs and may be initially successful, but, often enough and sooner or later, the addictive process will develop and progress in the direction of the full-blown picture. Therefore, the physician must be cautioned particularly about the use of any benzodiazepine (including alprazolam) in panic disorder and agoraphobia. Alprazolam can be helpful but not infrequently it leads to a "normal dose" dependency disorder where it is most difficult to get the patient off the drug and where, after a period of time, it can build up to a serious addictive disorder.[24, 25] If medications are to be used, the antidepressants such as the tricyclics or at times monoamineoxidase inhibitors should be considered. They are effective and are not addictive.

ALCOHOLISM AND ORGANIC MENTAL DISTURBANCES

Concerning the organic mental syndromes, they are for the most part covered in the chapter The Medical Complications of Alcoholism elsewhere in the book. They are the consequences of the effects of alcohol's direct neurotoxic properties and the nutritional deficiencies (avitaminoses, etc.) on the CNS. Insofar as they involve the higher functions, they can seriously interfere with the patient's participation in a treatment program.

It is important, in terms of prognosis, management, and treatment, to differentiate alcoholic dementias from other, unrelated dementias such as Alzheimer's, from unrelated CNS disturbances such as cerebrovascular accidents and tumors, and from possible consequences and sequelae of the alcoholism itself such as subdural hematomas, traumatic injury to the brain, Wernicke's encephalopathy, and Korsakoff's syndrome. The alcoholic dementia does not show clouding of consciousness and can show slow improvement on abstinence beginning anywhere from 3-6 months; sometimes such improvement is not noticeable for up to 1 year.

The full-blown picture of alcoholic dementia or of Korsakoff's syndrome may not be present, but one may still find cognitive and memory deficits. Such difficulties are not infrequently found extending along a continuum at the polar ends of which are the full-blown pictures of alcoholic dementia on the one hand and Korsakoff's syndrome on the other. Many alcoholics, after the acute or subacute detoxification phase, show disturbances in memory, in visual spatial skills and abstracting abilities, in sensorimotor performance, and in perceptual capacities. Verbal functions are less affected but performance intelligence such as shown in nonverbal abstraction and others of the aforementioned functions is more severely involved. New learning of a verbal nature may be more severely impaired immediately postdetoxification but it recovers rapidly, whereas new learning of visual spatial information tends to stay impaired for much longer, in terms of months, much more so in older alcoholics with longer drinking histories than with younger alcoholics. Short-term memory may well return to normal but long-term memory as well as visual spatial functions tend to show deficits even after years of abstinence. Interestingly enough, even heavy social drinking can show some impairment.[26]

The degree of disturbance seems to be more related to the amount of alcohol consumed at a sitting or during a bout rather than the frequency of drinking. Long-term recovery, however, may occur and rehabilitative training may well hasten and improve the recovery process. Pathologically one sees signs of general cortical atrophy (such as fewer and more shallow sulci, etc.) but CT scans reveal anatomic improvement increasing from 3-6 months after cessation of drinking (even at times to the point of complete recovery from the defect). This finding is correlated with the clearing of the EEG, the clinical evidence of intellectual improvement, and the disappearance of acidosis of the cerebrospinal fluid.[26] There appears to be no more reason to write neurologic funeral orations than to write psychologic ones when it comes to the usefulness of sobriety and abstinence on alcoholic neurologic and psychiatric disorders.

REFERENCES

1. Schuckit M: Alcoholism and other psychiatric disorders. *Hosp Com Psych* 34:1022–1027, 1983
2. Solomon J: Alcoholism and clinical psychiatry, in Solomon J (ed): *Alcoholism and Clinical Psychiatry*. New York, Plenum, 1982
3. Ramsay A, Vredenburgh J, Gallagher R: Recognition of alcoholism among patients with psychiatric problems in a family practice clinic. *J Fam Pract* 17:829–832, 1983
4. Vogel C, Blom M: Retrospective study of alcohol use by VA patients. *Hosp Com Psych* 36:287–290, 1985
5. Blumberg A, Cohen M, Heaton A, et al: Covert drug abuse among voluntary hospitalized patients. *JAMA* 217:1659–1661, 1971
6. Cotton N: The familial incidence of alcoholism: A review. *J Stud Alcohol* 40:89–116, 1979
7. Bleuler M: Familial and personal background of chronic alcoholism, in Diethelm O (ed): *Etiology of Chronic Alcoholism*. Springfield, IL, Charles Thomas, 1955, pp 110–166
8. Rimmer J, Jacobsen B: Alcoholism in schizophrenics and their relatives. *J Stud Alcohol* 38:1781–1784, 1977

9. Kindler K, Gruenberg A, Tsuang MT: Psychiatric illness in first-degree relatives of schizophrenic and surgical control patients. *Arch Gen Psych* 42:770–779, 1985
10. Schuckit M: Genetic and biochemical factors in the etiology of alcoholism, in *Psychiatry Update, Vol 3*. Washington DC, American Psychiatric Press, 1984, pp 320–328
11. Gottheil E, Waxman H: Alcoholism and schizophrenia, in Pattison EM, Kaufman E (eds): *Encyclopedic Handbook of Alcoholism*. New York, Gardner, 1982
12. Kesselman M, Solomon J, Beaudelt M, et al: Alcoholism and schizophrenia, in Solomon J (ed): *Alcoholism and Clinical Psychiatry*. New York, Plenum, 1982
13. Freed E: Alcoholism and schizophrenia: The search for perspectives. A review. *J Stud Alcohol* 36:853–881, 1975
14. Shan-Ming Y, DeZhao X, Yuzhen C, et al: The frequency of major psychiatric disorders in Chinese inpatients. *Am J Psychiat* 141:690–692, 1984
15. Opler M: Cultural differences in mental disorders: An Italian and Irish contrast in the schizophrenics, in Opler M (ed): *Culture and Mental Health*. New York, Macmillan, 1959, pp 425–442
16. Serban G: *Adjustment of Schizophrenics in the Community*. Jamaica, NY, Spectrum, 1981
17. Fruensgaard K: Withdrawal psychosis: A study of 30 consecutive cases. *Acta Psychiatr Scand* 53:105–118,1976
18. NIAAA: *Alcohol and Health*. Fifth special report to the US Congress, from the Secretary of the Department of Health and Human Services, GPO, 1983, pp 112–113
19. Kofoed L, Kania J, Walsh T, et al: Outpatient treatment of patients with substance abuse and co-existing psychiatric disorders. *Am J Psych* 143:867–873, 1986
20. Keeler M: Alcoholism and affective disorder, in Pattison EM, Kaufman E (eds): *Encyclopedic Handbook of Alcoholism*. New York, Gardner, 1982
21. Goodwin D: Alcoholism and affective disorders, in Solomon J (ed): *Alcoholism and Clinical Psychiatry*. New York, Plenum, 1982
22. Winokur G, Cadoret R, Baker M, et al: Depressive spectrum disease vs. pure depressive disease: Some further data. *Br J Psychiatr* 127:75–77, 1975
23. Rada R: Alcoholism and sociopathy: Diagnostic and treatment implications, in Pattison EM, Kaufman E (eds): *Encyclopedic Handbook of Alcoholism*. New York, Gardner, 1982
24. Noyes R, Clancy J, Coryell W, et al: A withdrawal syndrome after abrupt discontinuation of alprazolam. *Am J Psychiatr* 142:114–116, 1985
25. Mellman T, Uhde T: Withdrawal syndrome with gradual tapering of alprazolam. *Am J Psychiatr* 143:1464–1466, 1986
26. NIAAA: *Alcohol and Cognitive Loss*. Special supplement from the Department of Health and Human Services, Sep 1984, pp 1A–4A

10

Implications of the Disease Model for Psychotherapy and Counselling

Herbert S. Peyser

The disease concept of alcoholism emerged almost two centuries ago, set forth by physicians Benjamin Rush in the United States and Thomas Trotter in England. It was part of the developing worldwide trend toward regarding medical disorders in general and, more specifically for our purposes, the major psychiatric and behavioral disorders as well, as diseases of the body, located in the organs of the body. They were no longer regarded as states of possession by spirits and demons, as weakness of character or sinfulness, as punishments by God, criminal acts of an untamed wild beast, or the abnormal distribution of humors and temperaments. These being medical disorders, those afflicted would be examined and treated rather than punished, purged, bled, exorcised, or confined. Accordingly, in the last decade of the 18th century, Pinel struck the chains off the inmates of the madhouses in Paris while Chiarugi in Italy and Tuke in England were doing similarly in their countries.

ALCOHOLISM:
A Practical Treatment Guide
ISBN 0-8089-1912-1

Thus the disease model arose initially as a change in philosophic outlook and world view rather than as the result of scientific discovery. Changes in philosophic outlook occur before and prepare the way for scientific discovery. It was first necessary to regard these people as patients, as ill, before one could begin to deal with them humanely, objectively, and medically and seek causes and treatments.

As physicians and others searched for the etiology of these disorders, they followed at first the single pathogen, single cause model of the medicine and the biology of the 19th century. They looked for the external agent that, taken inside, would cause the disease in the organs of the body. For example, the tubercle bacillus was understood to be the sole cause of tuberculosis, but as medical science moved into the 20th century, it became apparent that such a model was inadequate. The tubercle bacillus was only a necessary but not a sufficient cause. The amount of money one had, where one lived and how one lived, the phenomena of overcrowding, of nutrition, of exposure to sunlight, of inherited resistance, and so forth were also causes of the disease. Indeed, this all showed itself in the sanatoria beginning to close before the development of antibiotics specific for the bacillus; the closings were, instead, the results of social engineering. A multifactorial model of disease, of its etiology and treatment, had emerged to replace the single pathogen model, and this changed the disease concept of the psychiatric and addictive disorders as well, both in terms of etiology and therapy.

ETIOLOGIC FACTORS

Insofar as alcoholism is a disease, it must therefore have a number of factors in its etiology.

Predisposing Factors

1. These include *genetic factors* that increase the risk of the disorder as determined by family, twin, and adoptive studies. It has been found, for example, that male offspring of alcoholic fathers are at high risk.[1] Other work has been devoted to the discovery of cognitive, neuropsychologic, and biologic markers of inherited risk. Such markers are being searched for and found in electroencephalographic and event-related potentials or average evoked responses to repetitive sensory stimuli, and in prolactin and cortisol responses to alcohol challenges in high-risk individuals.[2] These findings, incidentally, strongly point to the disease model as opposed to a purely learning theory model.
2. There may be other *biologic and constitutional factors* as well. These may involve neurophysiology and neurotransmission across the synapse, the chemistry of the metabolism and detoxification of alcohol, the capacity to develop tolerance, the capacity to recover from the sedative hypnotic effects, and so forth. As yet one cannot be more specific, for these factors are not clearly delineated as causal at this time. Research is, however, very active in these areas.[2]

3. There are definitely *sociocultural factors* even where one is dealing with genetically predisposed individuals. For example, the Irish have more alcoholism in general as do the Russians, the Poles, and so forth. The Chinese do not drink anywhere as much and neither do first-generation Jews in the United States. As the latter become more assimilated, however, the social prohibitions in the form of the degree of the disgrace of drunkenness diminish, the rates rise, and the hidden alcoholism comes out of the woodwork as well. It is not a matter of the availability of alcohol alone for in two wine-drinking countries, France and Italy, the incidence of alcoholism is far higher in the former than in the latter. It appears that the incidence of alcoholism may have more to do with very severe social disapproval and this may account for the formerly lower rates in women (as in Jews) and the increasing incidence as discrimination against and oppression of women diminishes. However, the tendency for women to turn more secretly and seemingly with medical legitimation to sedative pills rather than to make the socially more shameful overt statement of alcoholism still exists.[3]
4. Finally there may well be *psychologic factors* such as identification with an alcoholic parent, learned or conditioned alcoholic drinking and behavior, oral fixations, cognitive deficiencies, and so forth. Although postulated and at times seemingly logical and even helpful, these factors have not been scientifically proven or clearly delineated in terms of predisposition. Their possibility, however, cannot be dismissed, for the existence of such etiologic factors is too often a deep clinical impression.

Precipitating Factors

The onset of the disorder may be *insidious or acute* and fairly well demarcated. In the latter instance it often seems reactive to certain events that trigger the emergence of the latent disorder. Such events may involve a threat to one's health, physical or mental, to one's life, one's work, or one's job, school, or career. They may involve a painful loss in work, love, or social situations, in one's family or personal life. On the other hand, they may involve, paradoxically, what appears to be a success or accomplishment, but which is really an *unconsciously* forbidden achievement in any of the above areas, a situation where one is "wrecked by success."[4] The latter type of precipitating event is not at all uncommon in psychiatry, especially among people with masochistic neuroses and neurotic character structures. Depressions, psychotic states, or, if one is so predisposed, alcoholism or other drug dependency can be kicked off by such events. In other instances one may not see a specific causal event and the illness may appear to emerge without apparent precipitation.[5]

As noted elsewhere in this book, the sedatives and narcotics, whatever their effects may be at the synapse, are, among other factors and at a higher level, central nervous system (CNS) depressants, particularly of the reticular activating system, an arousal system. They thus serve, among other functions, the functions of diminishing alertness and awareness and of disinhibition. They can therefore diminish superego signals, so to speak, can decrease impulse controls, and can blunt awareness of noxious memories, perceptions, ideas, feelings, and thoughts, also signals for repression and inhibition, thus apparently "freeing" some inner aspects of the self.[5] It is for this reason that at A.A. meetings one will often hear how "I used to be unable to speak to people of the other sex. . .to dance. . .to go to parties. . .to have sex. . .to speak to my boss. . .to speak up in class. . .etc. . . .but when I had a drink, . . .a pill. . .a shot. . .whatever. . .I could." Of course a drink or other such drugs can do this for anyone, but the patient predisposed to an addictive disorder will go on with loss of control; the clinical picture will then develop and progress. This is the manner in which the more insidious onset type of alcoholism may present itself. It is important to keep this in mind in treatment for it is not enough to stop drinking; one must effect a change within the patient so that the alcoholic or other drug dependent patient can achieve at least some of the freedom (disinhibition) he or she has been searching for , but, now without the alcohol or drug. This is "sobriety" as opposed to merely being "dry," with internal unity and intrapsychic harmony existing instead of the individual being torn by conflict and struggling to contain his or her damned-up, thwarted desire and strivings. A person must find at least some fulfillment in work and/or love in order to be truly sober. Some of the psychologic aspects of the pressure to drink will then be decreased; some if not all of the pressure, for one must continue to be on guard against the possibility of a more biologically based and nonpsychologically meaningful need to drink or take drugs.

In this latter regard, it is not unusual for some alcoholics to recollect, after the recovery has begun, that very early in life, even in childhood, he or she would surreptitiously empty the parents' and guests' liquor glasses after the party was over or sneak drinks from the family liquor cabinet or pills from the medicine chest. It is not yet clear what psychobiologic condition predisposes to this behavior but it is certainly very early in onset and not necessarily psychologically purposeful.

Autonomous Self-Perpetuating Factor

There is in addition an autonomous, self-perpetuating factor that shows itself when, no matter what precipitates the disorder, it now goes on of its own accord, regardless of the consequences and often without any sensation of gratification from the alcohol or the drug. This is the "loss of control" factor, the essence of the disease model as opposed to a learning or conditioning model in which the feedback from the consequences, the dysphoric state, the damage to one's life, and so forth would affect the continuation of the drinking or drug taking. But it does not do this in persons with the disease for he or she will go on drinking or drug taking regardless of the consequences. The psychobiologic basis for this factor is, as noted, unknown but is being searched for. It has been thought that it may have some relationship to the second phase of the physiologic effect of the intake of alcohol or sedative or narcotic drugs. This is the hyperexcitable phase that follows the CNS depressant phase and that presses for more sedation (with consequent increase in hyperexcitability and so on) or at least for the homeostatic need for more of the drug that set off the change in the neurophysiologic state. It may be related to the effects of the drugs or alcohol on the neurotransmitters, their release and uptake, the altering of the density and/or sensitivity of their receptors, or other such neurobiologic phenomena.[1,3]

However, this autonomous factor, regardless of its origin, is the reason that the addiction itself must receive the primary attention. No discussion of any psychologic or situational factors in psychotherapy, no matter what etiologic role they might have played, can be of avail as long as this self-perpetuating, autonomous factor is in operation, at least in most instances. The reason is that once it has begun, regardless of his or her excuses and rationalizations, the individual now drinks or takes the drug to drink or take the drug, and not for any other reason. Psychotherapeutic intervention awaits the doing away with the drinking or drug taking and the erection of an internal barrier to the use of alcohol or drugs. Only then can one engage the patient in a serious discussion as to other psychologic or situational factors in his or her disorder.

It is interesting to note that there are other nonchemical, nonpharmacologic addictions and impulse disorders with this autonomous factor—compulsive gambling ("chasing one's money"), bulimia ("binge eating"), and so forth—and they have to be approached similarly. Their existence suggests additional, nonphysiologic but, rather, psychologic considerations, where this factor is concerned.

THE MANNER IN WHICH PSYCHIATRIC DIFFICULTIES PRESENT THEMSELVES

Another and more psychologic way of looking at this autonomous factor can be seen in the manner in which the problem presents itself to the therapist or clinician. Psychiatric difficulties tend to fall into three groups:

1. There are the *ego alien problems*, those felt to be outside the person's ego and instead felt to be inflicted upon the self (although in reality made up *unconsciously* by the individual). Such conditions exist in phobias, compulsions, hysterical and psychosomatic symptoms, and so forth. Because of the nature of the situation the patient's unconscious forces for health are at once allied with the therapist in opposing the symptoms and the unconscious forces that put them in place and keep them going. Psychotherapists do best with such people for obvious reasons.
2. There are the *ego syntonic problems*, mostly character and personality traits, operations, and methods of dealing with people and situations. These, too, may have been developed to deal with internal conflicts. Modesty and meekness, for example, are characterologic methods of suppressing and defending against assertive and exhibitionistic tendencies that are felt to be dangerous or forbidden, while stage fright or the sudden loss of memory or voice when about to speak in public represents a symptomatic defense against the same tendencies. The former, it can be seen, are aspects of the self, ego syntonic, legitimized, "egotized." In opposing these traits of

character, the therapist seems to be opposing the very ego and self system of the patient himself or herself. Therefore, the therapist must work first to help the individual to isolate and objectify these character traits and to see them as the problem, just as though they were symptoms. This is much more difficult to do and there is much greater resistance to cure here than with the ego alien symptoms, and many more relapses back into old, neurotic ways.

3. Finally there are the *immediately gratifying, tension-relieving or need-consumating problems*, gratifying, relieving, and consumating in the real world and not merely symbolically. This situation can also be seen in the impulse disorders that have similar qualities such as gambling, bulimia, kleptomania, pyromania, impulsive acting-out, compulsive self-mutilation, masochistic love attachments, in paraphilias, and in the situations of great secondary gain (e.g., "compensation neuroses"). In all these the patient's attachment to the drink, the chemical, the food, the money, the object, the fetish, the lover, the situation, the fantasy, the action, or whatever, is so intense and the possession of it so needed and highly valued that the therapist appears to be opposing that which is essential to life itself. The therapist appears to be trying to take away what the patient feels he or she cannot live without. Even if there is no pleasure at all derived from it, there is enormous relief in its possession.

The needed drug, object, person, and so forth is loved (even if masochistically loved) and is treated in a manner reminiscent of the early attachment to a transitional object, which, indeed, Winnicott proposes as the developmental origin of these conditions.[6] He suggests that the addictions, the fetishes, and so forth are all successors to this normal phenomenon. The child, he states, chooses and creates an object or situation out of the transitional world of experience, of sights, sounds, and smells, and so on, that exists between his or her own world of needs and desires and the external world of satisfactions and gratifications (e.g., mother). This transitional object will not desert him or her. It is the child's own creation and possession, more or less under his or her control, and it can be relied on. It is a response to his or her awareness of the helplessness, powerlessness, loneliness, and the ambiguity and uncertainty of existence. It reassures and relieves the child who becomes terrified of giving it up.

It thus assumes a primacy and its possession seems to protect the child against interpersonal dangers. The mother herself, a creature who comes and goes, cannot console the child for the loss of the far more permanent and controllable transitional object. It represents as well, therefore, the child's solution to the internal conflict between his or her needs for security, to hold onto the mother, and his or her developmental needs that are pushing the child to separate from the mother and to grow. If this theoretical formulation is accurate, one can readily understand some of the intensity of the psychologic resistance of the patient to giving up his or her chemical, fetish, or whatever.

THE PHASES OF THE PSYCHOTHERAPEUTIC OR COUNSELLING PROCESS

This accounts for some of the problems patients with these disorders present to the psychotherapist and why some other activity, what is described in this book, must take place before further psychotherapy can proceed. The therapist or counsellor will find the psychotherapeutic process as a rule tending to move through a series of phases similar to the phases of the development of any relationship and perhaps of life itself. The first is the autistic phase, a phase of relative unrelatedness, of defense against involvement, a phase of magical, narcissistic, and omnipotent self containment aided and abetted by the alcohol, the drug, the fetish, or whatever. As the individual begins to enter into a relationship, such a relationship first assumes a highly narcissistic quality, the patient (for self-protective purposes) identifying with and incorporating into himself or herself highly overestimated and idealized abilities and qualities needed or valued by the patient and attributed to the therapist or group. The therapist (or group) then takes over the function of the chemical, the fetish, or whatever.

There is a great vulnerability in surrendering to and giving oneself to a relationship (with an individual or group) that one does not control. The patient does this slowly and hesitantly, first searching out the group or individual therapist to reassure himself or herself as he or she goes. As the patient slowly gives up the drink, the fetish, or whatever magical object he or she has hidden behind to remain "secure" in the autistic phase, he or she may enter for a while a phase of intense, clinging, helpless, clutching, perhaps symbiotic attachment. Out of this will emerge the phase of narcissistic identification noted above. Only after this phase has developed can the patient move in the direction of a more equal dyad and begin a dialogue with a more mature transference and a therapeutic alliance. This is then followed by phases of development and change, working through, resolution of conflicts, separation, individuation, and termination.

All this has been described here in a necessarily abbreviated and truncated manner, but it can be seen that the possession of a magical object or situation, the alcohol or drug, the lover, the fetish, the money, or whatever (i.e., a kind of derivative of a transitional object) will hold the patient back from moving out of the first, autistic phase into a phase of beginning relatedness. This latter phase is the prerequisite for therapy, for therapy is not solely a heuristic, intellectual endeavor. It requires the patient's active emotional, interpersonal, transactional participation. The overcoming of the obstacle of the alcohol or other drug is a major early task of A.A. and the other 12-step self-help recovery programs, particularly in terms of the first three steps (see elsewhere in the book for the exposition of the 12 steps of the A.A. program.) This will be discussed later.

THE STAGES OF THE OVERALL THERAPEUTIC PROCESS IN ALCOHOLISM

The approach to the alcoholic or other substance-dependent patient must move through the following stages:

1. The *recognition and diagnosis* of the disorder. This has been discussed elsewhere in the book as well as in the chapter on Alcoholism and Clinical Psychiatry where the dangers involved in too early a diagnosis of a primary or even concurrent psychiatric disorder were pointed out. Other dangers associated with the problem of diagnosis involve the use of addicting psychotropic medication for the chronically suffering patient, medication that might initiate a drug dependency in such a patient. Another danger is the lack of awareness of the possibility of the patient's clandestine use of alcohol or other drugs should the therapist not prescribe them; the patient may seek them on the street, in the bar, from other physicians, or elsewhere. In this instance many of the presenting symptoms of anxiety, an increase in phobias and obsessional fears, psychosomatic difficulties, dysphoric states, and cognitive difficulties may be secondary to the addiction and not primarily psychogenic.[5,7]
2. *Motivating* the patient for treatment. This too has been covered elsewhere in the book. In essence it means looking about for one's leverage, usually in one of the three main areas of life that the addiction to alcohol or other drugs begins to encroach upon. These are the areas of (1) physical and mental health, (2) school, career, and job, and (3) social, sexual, and intimate relationships. It is the impingement on one or more of these areas that constitutes the basis for the diagnosis of an addictive disorder and therefore is the area of leverage for motivation. It is only when the patient becomes aware that the negative aspects of drinking or drug taking outweigh the positive with particular attention to any or all of these three main areas of life that he or she will begin to work toward sobriety and health. This is the basis for the first part of the first step in A.A.'s 12-step program: "We admitted that our lives were unmanageable because of..." It is this that the therapist must work to bring about rather than passively waiting for the patient to "hit the bottom." Perhaps something can be done *before* the liver is destroyed, the mind irreparably damaged, the marriage or job gone down the drain, a life thrown away.

   This is done by manipulating one or more of the three areas already mentioned. Clearly, job-based programs can be effective in this regard with their threat of firing or at least not promoting the patient. In another instance, the physician's warning of the threat to health on the basis of physical examination or laboratory findings could help. Working with significant others to detach from the patient's addiction can help here as well but can also present serious problems where the relationship between them and the patient is not a mature one but is one of fusion or symbiotic attachment. Such programs as Al-Anon, and so on can be helpful to teach the spouse, parent, or whomever to "detach with love" and to cease "enabling" and rescuing the patient from the consequences of his or her addiction (such consequences must be faced if the patient is to recognize how the drug has made life unmanageable). This is also the role of therapy or counselling of the significant others where the previously mentioned deeper and more intense symbiotic or masochistic attachments exist. Formal structured interventions, involving family, friends, associates, coworkers, and so on may be organized by clinicians or, better, by therapists, groups, or institutions trained and experienced in this procedure. Here the positive is emphasized ("We love you and cannot see what is happening to you...") but at least implicit threats of withdrawal and loss are present. The professional intervenors work with the participants beforehand and aid in the active follow-through work afterwards.

3. *Detoxification, management and treatment of the medical complications, rehabilitation centers and hospital services, halfway houses, and therapeutic communities.* These have also been covered elsewhere in the book.
4. *Long-term management.* This has been discussed in part in another chapter. In this chapter the psychotherapeutic and counselling tactics will be gone into in more detail.

THE ORIENTATION OF THE TREATMENT PROGRAM

The treatment program is oriented in the following directions: (1) the addictive disorder is a disease in itself and, except where there exists an acute medical or psychiatric emergency (i.e., suicidal trends or danger to others), it requires at least equal and usually primary attention; (2) medication is not to be used unless absolutely necessary, and never an addictive medication; (3) the aim is abstinence, for although there may be some patients who can return to social drinking, there are not many and the risk of loss of control and relapse into alcoholism or drug taking is much too great; (4) in the place of the alcohol or other drugs one must supply interpersonal relationships, either in the therapeutic or counselling dyad, in professionally led or self-help groups, or in the fellowship of a self help program, or any combination of these. If one takes something away from someone, one must provide something else in its place. Through these relationships one attempts to erect a barrier against drinking and drug taking, to change and to develop new, nonchemically-dependent relationships and modes of living and coping. The discussion of inner conflicts and underlying psychologic problems is considered in this treatment program to be secondary to the concentration on the impulse to drink or take drugs and must await the construction within the patient of a solid internal opposition to the impulse. Such inner conflicts and problems, however, must be discussed insofar as they constitute resistances to the development of that barrier and the new, nonalcoholic and nonsubstance-dependent ways of living, and resistance as well to the giving up of alcoholic and other pathologic relationships and the development of new and healthier ones.

In this procedure, the treatment program will use encouragement, acceptance, advice, direction, common sense, conscience, morality, religion, expiation, sympathy, empathy, the support of a surrogate family, work with the real family and social and work environment, and a kind of conversion experience. The concentration on insight and underlying conflicts and problems too early may even be dangerous, for just as in obsessional patients, these patients may well be all too willing to discuss such conflicts or problems in order to avoid facing the necessity of giving up the addiction. An empty ritual can be made out of the treatment process: "See, I am working on it, so I need not do anything more such as giving up the alcohol. . ." Or else: "See, I am working on my problems and when I uncover the reasons then the wish to drink or take drugs will go away. . ." All this may well constitute professional "enabling." Indeed, the entire notion of the unconscious may be similarly misused: "See, it is my unconscious and I am not responsible for that." This is, of course, not so. The unconscious is as much a part of the patient, perhaps even more so, than his or her conscious ego. Freud wrote a paper on the "Moral Responsibility for the Content of Dreams"[8] wherein he observed: "Obviously one must hold oneself responsible for the evil impulses of one's dreams. In what other way can one deal with them?" And similarly with our unconscious. Repression is a form of disavowal of responsibility and avoidance of the hard work, effort, and persistence required in dealing with such impulses and problems. The notion of the unconscious may be misused to serve the purpose of disavowal and avoidance as it often is with obsessionals as well as addicts.

On the other hand, the therapist must recognize that there are exceptions to this rule. For example, there is the case where the use of alcohol enables a patient to carry out a perverse, masochistic game without which he or she can have no sexual life and where that patient has no other gratifications in work and so forth. In such a situation the therapist must acknowledge this and work through these matters psychotherapeutically in order to help the patient to be able to participate in the treatment program. This might well mean going into unconscious material, but only to enable the treatment program to proceed.

THE PSYCHODYNAMICS OF THE RECOVERY PROCESS

Treatment can take its cues at least in part from the experience of A.A. and the other 12-step self-help recovery programs. As can be seen, these programs attempt to deal with the various issues discussed earlier. The first step (see the statement of the steps in the chapter on Long-Term Management) confronts and accepts the fact of the illness and what it has brought the patient to. The rest of that step and the next two steps attempt to overcome the block to the full emotional participation in the recovery program as discussed previously. It is not enough to come to the group, the counsellor or psychotherapist, the meeting, and so forth. One must decide freely to become part of them, giving up one's autonomy at that level in search of a higher, truer autonomy with freedom from the addiction and development of mastery of oneself and one's life. This decision is a free act and no one can make one give oneself to the process. The therapist, just as A.A., can only make the patient come, bring in the body, and go through the motions. But only the patient, in his or her own time, can decide to "surrender" instead of merely complying with the program.[9] The process is couched in religious terms but one need not be religious, only "spiritual" (in the sense of transcending the immediate, the material, and the egocentric). One can surrender to the program, to the group, to a higher purpose as well as a "Higher Power."

After this the patient must begin to recognize and oppose the denial, the ploys and mental maneuvers he or she has used to defend and perpetuate the addiction. This is what the rehabilitation centers work on for the most part. The defiance, narcissism, grandiosity, and omnipotence must be given up. In order to combat this A.A. uses the "spiritual" approach. (In psychotherapy it can be seen that all this recapitulates earlier struggles with reality, parental authority, and the world in terms of toilet training and other behavior, masturbation and sexual freedom, identity and values, occupation and love life, etc., and there it must be worked out psychotherapeutically. Ultimately the patient must freely decide to recognize historical necessity and move beyond such struggles to a more advanced level of development, with maturity in activity and responsibility.)

In doing this, the program—or the therapist—attempts to help the patient overcome Western civilization's excessive commitment to strict Cartesian dualism, for Western epistemology delineates and separates out a sense of "self" that is separated and isolated from all the rest of the unconscious thinking, feeling, acting, and deciding processes, and from all the internal and external informational pathways relevant at any moment to any given decision. Such an individual self, according to Bateson,[10] has in the West been reified, personified, endowed with pride, even arrogance, with narcissism and the illusion of "self control"; the illusion of control, that is, over the entire system of interlocking processes of which it is in reality merely a small part. By requiring surrender to the total system in which the self, as popularly conceived, is embedded (i.e., surrender to the "Higher Power"), A.A. and the psychotherapeutic process returns the focus of alcoholism to within the full self where it can be dealt with.

Once this step has been taken the patient is then ready to look into himself (the fourth step), his or her idiosyncrasies, his or her methods of dealing with people and with life, his or her traits of character, . . .shortcomings, . . . wrong-doings, and "character defects." These are then (the fifth step) spoken out loud to another, a procedure so essential to the psychotherapeutic process as well. It is only when it is said out loud to another, placed "out there," equidistant between the two or more people in the dialogue, that it becomes truly real, objectified, isolated, and available for change. (There are elements of the usefulness of the confessional process here as well.)

Then one prepares to change, for it is not enough not to drink ("dryness"); one must change the personality and coping methods that have been tied in with the solution to life's problems by drinking or taking drugs ("sobriety"). There is to be the death of an old way of being and a rebirth and beginning of a new way, in a new and different community of people. The addiction has been interwoven with the entire personality and has been part of the individual's total adaptation. New adaptive mechanisms must be worked out.

One then avoids the obsessional defense against such action by the splitting of word and deed, which one does by reuniting them. Therefore, one must make amends to the others one has harmed in one's illness (the eighth and ninth steps). All this is to be continued (the tenth and eleventh steps) as a permanent ongoing process, carried on within the self, between the self and another, or between the self and the group. The message will be carried by the patient to others (the twelfth step). The patient's story will be told again and again, for the patient's own sake, to keep it all in mind and keep one's awareness of and one's guard up against the return of the disorder, and perhaps to expiate as well. In addition, in telling one's story one reaffirms the positive meaning and direction that the recovery process has given to one's life, so negative and apparently meaningless before. Meanwhile factors and situations that predispose to relapse are identified and methods of counteracting them are worked out (e.g., "H-A-L-T: don't be hungry, angry, lonely, or tired"). Early warning signs of relapse are recognized and therapeutic measures developed.

The patient must continue through attendance at meetings and through the twelfth step to counter denial and rationalization. In this movement of change in the personality, negative reasons for sobriety are in the process of being converted into positive and, hence, more lasting ones. Old modes of being are to be replaced by new ones. This is the conversion process as exquisitely described by William James,[11] and the therapist's task is to uncover the resistances to this process, conscious and/or unconscious, and work with them as intensively and as deeply as necessary to enable the process to go on.

At the same time the concentration on the disease aspect as well as the sharing with others will help to overcome the problem of shame over the loss of control, so common in these disorders, as it is in life itself. Shame over loss of control is ubiquitous and may well go back in its origin to the first years of life and the conflicts over establishment of control and discipline over all aspects of behavior, including, of course, the excretory functions, the first concerns over control. The notion of a disease moves the patient away from regarding himself or herself as bad, weak, sinful, criminal, stained, or blemished. This is the phenomenon that took place in general psychiatry when Pinel struck the chains off the mentally ill in Paris at the end of the 18th century and that found its expression in alcoholism in the ideas of Benjamin Rush in America and Trotter in England. It is accepted almost everywhere now. The patient who fails to accept the disease concept will find it much more difficult to enter a program leading to sobriety and must be worked with around his or her need for control and sense of shame. As noted, the first three A.A. steps attempt to deal with this.

OTHER IMPLICATIONS OF THE TREATMENT PROGRAM AND THE DISEASE CONCEPT

The usefulness of the program is so great that it has been adapted to overeaters (OA), to gamblers (GA), and to others. It remains to be seen whether this kind of program can be extended to other groups mentioned in this connection: paraphiliacs, masochistic lovers, and so forth. Only after this 12-step program or something similar is deeply worked upon in all its phases is a firm opposition to drinking or drug taking created within the individual, and only then can further treatment take place. The alcoholism or other drug dependency must always, however, remain primary during psychotherapy. Should the addiction return, treatment must shift away from whatever it was dealing with back to the addiction until it is under control once again.

The above is the process of treatment on the part of the 12-step self-help recovery programs. The psychotherapist or counsellor must understand this program in depth (best done by attending meetings even if he or she is not a "recovering alcoholic"), and must work in conjunction with such a program and even use its techniques and approach in the therapeutic and counselling process. If the patient will not go to A.A., N.A., or whatever because of shame, great needs for privacy, or other such personal inclinations, then the therapist or counsellor can bring the program to the patient. In doing so, the therapist can follow the general strategies already outlined with whatever parameters or alterations are required, based both upon the patient's needs and upon the therapist's orientation and training.

The therapist must, however, be flexible as in all counselling and psychotherapy. For example, although the odds strongly favor the A.A. program, the therapist should not rigidly demand strict adherence if all is going well anyway. After all, people vary, not all alcoholics are the same, and the therapist does not absolutely know all the answers. The patient must be helped to find his or her own unique way to sobriety, which may or may not involve A.A. All the therapist or counsellor can do in this regard is to point out the odds, make suggestions, warn about self deception and other dangers, and support the patient on the way to recovery. Whatever works, works. Often the therapist will find continuing contacts with the patient's family and significant others (network therapy) to be a valuable addition to the treatment process, for intervention, support, monitoring, and follow-up.

The very essence of the disease in this disease model of alcoholism and other drug dependencies is as yet undetermined. The work on the psychologic match between the needs and mood states of the patient on the one hand and the effects of the different drugs on the other can account for only a small and certainly not the essential factor in the etiology of these disorders. Similarly the work on the neurochemical and synapse physiology level is in its earliest phases and is hardly clear. The sociologic factors, powerful as they may be, are not specific enough. In addition it should be noted that addictions are transferable. The smoker who stops cigarettes will usually gain weight as will the alcoholic who stops drinking, a food addiction tending to replace the other addiction. At A.A. meetings one sees clouds of smoke and a crowd around the coffee machine. Hence the disease is not as specific as one might think, and its essence may well lie in the addictive process itself rather than the specific agent.

There seems to be much more polypharmacy today and much less specificity of choice of drugs. We saw the patients of the 1960s, 1970s, and 1980s switching from drug to drug, category to category, following the fad of that particular era:

hallucinogens to narcotics to sedatives to stimulants, back to hallucinogens, then cocaine. The addictive process may be fundamentally psychobiologic but the choice of drug is strongly sociocultural. Although the etiology remains obscure, the phenomenology and the broad outlines of the treatment program are clear.

For special groups there will be different factors in the therapeutic approach. Those involving women and the economically and culturally disadvantaged are discussed elsewhere in this book. Other special groups involve the aged and homosexuals. Such treatment programs must have therapists with whom the patient can identify—alcoholic women, blacks, Hispanics, Native Americans, the poor, the aged, homosexuals, and so on—for each of the categories.

SPECIAL NEEDS FOR SPECIAL GROUPS

Special needs must be addressed. With the aged one must be careful about their physicians over-sedating them and must make sure that the patients are informed about their medications and how to carry out the medication instructions. The therapist must take an active role in these matters, perhaps contacting the physician or, on occasion, the pharmacist when the patient is going to a number of physicians. The benzodiazepines and other sedatives crossreact with and, as many drugs do, potentiate the effects of alcohol, and one must be careful about these matters. Furthermore, the aged are extremely sensitive to such medications and must be given them in low doses, if at all. Indeed, some are given benzodiazepines for sleep difficulties (temazepam, flurazepam, triazolam) or depression (alprazolam) and slowly develop drug dependency at even low dosages; sooner or later withdrawal symptoms of agitation, worsening of depression and sleep disturbance, autonomic system difficulties, and so on appear and the patient has to be slowly (perhaps up to a couple of months) detoxified before any other psychiatric treatment can take place.

As for the homosexuals who meet their partners in bars, they may have to have a nonalcoholic place to meet them instead, and this can be provided by certain A.A. groups. Otherwise they will be exposed to a heavy environmental pressure to drink again, perhaps before they have developed a solid recovery. (Such groups, as a by-product, might serve a useful function in protecting against AIDS as well.)

In general, regardless of whether the patient is heterosexual or homosexual, it is best to discourage much involvement in love and sexuality, especially serious involvement or where much anxiety is involved, for a while, perhaps for the first year of recovery. Sobriety must have the priority among the individual's concerns, and other goals and activities must be secondary until the sobriety is solid. This is particularly true where the patient's sexuality is unclear, such as in the case of the married man who when drunk engages for the most part in homosexual acts. Ultimately, he may have to face this problem in psychotherapy, but during the early period of recovery he must put it off. Indeed, a patient must put off all such major decisions for if he is conflicted over a marriage or over homosexuality, change may increase anxiety before he is ready to tolerate it and may push him back to drinking or drug taking.

In general, as the illness of alcoholism and other drug dependencies progresses, sexuality diminishes, especially in terms of the ability to perform. Sobriety can, but may not, restore that. In some instances sobriety may even take away some of the ability to perform that had been accomplished only under the disinhibition of the alcohol or other substance. (In such cases further psychotherapy in the direction of reevaluation and reorganization of the superego and other inhibiting forces may be necessary to help the patient obtain the gratifications he or she was seeking through the drug; without such a change, full sobriety cannot be attained, for the patient will be pushed back toward the chemical to obtain those gratifications.) In other instances, and more commonly for a short time after sobriety begins—a matter of months—sexual passions disappear, but they reappear later as the recovery process continues. The therapist can make no promises to the patient as to full return of function, but he or she can assure the patient that continued intake of alcohol usually leads to further sexual hypofunction, sooner or later.

Similar caveats concerning major changes exist where it comes to work, jobs, or choice of career, unless, of course, the job is tending bar or similarly dangerous activity. The therapist should oppose any major changes until sobriety is strongly entrenched and even then keep his or her eyes on the anxiety level and the tendencies to slips and recidivism. The therapist furthermore must not permit the patient to use his or her worries over sexuality, career, or such as an excuse to drink or even to direct the therapeutic attention away from the primary task at hand, the dealing with the addiction. The other work will come later.

The subject of methadone maintenance for opiate addiction has not been addressed in this book, for the book concerns itself with alcohol and related drugs, not the injectible opiates. They often present quite a different problem, requiring much longer treatment (e.g., a year or more in a therapeutic community) or even maintenance therapy. There is no maintenance therapy for alcoholism and sedative drug disorders; the oral narcotics (e.g., oxycodone, pentazocine, propoxyphene) can often be handled similarly in an abstinence, drug-free program. Where the patient has a major, serious opiate dependency disorder, however, one that seems to require methadone maintenance, he or she in such a program may, blocked from a narcotic "high," move over to the alcohol-sedative or, possibly, stimulant category. Should such patients subsequently come into an alcohol or other drug-free, abstinence-oriented program while on methadone maintenance, they would present serious problems for such a program. Only a special program, specially set up for just that purpose, would be able to handle them. Therefore, it would be advisable for the usual abstinence-oriented programs to avoid dealing with such a problem. As far as they are concerned, methadone maintenance is a legitimate treatment and a useful one in certain situations,[12] but it is not sobriety in their sense of the term. The methadone maintenance program would tend to be seen by them as a kind of "holding operation," on practical grounds for practical reasons, until the patient can, if possible, be weaned away from the drug and helped in the direction of full sobriety. Sobriety is the goal wherever possible.

The very essence of sobriety here, just as in the treatment of any other psychiatric disorder, is the development of the capacity for love and work, for achievement and enjoyment, without resorting to alcohol or other such drugs. Ultimately, the acquiring of friendships and partners in love and in life, the carrying out of the act of love, the attaining of goals, the assertion of the self—all without recourse to alcohol and other drugs—are the tasks of the treatment process.[9] All psychotherapy must be conducted in the light of this. This is the goal. All else is secondary.

REFERENCES

1. NIAAA: *Alcohol and Health.* Sixth special report to the US Congress, from the Secretary of the U.S. Department of Health and Human Services, 1987, pp 28–43
2. Watson R, Mohs M, Eskelson C, et al: Identification of alcohol abuse and alcoholism with biological parameters. *Alcoholism Clin Exp Res* 10:364–385, 1986
3. Heath D: Sociocultural variants in alcoholism, in Pattison EM, Kaufman (ed): *Encyclopedic Handbook of Alcoholism.* New York, Gardner, 1982
4. Freud S: Some character types met with in psychoanalytic work: (II) Those wrecked by success, in Strachey J (ed): *Standard Edition of the Complete Psychological Works of Sigmund Freud,* Vol 14. London, Hogarth, 1958
5. Peyser HS: Stress and alcohol, in Goldberger L, Breznitz S (eds): *Handbook of Stress.* New York, Macmillan-Free Press, 1982
6. Winnicott DW: Transitional objects and transitional phenomena (1953), in *Collected Papers: Through Pediatrics To Psychoanalysis.* New York, Basic, 1958
7. Noyes R, Clancy J, Coryell W, et al: A withdrawal syndrome after abrupt discontinuation of alprazolam. *Am J Psychiat* 142:114–116, 1985
8. Freud S: Some additional notes upon dream interpretation as a whole: (B) Moral responsibility for the content of dreams, in Strachey J (ed): *Collected Papers of Sigmund Freud,* Vol 5. London, Hogarth, 1950
9. Tiebout HM: Therapeutic mechanisms of Alcoholics Anonymous. *Am J Psychiatr* 100:468–473, 1944
10. Bateson G: The cybernetics of "self": A theory of alcoholism. *Psychiatry* 34:1–18, 1971
11. James W: *The Varieties of Religious Experience.* New York, New American Library (Montor), 1958
12. Dole VP, Nyswander M: Methadone maintenance treatment: A ten year perspective. *JAMA* 235:2117–2119, 1976

11

The Woman with Alcoholism

Lynne Hennecke
Vernell Fox

It is difficult to find in the vast literature on alcoholism any studies done on the alcoholic woman before the 1960s. Even today, many publications fail to make clear until the last paragraph that conclusions are based on all male samples.[1] The implicit notion, then, is that there is little if anything that differentiates the alcoholic woman from the alcoholic man and that research findings can simply be extrapolated to include her. Too often this assumption has led to an insensitivity to the special treatment needs of the alcoholic woman. When these needs are appropriately addressed in treatment, the usual assumption of a poor prognosis diminishes considerably.

Although the ratio of women alcoholics to men alcoholics is not known with any precision, estimates vary from 1:4 to 1:2.[2] A recent study has attempted to relate this ratio to a genetic paradigm for transmission of alcoholism.[3] We do know that drinking for women has increased as society has become more permissive of her drinking behavior, for example, drinking in public. This permissiveness, however, has not extended to a relaxation of social attitudes toward women's drunkenness. Studies[4-6] indicate that not only do both sexes report more in-

ALCOHOLISM:
A Practical Treatment Guide

ISBN 0-8089-1912-1

tolerance towards female drunkenness but even among alcoholic women the attitude expressed is one of disgust. The negative evaluation concerns the area of social roles, that is, the drunken woman unable to provide nurturant behavior and unable to employ the customary sexual restraints. The notion of moral weakness, therefore, is more explicit for women than it is for men. These attitudes have both helped to reinforce the alcoholic woman's denial of her disease and diminish her chances of seeking or being offered treatment. Even the physician shares this negative attitude. A report[7] on physicians' attitudes towards the alcoholic woman notes that the physician "believes the alcoholic woman to be sicker than the alcoholic male." Most of the physicians reported their awareness of their patients' alcohol problems, although less than 15 percent came to him for that specific complaint. Unfortunately, many of the physicians were loath to deal with the alcoholism in any open and direct way.

PHYSIOLOGICAL CONSIDERATIONS

Recent research[8] indicates that women metabolize alcohol differently than men. A standard dose of alcohol per body weight under standard conditions produces higher and more variable peak blood alcohol levels in women than in matched male controls. This study shows that the premenstrual phase seems to be a particularly susceptible time for high level effects of the drug. Blood alcohol concentrations in women who drink are also affected by exogenous hormones, such as oral contraceptives; alcohol tends to clear more slowly from blood, allowing a longer duration of intoxication. Quantity of alcohol consumed has been used as a diagnostic criterion. When it is and when epidemiologic studies do not take these apparent hormonal factors into consideration and furthermore ignore the differences of body weight between the average man and the average woman important information is obscured.

Compared to men, women alcoholics ae more prone to develop liver disease at an earlier age even though quantity of alcohol consumed is less than men and the drinking history is shorter.[9] There also appears to be a higher mortality rate in women once liver disease has developed.

Recent interest in bulimia has produced studies[10,11] that have revealed a relationship between that disorder and alcoholism. Almost a third of patients in treatment for bulimia report a history of drug/alcoholism treatment.

A number of gynecological-obstetrical problems, such as infertility, miscarriages, and hysterectomies, have been associated with alcoholism in women.[12] The incidence of congenital abnormalities in the offspring of heavily-drinking women is estimated to be about 32 percent.[13] About a 12 percent risk factor has been estimated for all pregnant women (alcoholic or not) if they drink during the first trimester. The critical amount of alcohol that would elicit the full spectrum of congenital abnormalities known as the fetal alcohol syndrome

(FAS) has not yet been determined. It is likely, however, that a relatively modest amount of alcohol ingested during the first seven weeks of pregnancy (the very period during which women fail to recognize that they have conceived) might result in the FAS. FAS is thought to be the third most common congenital defect (Downs Syndrome = 1:600, Spina Bifida = 1:1000, FAS = 1:2000) and the leading preventable one.

Difficulties and risks persist after the birth of a child.[14] There is a higher incidence both of postpartum death in drinking mothers and in deaths of the newborn than in the general population. Raising a physically handicapped child presents problems, particularly to a mother who cannot cope with her own problems. The irritability of the child and the disease of the mother makes early bonding difficult.

Survey statistics have indicated that physicians prescribe psychoactive drugs for women at about twice the rate they do for men.[15] Too often the physician is unaware of the patient's alcoholism.[16] Thus, many alcoholic women today suffer from cross-dependence. It is estimated that between 30 and 50 percent of alcohol-related hospitalizations are for combined drug problems. Cross-dependence and ignorance of the dangers of combining drugs have led in part to the alarming fact that rates of both attempted suicide and completed suicide are higher among women alcoholics than among male alcoholics or the general population.[17]

TREATMENT CONSIDERATIONS

The above-mentioned physiologic factors give rise to certain treatment considerations. For example, education about effects of alcohol on the neonate should be part of the prevention strategy for controlling congenital abnormalities. The majority of alcoholic women, perhaps because of the high value they place on motherhood and nurturance,[18] respond to this information and either significantly reduce their alcohol intake or stop drinking altogether.[19] However, for the alcoholic woman who has not stopped or will not stop drinking, abortion may well be indicated or at least seriouly considered. The guilt surrounding this issue, either about a possible abortion or about a child with congenital abnormalities, requires particularly sensitive attention.

Another physiologic factor that has specific treatment considerations is the observation that some alcoholic women relate drinking episodes to their menstrual cycle, particularly the premenstrual period. An alert therapist should consider this phenomenon, particularly if the patient is prone to "slips." Strategies such as ibuprofen therapy for the prevention/relief of dysmenorrhea,[20] extra A.A. meetings, telephone contact, etc., should be planned to help her negotiate this difficult period.

Generally speaking, a certain telescoping of the disease of alcoholism, that is, later onset and more rapid progression, differentiates female from male alcoholics. Later onset can be explained in part by the differential socialization process for males and females. The literature suggests that sex-role conflict *per se* may be the important stress factor contributing to women's alcoholism regardless of the direction (masculine or feminine) of the desired sex role identification.[21,22]

Parents and society as a whole tolerate nonstereotypic sex role behavior during childhood and adolescence in females but not in males. This latitude of behavior is allowed until the female is of marriageable age when her role becomes more stereotypically defined. Alcoholic drinking for women often begins with specific situational factors, some acute threat to her feminine adequacy such as marital or interpersonal relationship problems, a miscarriage, or children leaving home. This is not to imply that she had not been drinking, perhaps heavily, prior to this. Most likely she had, alcohol being an important part of her life and probably a major coping mechanism. The situational factor adds considerable weight in breaking her tenuous hold on controlled drinking or converting a latent or covert illness to an overt phase.

What is perceived as more rapid progression of the disease in females may be due in part to the previously mentioned harsher judgment of women's drunkenness. Alcoholism in men may seem to progress more slowly simply because society views much of his drunken behavior more benignly than that of the woman alcoholic. More rapid progression, however, will perhaps be linked in part to the differential rate that women metabolize alcohol.[8]

Both men and women alcoholics are isolated, but the isolation of women alcoholics differs somewhat from that of men. Except for the early stages of her disease, the alcoholic woman is rarely a "bar drinker." She prefers to do her drinking alone, whether she is a housewife or a career woman. She is aware of society's (and her own) view on drunkenness in women and she feels "safer" drinking alone. Moreover, a difficult and problematic identification with the mother[23] (indicated by role conflict as seen in the higher scores on "femininity" scales and "masculine" oriented sex role preferences[21,22]) contributes to this extreme isolation by interfering in close relationships with other women. She becomes further isolated by either an overprotective family, friends, and community, or sometimes by a spouse who uses her alcoholism as an excuse for his extramarital affairs. If she happens to be working, her problem is dealt with by dismissal rather than confrontation. Even if her physician is willing to suggest that she may have a problem, he will often offer her valium or other psychotropic drugs as a substitute to help her with her "nerves."[15,16]

The double stigma of alcoholism and alcoholism in a specific person (woman, Jew, cleric, physician, etc.) presents a major obstacle to recovery unless the dignity of the disease concept is projected to the patient by the physician.

TREATMENT

Breaking isolation is the key to recovery from the disease of alcoholism. For the alcoholic woman, this is most successfully accomplished not only through some combination of psychotherapy and active membership in A.A., but with an on-going participation in a women's group as well. The development of a new and better (more gentle, loving, or benign) sense of self is facilitated by a new set of "parents" (the therapist, members of A.A., and, especially, members of the women's group) who love her as she is, and are prepared to stand by her as she explores who she wants to grow up to be. To facilitate the expression of her feelings of empathy, without confusion and resentment, the alcoholic woman must establish her autonomy, understanding both her right and her responsibility to accomplish this task. All treatment modalities are sources of support to this newly emerging sense of autonomy, but it is in the women's group that she will feel most comfortable to explore honsetly and openly such sensitive areas of life—sexuality, extramarital affairs, child abuse, abortion, prostitution.

The severe ego devaluation suffered by the alcoholic woman can be helped by the joint efforts of the women in the group to attempt to remove sex role stereotyping, sex bias, and double standards. Women's groups are particularly sensitive to such symptoms of subclinical depression as needing to please others, not ever getting angry, and the underlying feeling of hopelessness and helplessness—"I can't help myself; you must take care of me and then I'll resent you for it." They learn that they are not alone in their wants and needs.

A two-year followup study[24] showed that the initiation of a women's group in the treatment process was a key factor in turning a virtual no success rate into a success rate that exceeded the rate for men. For about 20 years, Gitlow has used a leaderless women's group as a mechanism through which to achieve an improved incidence of long-term recovery.

Although it is critical that the patient's consort become involved in the recovery and growth process, experience with women patients is that the accomplishment of this component of treatment is especially difficult. It is often impossible to involve the husband in the recovery process. Rarely do they come in, call, or otherwise complain (as do their female counterparts attached to male patients). Thus, there are fewer opportunities to relate spontaneously to their needs and involve them. When it is suggested that the woman might directly request that the partner participate in her treatment, her anxious response is often that he "would not be interested" or "has already been bothered too much." In contrast to the stability of marriages between an alcoholic male and his female spouse, a vast majority of husbands leave their alcoholic wives.[25] After some months of treatment, some women gradually begin to disclose the relationships of their husbands' psychosexual pathology and their resistance to the patient's change, especially to the concept of their total abstinence. In these instances, it is well to direct and support the alcoholic woman in the necessary divorce proceedings or termination of the destructive relationship. Again, the group can provide shared experience. Divorce, after the initiation of treatment and abstinence, tends to correlate with long-term recovery.[26,27]

Although active participation in A.A. will be an important component in the recovery and maintenance process, some women are especially vulnerable to seeking dependent relationships with males in this group. What appears to be a familiar avenue (men) to some sense of self worth and thus a solution to her problems of self esteem can often prove disastrous or at least threatening to her sobriety when there is trouble in the relationship. A healthier alternative for her would be to develop and strengthen her autonomy and independence.

Most often, the alcoholic woman, not unlike other women in our society, primarily defines herself by her affiliative relationships. This limitation on her self definition can be dangerous to establishing her sense of autonomy (a necessary antecedent to identity achievement) particularly when there have been problematic identifications in childhood that distort relationship expectations.[23] It often takes several years of recovery before she is able to attain a realistic evaluation of these expectations. It is important, therefore, that she have an alternative, healthier avenue to defining herself and improving her self-esteem.

Recent studies[28] have shown that a career is the primary way in our culture to manifest one's self concept. "I am a physician" really claims "I am an intelligent and caring person." Since the alcoholic woman's role preferences are often in the "masculine" direction,[21,22] she must be encouraged to develop those that are pertinent to her self concept rather than be made to feel that these preferences are deviant.

Even if the alcoholic woman is currently working outside of the home her career or job choice (often chosen for its drinking opportunities or environment) should be reassessed as to its congruence with her self-concept. Exploring abilities and strengths for career possibilities will counter feelings of inadequacy, confusion, and low self-esteem. A firmer sense of identity will thus be established.

Immediate practical needs might well dictate the necessity of getting a job—any job—during the first stages of recovery. One therapeutic benefit from her working early on in her recovery is that work structures time and is, therefore, an anxiety binder. If the alcoholic woman goes back to the unstructured world of housework and childcare, which may induce feelings of boredom, inadequacy, and dangerous isolation, she runs a greater risk of recidivism.

Educational goals that will help facilitate a career choice or change should be explored. Consideration of her personal potential serves as a useful mechanism for exploration of her dependency needs and willingness to undertake responsibility. Obviously the therapist should avoid entering "test situations" in which the effort to develop a meaningful career becomes the means by which the patient demonstrates her ultimate inadequacies.

Although children can be an effective leverage to motivate the alcoholic woman to seek treatment, they can also be an obstacle when there is no available child-care resource[16] or when they feel a threat of losing custody of their children by admitting their alcoholism by seeking treatment.[29] This problem can be particularly difficult if she needs hospitalization for detoxification or long-term residential rehabilitation. Some knowledge of and guidance to appropriate community services are important in planning her treatment.

Unfortunately, the literature frequently quotes a few limited studies that have found that women do not do as well in treatment as men. It is gratifying to note that a recent analysis of treatment-outcome studies shows that results with women patients were generally good.[30] Experience has been that when the specific needs of women with alcoholism have been addressed, the women themselves reach out to other women in and out of treatment (the majority of women enter treatment referred by other women patients), and the prognosis for recovery of women becomes as good, or perhaps better than, their male counterparts.

REFERENCES

1. Vanicelli M, Nash L: Effect of sex bias on women's studies on alcoholism. *Alcoholism: Clinical and Experimental Research* 8(3):334–336, 1984
2. NIAAA: *Alcohol and Health,* first special report to the US Congress on, from the Secretary of DHEW, GPO, 1971
3. Spalt L: Alcoholism—evidence of an X-linked regressive genetic characteristic. *JAMA* 241:23, 1979
4. Lawerence JJ, Maxwell MA: *Society, Culture and Drinking Patterns.* New York, Wiley, 1962
5. Knupfer C: Female drinking patterns. *Soc Prob* 12:224, 1964
6. Curlee J: Alcoholic women. *Bull Menniger Clinic* 31:154, 1967
7. Johnson MW: Physicians views on alcoholism with special reference to alcoholism in women. *Neb State Med J* 50:378, 1965
8. Jones BM, Jones MK: Women and alcohol: Intoxification, metabolism and the menstrual cycle, in Greenblatt M, Schukitt MS (eds): *Alcoholism Problems in Women and Children.* New York, Grune & Stratton,1976, pp.103–136
9. Hill SY: The biological consequences of alcoholism in women. NIAAA Workshop of alcoholism and alcohol abuse among women, Jekyll Island, GA, April 2–5, 1978

10. Mitchell JE, Hatsukami D, Eckert ED, Pyle RL: Characteristics of 275 patients with bulimia. *Am J Psychiat* 142(4):482–485, 1985
11. Brisman J, Siegel M: Bulimia and alcoholism: Two sides of the same coin? *J Substance Abuse Treat* 2:113–118,1984
12. Gomberg ES: Alcoholism in women, in KIssin B, Beigleter H (eds): *The Biology of Alcoholism.* Vol. 4, New York, Plenum Press, 1976, pp 113–118
13. Ouellette EM, Rossett HL, Rosman NP, Weiner AB: Adverse effects on offspring of maternal alcohol abuse during pregnancy. *N Engl J Med* 297:528–530, 1977
14. Fox, VL: Alcohol and pregnancy. Presented at University of Utah School on Alcoholism and Other Drug Dependencies, Salt Lake City, Utah, June 1978
15. Abelson HI, Fishburn PM, Cissin I: *National Survey on Drug Abuse.* Vol. 1. National Institute on Drug Abuse, US department of Health, Education, and Welfare, Rockville, MD, 1977, p102
16. Sandmaier M: *The Invisible Alcoholics: Women and Alcohol Abuse in America* New York, McGraw-Hill, 1980
17. Aldoory S: The chemical curtain: polydrug abuse among women. *Alcohol Health Res World* 3(2):28–36, 1978
18. Wilsnak SC: Sex-role identity in female alcoholism. *J Abnorm Psychol* 82:253–261,1973
19. Rossett HL, Weiner LW, Zuckerman B, et al: Reduction of alcohol consumption during pregnancy with benefits to the newborn. *Alcoholism Clin Exp Res* 4: 178–184, 1980
20. Pulkkuner MO, Csapo AI: The effect of Ibuprofen in the intrauterine pressure and menstrual pain of dysmenorrheric patients. *Prostaglandins* 15:1055–1062, 1978
21. Wilsnak SC: The impact of sex role on women's use and abuse, in Greenblatt M, Schukitt MS (eds): *Alcoholism Problems in Women and Children.* New York, Grune & Stratton,1976, pp. 37–63
22. Scida J, Vannicelli M: Sex role conflict and drinking. *J Stud Alcohol* 40:1,1979
23. Gitlow SE, Hennecke L: Etiology of alcoholism: A new theoretic mosaic. *Sem Adolescent Med* 1:235–238, 1985
24. Fox VL: Clinical experiences in working with women with alcoholism, in Burtle V (ed): *Women Who Drink.* Springfield, IL, Charles C. Thomas, 1979, pp 119–126
25. Lindbeck VL: The alcoholic woman: A review of the literature. *Int J Addict* 7:567–580, 1972
26. Gitlow SE: Personal communication
27. Knott D: Personal communication
28. Super DE: *The Psychology of Careers.* New York, Harper and Row, 1957

29. US Department of Hesalth, Education, and Welfare. *Services for Alcoholic Women: Foundation for Change*. Washington, DC, Superintendent of Documents, Government Printing Office, 1979
30. Corrigan EM: *Alcoholic Women in Treatment*. New York, Oxford University Press, 1980

12

Problems Peculiar to Patients of Low Socioeconomic Status

Marvin D. Feit

This chapter is designed to orient the physician to the management of low-socioeconomic-status patients who present a clinical picture of alcoholism. Upper- and middle-class patients usually present a resource-positive environment often compatible with the physician's personal background. Therefore it is quite easy for physicians to relate to these patients, to perhaps understand the presenting problems, and to develop traditional plans utilizing such patient resources as money, employment or marketable skills, and the support of family members.

The low-socioeconomic-status patients are a class of economically poor patients composed largely of minorities—blacks, Hispanics, Native Americans, poor whites, and others. These patients are typically quite different in lifestyle from the physician, come from and have different cultures, have virtually no money and practically no hope for long-term employment, are perhaps limited in formal schooling, and may have obscure family relationships. This group includes the homeless as well, with its subgroups of the dispossessed, the unemployed, the mentally ill, and the addicted.

These patients present special problems to the physician. Prescriptions and treatment plans often don't work. The patients are people with whom the physician is not only unfamiliar but who possess characteristics so different as to potentially arouse fear and distrust within the physician. June Christmas notes that

ALCOHOLISM:
A Practical Treatment Guide
ISBN 0-8089-1912-1

Table 12-1
Problems in Management of the Low-Socioeconomic-Status Patient

Estrangement and distrust in the therapeutic relationships (experiential differences→inability to identify with one another→fear)
Within patient
Within physician
Low resources
Lack of funds for treatment precludes certain services (private medical care, many inpatient rehabilitation facilities, etc.)
Lack of basic literacy, schooling, and job skills with which to find a place in the dominant culture, should such be desired.
Lack of opportunities for establishing ego strength, identity, and self-respect within the culture (work, housing, acceptance of culture variations, etc.)
Debilitating results stemming from the required assistance programs (welfare, etc.)
Lack of support by family members possessing the above resources

in such an atmosphere, professional despair, combined with a cultural connotation of chronicity, often defines the situation as inevitably hopeless.[1] In addition, patients bring to the therapeutic situation their own anxiety and distrust, compounding the alienation. See Table 12-1.

MANAGEMENT

There are ways physicians can manage low-socioeconomic-status patients. First, they have to recognize that the patient has a drinking problem; second, that the patient is different from the physician; and third, that the patient might require a different approach. Each of these—defining the diagnosis, therapeutic arrangement, and treatment approach—will present problems specific for this group of patients. The physician's approach not only must take these circumstances into consideration but must do so in a unified and integrated manner for greatest success. Every patient is unique, and treatment requires that the therapist identify this uniqueness. The problem in this group is the therapeutic distance from the patients, physician difference from them, and physician inability to see the unique qualities of patients that are so different from his own. The physician cannot use his own background and frame of reference for understanding and empathy here.

Problem Detection and Recognition

The methods noted in Chapters 1 and 2 pertain to these patients as well.

Physicians need to develop their listening skills when working with alcoholics; this is particularly necessary with low-socioeconomic-status patients. Quite often these patients are suspicious of formal institutions in a white, upper- and middle-class-dominated society, having experienced rejection or embarrassment one or more times. They often won't admit problems in formal institutions to physicians or other helpers who do not deal with them as individuals in their own right. Often these patients are outwardly compliant, say all the right things, and appear motivated when just the opposite is actually happening. Detecting double messages and hidden agendas and assessing the extent to which a patient "owns a problem" (i.e., accepts that he is indeed an alcoholic) requires the development of listening skills. Basically one has to listen to patients rather than tell them what to do.

The art of modifying learned cultural distrust by a correcting experience with the therapist is limited by several factors, one of which is the usefulness of such distrust—its defensive and protective aspects. The "niceness" on the part of the therapist may merely convince patients that the doctor is trying to manipulate them; they then feel threatened rather than convinced and will flee at the first advance. The physician *must not try to get so very close to the patient too quickly*, but must feel the way slowly, with patience and with respect for the differences between them.

Shift in Approach

Although all patients pass through stages of ambivalence regarding their desires to stop drinking and thereby change the very fabric of their lives (e.g., fearing loss of friends, activities, sometimes families and careers), it is usually possible to convince them of the disproportionate benefits likely to accrue from abstinence. Socioeconomically deprived patients, however, present a quantitatively different problem in that giving up alcohol and its related activities may involve social and human loss with relatively modest concomitant gain. For example, for many patients the world consists only of friends who drink, and they move within a system that includes hospitals, jails, shelters, flophouses, or single-room-occupancy (SRO) hotels. In this system, patients receive security, warmth, food, personal recognition, and attention to basic needs at critical moments. Not only does life without alcohol seem no better or even worse for these patients than life with alcohol, but the physician may also be unable to appreciate a clearcut advantage to abstaining. No physician who lacks such a conviction is likely to convince a patient of the need for sobriety. Such belief, easy with better-endowed patients, is especially difficult with the economically deprived. The doctor must therefore formulate for such patients realistic and achievable aims that represent clear and self-evident improvements.

Physicians, then, must be able to view the individual operating in a social context that is usually quite different from that which they know and with which they are familiar. In order to achieve this view, physicians must begin to ask more appropriate questions. For example, in the case of a "career" drinker it might be possible to identify people to whom the patient responds, such as certain policemen or room clerks. In any event, this individual's situation may not appear as hopeless as it first seems.

The Cultural Context

There are other areas of concern that might be useful for physicians to explore. One should minimally inquire about the individual's past experience in dealing with formal institutions, what he sees as problematic in relation to drinking and in life itself, what is acceptable and unacceptable drinking behavior in his culture and environment, how he feels about seeking help, and how he has arrived at the present situation or the "pathways" to treatment. This should not be interpreted as implying that the physician should utilize any psychodynamics so discovered in an early attempt to encourage intellectualization. Such an effort commonly diverts attention from the primary task of dealing with the drinking to the more "acceptable" one of an intellectual discussion requiring little, if any, change. Understanding the patient's illness is of value only insofar as (1) it increases the strength of the relationship between the patient and physician (therapeutic alliance), (2) it helps the doctor discover what actions may be needed for intervention, and (3) it may help the physician determine the most efffective means for increasing motivation (i.e., exerting therapeutic leverage).

Identification of the "pathways" to treatment can often serve to clarify the resources available to individuals and, in turn, suggest points of intervention in a treatment process. Usually these resources require physicians to look beyond their understanding of the formal or classical network of services. One cannot separate medical management from the milieu in which low-socioeconomic-status patients live or survive. For these patients, physician contact in formal institutions may be used only after their familiar network resources are exhausted. Native Americans, for instance, generally arrive in the mainstream health care system only after thinking through themselves, going next to their immediate families, then to the extended family (cousins, aunts, uncles) and social network, to the religious leader, and to the tribal council.[2] Effective management with Native Americans might necessitate continued communication as well as involving other Native Americans from the patients' own health care orientation, such as tribal leaders or healers ("medicine men"). A similar approach would need to be followed for other individuals with similarly specific characteristics.

In a cultural context, concepts vary and have different meanings and connotations to those involved. Consider the concept of family. The type of family studied most in America is the nuclear family, consisting of two partners and their children. This definition is inappropriate when applied to many of the ethnic and cultural groups comprising most of the low-socioeconomic-status patient category. For example, the one-parent family is today a rather significant part of American society, while Native Americans have a very broad definition of family, often with as many as 200 members, since they consider the extended family (aunts, uncles, cousins, grandparents, and so forth) and accept all born into such a family as full members. "Illegitimacy" and "orphan" are terms that in general mean nothing to Native Americans. Many blacks and Hispanics also tend to see the family as different from the nuclear concept of family most typically taught to professionals. Socioeconomically-deprived patients do indeed have families, but they are usually different from what physicians and other professionals are often taught. Once such families are identified, physicians will be quick to recognize that the familiar functions provided by all families will be present.

Locating individuals in their cultural context is therefore an essential component of managing low-socioeconomic-status patients. It is imperative that the helper know the culture and history of the patients, since they represent their resource-positive environments from which emerge the strengths physicians can build upon in the treatment process. Although this circumstance is universally true, the physician's own experience allows ready access to the cultural information about patients whose backgrounds are similar to his own (by identification); such is often untrue in regard to the socioeconomically deprived patient. The helper must not assume such awareness but must rather question the validity of initial interpretations. These patients must be viewed in relation to their own distinctive problems and not in a stereotypic and predictable manner. For example, "Latin machismo, the coping strengths of black women, and Native American adolescent strivings for consciousness of [tribal] heritage may not apply to each individual within his or her respective minority group, or may be manifest in ways that differ so widely that to be content with a label or slogan is to deprive the person of individuality."[1]

Treatment Planning

Development of a treatment plan is another area that can be used advantageously in patient management. Physicians might enlist the aid of patients in this process by asking them to identify their problems and how they think these problems may be resolved or alleviated. Here is a moment when physicians can test the reality awareness of their patients by assessing and discussing the extent to which patients can achieve their own goals. Moreover, physicians can use this time to ask patients how they and other helpers may be useful to them. This technique would be valuable in helping patients make better use of physician services.

It is important for physicians to explore the nature of the problem(s) presented by patients. Frequently professionals accept patient statements only to learn later that such statements may be inaccurate and not helpful. One should not easily accept a patient's view as not being able to obtain a job as the reason for drinking if past data and a few questions suggest that the patient has no real history of employment and has no apparent marketable skills. Yet a job to such a patient may in fact be possible to obtain—bearing in mind that a physician may see a job as consisting of a high degree of stability, full time and with regular hours, and with a regular income, but to the patient a "job" may mean securing odd jobs, much part-time work, hustling, and a host of other things, legal and illegal. Asking such questions as how one manages one's time and how one "makes it" financially allows patients to provide clear pictures of themselves in their own environment.

Treatment plans should perhaps be viewed not as prescriptions to be followed routinely but as growth documents against which patients can measure their achievements from time to time. It should be recognized that a treatment plan developed at one time probably will need to be modified or changed several times in the course of treatment. Physicians must accept that alcoholism, as a chronic relapsing illness, may run a recovery course replete with recidivistic complications that must be anticipated. The patient should be aware of the cost and potential dangers of such "slips," but a constructive plan for dealing with them might avoid excessive loss or demoralization with treatment. In other words, discuss with the patient the difficulties that emerge in the treatment process and what alternatives might be available to him.

A major consideration in developing a treatment plan is the recognition that gross cerebral changes may occur with chronic alcohol abuse (whether through trauma, avitaminosis, or toxicity of ethanol). Frequently these changes are not demonstrated by the mental status examination or traditional psychometric techniques. The cortical deficits produced by chronic alcohol abuse are similar to the effects of aging or Alzheimer's dementia, which means that complex integrative functions would be impaired intitially whereas simple sensory and motor functions and familiar learned patterns used over a lifetime would be retained until more severe stages of deterioration are reached. If alcohol use results in significant cortical damage as indicated by some research findings, it is possible that it may represent the source of loss of impulse control, inability to abstain from alcohol consumption, and difficulty in adjusting to a new psychosocial ambience. The reversibility of the alcohol-related cerebral dysfunction is ill defined, but evaluation suggests that at least 1 year of abstinence is essential for this process. It is necessary to appreciate the overt and subtle organicity that exists in this population: unrealistic expectations may only lead to a behavioral decompensation and readdiction, and abstinence from alcohol and adequate nutrition are the bases for treatment. (For further discussion, see the section on Alcoholism and Organic Mental Disturbances in Chapter 9.)

By their very label, low-socioeconomic-status patients present themselves as obviously in need of financial support. Such patients are usually referred to the state Department of Human Services, formerly called the Welfare Department, and if they meet the eligibility requirements for one of the various financial assistance programs they can receive monthly allotments.

The physician is generally not involved in establishing patient eligibility for Federal or state financial assistance programs; however, it is extremely important for physicians to understand some inherent strains on effective treatment plans and take appropriate steps with their patients. In effect, the social, psychological, and financial support systems of low-socioeconomic-status patients generally do not enhance the goals of the treatment plan. The usual treatment plan emphasizes support of a program aimed toward development of self-reliance and thereby self-esteem. This is not limited to retraining and other direct measures. Even that paramount therapeutic principle dealing with formulation of critical interpersonal relationships (see Chapter 7) serves ideally to promote such growth. The unresolved and problematic question is whether or not the development of a close therapeutic community and specific (narrow) societal relationships can result in self-esteem in the presence of continued dependence upon a "welfare system."

Treatment programs that address themselves also to improving the self-image of alcoholic individuals have a better chance of communicating effectively with their clientele. Such efforts need to be expanded, since these programs typically encourage patient participation in some form of social action. Physicians working in this atmosphere are often called upon to participate or to lead social political activities. The issue of whether or not such activity is appropriate for physicians depends on the setting, the administrators, the physicians themselves, and the patients. There is probably nothing worse than well-intentioned people acting inappropriately and missing the target.

Further, much research is needed to determine in which treatment programs low-socioeconomic-status patients recover best. For example, politically and socially active treatment programs may communicate effectively with their clientele, but to what extent does this improved communication result in greater patient sobriety? This and other questions suggest how much more knowledge needs to be obtained about a favorable response to rehabilitative efforts by alcoholic patients in general and low-socioeconomic-status patients specifically.

There are self-help treatment programs where professional help is not involved. Alcoholics Anonymous (A.A.) and the Nation of Islam are two such groups that involve peer assistance and improving one's self-image. Physicians have traditionally had a referral alliance with A.A. but not with other groups such as the religiously oriented Nation of Islam. Whereas A.A. often lacks appeal in poor and black communities, this latter group reports much therapeutic success and attributes it to the individual's conversion or change to a completely different way of life. Individual motivation and commitment to alter an existing lifestyle should never be minimized, and self-help treatment programs provide the atmosphere where such change can take place. Physicians can explore with their patients use of self-help treatment groups but must themselves be capable of understanding the life situation of patients and be able to recommend the more nontraditional helping group.

Organizational Support

Managing the low-socioeconomic-status patient must also include the development of supports external to the patient-physician relationship for the physician to be most effective. Physicians may rarely provide treatment by themselves for this group of patients. As part of a multidisciplinary team, and certainly as the key member, the physician ought to be quite vocal in ensuring the employment of highly trained and skilled counselors. Poor counseling can quickly undermine the developing patient relationship. One must keep in mind the past experiences of these patients to note their acute susceptibility to rejection and embarrassment. Just one negative situation may be all that is necessary for patient withdrawal to occur.

First contacts of any kind for low-socioeconomic-status patients are crucial in the treatment process. Intake may be one small part of the total program from the physician's perspective, but for the patients it is a time filled with extreme anxiety. How they are treated at intake often establishes how they perceive the staff and the program. It is often helpful for patients to see people with similar backgrounds during this phase of treatment.

Patient management is a responsibility of any physician. Clinical intervention by other professionals should proceed with the physician's being aware of what is happening to the patient. This is to suggest that simple referral to other professionals does not achieve effective patient management with this population. Low-socioeconomic-status patients can respond to physicians provided that they demonstrate an understanding of them, can determine their course of treatment, and ensure proper care. Indeed, these patients tend to regard a physician's words as extremely powerful and continually need to know that the physician is in control of the treatment process.

Physicians ought to be vocal in stating their need to be supported with a diverse staff. It is often comforting to patients to see people with similar ethnic and racial identities employed at all levels. Native Americans in Minnesota indicated a preference for securing health services from Native American workers.[3] They demonstrated this preference in the Minneapolis-St. Paul "Twin Cities" metropolitan area in relying upon Native American service agencies, while non-tribal health agencies located in the same community were continuously involved in strategies to recruit Native American clients.[4]

Staff development or training programs must become integral parts of treatment programs. Regular meetings of the staff, physicians, nurses, and counselors with varying social, ethnic, health, and economic backgrounds must permit candid discussions of not only the patients' but the staff personnel's relationships and feelings toward one another. Such staff activities need to be conducted on a regular basis with content being derived from the population served. For example, "pathways" to treatment and the community services that do exist for low-socioeconomic-status patients can be covered and would probably need to be updated periodically. Also, the resources within local communities, such as unions, houses of worship, and social clubs, ought to be involved in the training of staff and in developing more creative treatment situations.

CONCLUSION

Management of low-socioeconomic-status patients usually presents physicians with special problems. On one hand, the medical procedures, techniques, and diagnosis are the same as with all patients; on the other hand, low-socioeconomic-status patients are unique in that their lifestyles, values, culture, coping patterns, and norms are often quite different from those of the physician. Hence traditional treatment planning is not effective, and physicians have to do things differently in order to effect better management of these patients. Several suggestions were offered both in the context of the patient-physician relationship and in the organizational support system around the physician as a key member of the multidisciplinary team. Physicians must be aware that clinical interventions have powerful social and political consequences for their patients and should adopt a treatment protocol that accounts for this awareness. Effective management would allow low-socioeconomic-status patients far greater involvement in and exposure to the mainstream health care system, from which one could anticipate opportunities to yield more significant results with a population too often seen as hopeless. Physicians may have to get involved in extra-clinical concerns with these patients, refering them for help with financial, work, housing, medical, child care, legal, immigration, and other such matters in order to develop and maintain their sobriety.

REFERENCES

1. Christmas J. Alcoholism services for minorities: Training issues and concerns. *Alcohol Health Res World* 2(3):22-27, 1978
2. Red Horse J, Lewis R, Feit M, et al: Family behavior of urban American Indians. *Social Casework* 25(2):67-72, 1978
3. DeGeyndt W. Health behavior and health needs in urban Indians in Minneapolis. *Health Serv Rep* 88:360-366, 1973
4. Red Horse J, Feit D: Urban Native American preventive health care. Paper presented at the American Public Health Association Meeting, Miami Beach, October 1976

BIBLIOGRAPHY

1. Homelessness, Alcohol Health and Research World, Vol. 11, #3, National Institute on Alcohol Abuse and Alcoholism, 1987.
2. Westermeyer, J. The role of Ethnicity in Substance Abuse, in: Stimmel, B., (ed.) *Cultural and Sociological Aspects of Alcoholism and Substance Abuse*. New York, Haworth Press, 1984, pp. 9-18.

13

The Family in the Crisis of Alcoholism

James A. Knight

The story of alcoholism is the story of miscarried repair—a backfiring of the effort at maintaining equilibrium in one's life. While drinking to solve some problem, attain some goal, or accomplish some purpose, however major or minor, the person creates through the agent that he uses a problem greater than the original one.

Although knowledge of the causes and treatment of alcoholism remain limited, this knowledge is sufficient to encourage programs in prevention and treatment. It is often forgotten how frequently in the past major diseases were controlled with only fragments of knowledge. A good example is the control of cholera. This disease was prevalent in London in 1854. A careful epidemiologic study of the cholera patients by Dr. John Snow identified one common denominator among them: their use of drinking water from the Broad Street Pump. A rapid decline of the cases occurred after the pump had been removed. Although some living microorganism in the water was suspected as the causative agent by Snow in 1854, this was before the days of bacteriology. The causative agent, *Vibrio cholerae*, was not identified until 1883 by Robert Koch—29 years after Snow closed the pump and well on Broad Street and ended the 1854 epidemic of cholera. This example is cited only to show how absurd are the critics of many health programs who proclaim that little can be done until the total truth is known about an illness.

ALCOHOLISM:
A Practical Treatment Guide
ISBN 0-8089-1912-1

There is an old axiom about the family that describes it as an autocracy ruled by its sickest member. One may ask how the sick member attained such a role in the family. In studying illness, among the questions one must ask is what does this illness tell about the family from which this sick person comes? Life is filled with examples of families who have chosen one member to be sick or a scapegoat or a clown. At times, an individual family member chooses voluntarily to be sick in order to save the family. Usually the situation is less dramatic, with problems being brought by one or both partners in a marriage or with problems growing out of the marital interaction. When children come along, the family matrix may be such that it becomes productive of either health or disease. When confronted with an alcoholic patient, the therapist who asks what this illness tells about the family from which the alcoholic comes and who looks vigorously for answers will have begun the therapy of both the alcoholic and the family.

In discussing alcoholism in the family, there has been a tendency to think only of spouse or parent as the alcoholic, with little thought given to teenage sons and daughters as problem drinkers. In the United States there is an increasing incidence of new young drinkers. With an increasing prevalence of teenage drinking, there will be an increasing incidence and prevalence of teenage alcoholism, not to mention other drug dependencies.

While impulsivity characterizes much adolescent behavior, teenagers do attempt to learn self-control. In their effforts to attain maturity and independence and to work out their own philosophies of life, they rebel against most external controls, structure, or authority. Thus teenagers are a very susceptible population for alcohol use or abuse and the subsequent loss of impulse control. Therefore they may bring to the family the crisis of alcoholism with the same frightening fervor as that of an alcoholic parent or spouse. With the increasing availablity of alcoholic beverages to youngsters, the problem of teenage alcoholism promises to grow substantially. Prevention and early intervention hold greater promise than treatment. It is not easy to entice teenagers into treatment with professionals whom they view as authority figures.

PSYCHODYNAMIC CAUSATION IN ALCOHOLISM

In an effort to understand the family in the crisis of alcoholism, the therapist must have some understanding of psychodynamic causation in alcoholism. The theories of causation can be broken down into a number of categories.

1. The Freudian view contends that alcoholism results from one or more of three unconscious tendencies: self-destruction, oral dependency, or latent homosexuality.
2. Close to the Freudian view is the concept that alcoholism develops as a response to inner conflict between dependency drives and aggressive impulses.

3. Sharing much in common with the above theoretical views is the Adlerian view that alcoholism represents a striving for power that compensates for a pervasive feeling of inferiority. Alcoholic persons turn to alcohol to enhance their feelings of self-esteem and prowess.

David McClelland, the motivational psychologist, and his associates have extended the Adlerian theory in their research and have declared that the abuse of alcohol by many is motivated by unfulfilled power needs.[1] McClelland and his associates suggest that frustrated ambitions may play a role in the development of an alcohol problem. It is suggested that alcoholics may have enhanced needs for power but find themselves inadequate to achieve their goals. They resort to alcohol because it provides a sense of release and power and feelings of achievement. Since overindulgence in alcohol precludes an effective coping with the problems needing solution and leads to additional problems, this vicious cycle results in confirmed alcoholism.

Thus when persons provide themselves with drugs such as alcohol that change their pain to pleasure, depression to elation or an increase in self-esteem, impotence to omnipotence, the first step in addiction has occurred. This sudden change from frustration to gratification can be reminiscent of the experience of childhood when the mother attempts to keep the baby's frustration to a minimum by anticipating and gratifying all wishes. A little cry from the baby immediately brings everybody in the environment to identifying and responding to the baby's wishes. It is this regression, a return to the state of security and freedom from fear, that revives the old childhood wishes that never die. This is the latent and universal wish in the individual—to be taken care of and mothered.[2,3] The fact that alcohol can bring such a wish fulfillment is illustrated in such statements as, "Now I am not afraid of anything or anyone." "I can do anything I wish." "Nothing can happen to me."

With theories and psychodynamics in mind, one factor stands at the forefront: alcoholism is self-destructive behavior or at least represents a self-destructive tendency. Alcoholics appear to be willing actively, consciously, unconsciously, and repeatedly to damage themselves. The self-destructive drinking is a deliberate, strategic maneuver to accomplish certain ends. Exploration to find out what these are is a major part of the therapeutic endeavor.

According to Aristotle, the plot of a good tragedy contains three parts: prologue, climax, and catastrophe. These three stages correspond to the onset, course, and outcome of the disease of alcoholism. The prologue in the alcoholic's life may be childhood and the development of certain personality traits or a self-destructive lifestyle. The climax is the period in adulthood when the alcoholic struggles against the control of the developing illness and the loss of autonomy. The battle is between two forces—the self-destructive tendency and the wish to avoid the catastrophe. The climax yields, often suddenly, to the catastrophe, when the person relaxes the battle against the self-destructive tendency and surrenders to the bondage of alcoholism. (See Chapter 10 for further discussion of the psychodynamic factors.)

FAMILY DYNAMICS

Role Assignment or the Projection Process

All kinds of role assignments are made in families in order to make a family member appear to be someone different from who he is or to serve some particular purpose in the family.[4] This is a fascinating aspect of family dynamics and enhances our understanding of both illness and health in a family. As has already been mentioned, families choose a member to be sick, to hold the marriage together, to be the black sheep, clown, or scapegoat. We do not understand the many complicated factors that determine whether a given family member accepts the designated role, fights it, internalizes it, pretends to accept it, flees from it, or is in conflict with it. Some symptoms are developed as a function of efforts to escape the role assignment and others as reflections of the designations. Some symptoms are manifested only within the family culture, while others come into play only outside the family. A family member is often heard to say, "When I am not with my family, I am an entirely different person."

Also, the family projection process can diagnose, classify, and assign characteristics to certain family members. A wife may label her husband (a moderate drinker) as alcoholic. The wife's label is accepted by the children and transmitted to the grandchildren. The concept described here should be kept in mind when working with the alcoholic and family. The illness may contribute profoundly to both the family's equilibrium and disequilibrium.

Role Reversals in the Family

Karpman writes that only three roles are necessary in drama analysis to depict the emotional reversals that are drama—Persecutor, Rescuer, and Victim.[5] Drama begins when these roles are established or anticipated. The real drama relates to the switch in the roles. Fairy tales are simple but excellent examples of the switching in action roles. Think of Cinderella, Little Red Riding Hood, or the Pied Piper. The Pied Piper begins as Rescuer of the city and Persecutor of the rats. He then becomes Victim of the Persecutor mayor's doublecross (fee withheld) and in revenge switches to the Persecutor of the city's children. The mayor switches from Victim (of rats) to Rescuer (hiring the Pied Piper) to Persecutor (doublecross) to Victim (his children dead). The children switch from Persecuted Victims (by rats) to Rescued Victims to Victims Persecuted by their Rescuer.

Think now of the family in which the illness of alcoholism resides in one or more of its members. Picture the numerous circumstances or changes that precipitate a role reversal. Most likely the alcoholic will switch periodically from victim to rescuer to persecutor—and likewise there will be reversals in the roles of the other members of the family, especially the spouse. Also, there will be reversals in the role of the therapist.

Do Alcoholics' Self-destructive Lifestyles Originate in their Early Years in their Families?

The alcoholic in his drinking behavior is following a self-destructive path. How one tries to determine why the alcoholic is self-destructive will depend on one's conceptual framework and therapeutic persuasion. It is tempting to believe that the alcoholic's lifestyle is the living out of a parental injunction or message from in childhood, such as, "Don't be," or, "Don't be important," or, "Don't belong." Of course, there are many ways of being self-destructive; thus a number of other factors contribute to the use of alcohol when it is chosen as the agent of self-destruction.

The parental message brings to mind a patient who sought help because he was hearing voices. There were two voices—a male and female. The male voice usually spoke harshly to him and commanded him to do something detrimental to himself, such as, "Step in front of that moving car." The male and female voices often spoke to one another. If the male voice said, "Let's kill the son-of-a-bitch," the female voice would advise caution, "We better not; we could get into big trouble." While the male voice was openly hostile and destructive, the female voice generally cautioned restraint, not for the patient's sake but for their own protection. The patient found relief from these voices by reading the Bible. He would read until he came to an especially powerful verse. At that point the voices would scream, "Let's get the hell out of here before we get into trouble." This patient was an alcoholic, which he was slow in revealing. He had a bout of "intestinal flu" and could take essentially nothing by mouth for several days, including alcohol. By the time he recovered from the "flu," he was hallucinating. A review of his family history revealed that his mother was pregnant with him at the time of marriage. His parents did not want him and communicated this message to him throughout his years of dependency on them. Further exploration identified many other traits, and the family sources of these, seen frequently in alcoholics.

This patient's case history is mentioned only to raise the issue of when and where the alcoholic's self-destructive lifestyle originated and to encourage the therapist to look at the family as the possible source. Of course, why alcohol is chosen as an instrument to feed the self-destructive tendency deserves continued study. No single factor will emerge in answer to the *why*. Availability of alcohol, family and subculture's attitudes toward alcohol, personality makeup, aspirations, and numerous significant life history events are among the relevant variables.

General Systems Model

General systems theory is having considerable impact today on group and family therapy. The systems approach conceives of the individual as a dynamic system in constant interaction with an ever-changing environment.

Altering the family system, and hence the transactions between the persons (subsystems) who are part of the larger system, results in changes in the individual. Thus change at any point in the system may well affect any or all of its components. In other words, transactions within the family system are major determinants of individual behavior. Also, a change in the functioning of one family member is automatically followed by a compensatory change in another family member.

Much of the alcoholic's behavior and symptoms are products of family processes, which influence and are influenced by each family member's intrapsychic dynamics. Accordingly, processes and changes in the family, rather than insights alone, are seen as the major change-producing agents, although techniques for achieving such change vary greatly.

Thus the general systems model considers the alcoholic and his symptoms as part of communication within social systems (like the family or other units). The alcoholic may be seen as playing a symptomatic role that the family needs. Individual diagnosis may be a stigma that once stated or publicized immediately effects a change in family relationships, or it may constitute a self-fulfilling prophecy, thereby becoming part of treatment rather than merely of evaluation.

THERAPY WITH THE FAMILY

Combinations of individual and group therapy—involving many types of therapies—have proven to be effective in the treatment of alcoholics and their families. Space does not permit a discussion of these modalities or the new developments in them as described in books such as *Progress in Group and Family Therapy*, edited by Sager and Kaplan.[6]

If the alcoholic is married and has children, in each stage of recovery the interactions with spouse and children change. At times these interactions become so complex and intense that the members of the family not only expect, but almost seem to wish, that the alcoholic would resume drinking. This phenomenon is more easily understood if one views alcoholism in the conceptual framework of transactional analysis: alcoholism is a game, and a game requires several players in order to be sustained.[7] The spouse and children of the alcoholic, participating at some level in the alcoholic's behavioral patterns, feel a vacuum in their lives when the alcoholic stops drinking, equal to that felt by the alcoholic. Thus alcoholics in families may feel even stronger urges to drink because, in addition to their own internal proclivities, they will feel the pressures applied from the families. Since treatment of married alcoholics requires bringing about change in two or more people, it may appear at times that single alcoholics have better prognoses in treatment. This added burden of treatment by the presence of a family is usually overshadowed, however, by the positive influence that families are able to provide. While thinking at times that a certain alcoholic might profit by a separation or divorce because of the difficulties mentioned above, one usually finds that if this difficulty is worked through, the family is a great adjunct to the patient's health as a source for fulfillment of many needs and as a basis for existential meaning.

Initial Approaches with the Family

The health of each member of the alcoholic's family should be checked. Any member of the family could be physically or emotionally ill.

All family members should make in-depth appraisals of themselves, their positions in the family, and the character of relationships within the family.

Discuss without delay the family's drinking problem. Find out how it affects each member of the family and how the individual members of the family and the family as a whole affect the alcoholic's drinking.

Try to identify the strengths in the family and help the family mobilize these strengths in a positive direction.

Honestly examine one's own feelings and attitudes about drinking, drunkenness, and the family. The therapist's value system should not dictate the goals for the family, but the therapist can help the family identify and clarify its own goals.

The task of therapy is to create an environment for change, an environment where each family member can make a decision to change his life, to act the part of an autonomous person.

The therapist is an expert in human behavior disturbance and its remedy. With the family in the crisis of alcoholism, the therapist should be *active* in helping all family members discover their problems. (One can overdo the technique of letting patients discover their own problems.) Self-discovery can be awfully slow at times. Why not identify the problems of the family and its members as quickly as possible and get to work on them?

Therapy with the Family Unit

Since the patient's illness is often symptomatic of family psychopathology, some of the problems are more easily worked through with the total family unit rather than on an individual or couple basis. Family therapy is a growing area for exploration. Many clinicians have found that individual therapy can be accelerated by complementary conjoint family therapy. Although the members of the family indicate that they want the patient to get well, "well" means different things to the patient, to the relatives, and to the staff. Often the concept of being well on the part of the relatives means that the patient is to function much like a puppet, carrying out both the expressed and the unexpressed wishes of the family members without observable behavioral disruption. The family may see the hospital or clinic role to solidify and replaster the quality of relative-patient fusion as it was prior to the alcoholic disorder. Also, there may exist a common delusion, shared by both the patient and the family and reinforced by years of living together, that emotional separation and growth can lead only to eventual destruction.

In the treatment of the alcoholic and family, the therapist must not forget the axion about family dynamics mentioned above: "A family is an autocracy ruled by its sickest member." The situations in which one family member is put forth as the ostensible patient are really special cases in which the real patient may be reluctant to ask for help or to face what is bothering him. Thus the patient seeks help in a disguised and more acceptable way. While the request or call for help is the essential feature of a person's becoming a patient, it is a call that is often muted, disguised, or alloyed with ambivalence. One of the oldest techniques for a family to get help is to choose, and offer as the patient a family scapegoat, with the hope, often unconscious, that the scapegoat will lead the therapist back to the sick family.

Treatment of Couples

Because of the factors previously emphasized, group therapy with married couples has proven to be quite an effective treatment modality.[8] In such treatment programs the goals are (1) penetration of the patient's severe denial mechanism in association with the goal of abstinence, and (2) helping the couple to develop a satisfactory living experience in their marriage. In group meetings the "here and now" approach to treatment is greatly emphasized. Honest, direct impressions of other patients in the group are consistently requested of the couples. These involve opinions regarding improvement, attitudes toward spouse, identification of destructive or constructive behavior, and so on.

Group therapy involving married couples is usually successful because of a number of factors. The spouse of the patient helps in "pulling" the patient back to treatment, and the dropout rate is lower as a result of the spouse's cooperation. (Neither the patient nor the spouse can say, "I am the only one who is trying in the marriage.") There is a common goal of abstinence to unify the group. (After abstinence, the next goal is to have the couples work on their marital problems.) Both therapists and group members get a more realistic view of the home life of each participant by observing the marital interactions, verbal and nonverbal communications as well as feelings and mood. The therapists and group can refuse to accept the distortions of both husband and wife and thereby aid in the correction of the neurotic interaction.The initial neurotic needs that may have attracted the partners to each other in the hope of gratifying dependent or narcissistic tendencies can now be faced and treated in an open manner. With both marital partners present, minor bickering is eliminated and the crucial and urgent problems of the couple are directly faced. In individual therapy, minor bickering can consume the greater part of therapy, consisting usually of perpetual complaints about the spouse. All of the expected problems associated with recovery emerge in the group discussions and can be dealt with effectively and together.

In the group one often sees the psychodynamics of the spouse unfold in dramatic self-relevation. One gets a new appreciation of the spouse types such as the parental type or "mama or papa with sex," the managerial type, the martyr, the child type, the rescuer, etc. Let us look at some of these types as manifested by female partners, although they apply equally well to males.

The motherly type is competitive with her own mother and guilty about her femininity and about expressing it. This probably grows out of an old oedipal conflict in which she competed with her mother for the love and attention of the father. At the same time, she can offer sex plus what every mother usually offers. The motherly type is a controlling type who creates exactly the kind of home she wants, although it may be quite different from what her husband or children want. In the novel *The Pleasure of His Company* by Samuel Taylor and Cornelia Otis Skinner, Mackenzie Savage, the father, is quizzed by his daughter: "You were never very happy with Mother, were you?" He replies, "Your mother was a saint, who made our home an outpost of heaven. It's why I spent so much time in saloons."

The managerial type dominates every aspect of the marriage. (At other times she is forced to be managerial because of her husband's alcoholism.) The marriage may be only a vehicle for expressing the wife's distrustful, resentful attitudes toward men in general. In her view of life, men have the advantages. Why risk marrying one over whom you do not have some advantage? Therefore her husband's ineptitude is not only acceptable but even gratifying—up to a point. This type of woman often marries a person she perceives as inadequate, a cripple. She tends to be coldly angry in presenting her complaints about her husband's problems, and there is a quality of hardness and unforgivingness in her manner of expressing criticisms. Such a woman rejects her femininity, is distrustful of human relationships, and grasps for advantage or superior position in all her dealings with the world around her. When a therapist looks beneath the surface of this type of woman, he sees her fearfulness, her anxiety, and her strong dependency needs. When she feels secure with the therapist, she musters the courage to examine her feelings.

The martyr type is actually a sadomasochistic person. The masochistic side of the wife suffers the spouse's alcoholism. The sadistic tendencies in the same type of wife cause her to strike out at the alcoholic when he is drunk. Thus the wife is someone to scold him when he is bad, to think and plan for him when he is puzzled, to extricate him from his binges, and, above all, to worry and suffer over him.

The child-wife may be young chronologically or emotionally. Since both partners may be children emotionally, they cannot fulfill one another's needs.

The rescuer type of wife will be found among those women who repeatedly choose alcoholic, impotent, or unfaithful husbands. In many of these women, there is the history of an alcoholic father. On analysis it becomes clear that the unconscious goal of the marriage was to cure the father's alcoholism in effigy, thus winning back the lost affection of the alcoholic father, while proving at the same time that she could do a better job than the mother. The need to rescue may have other dimensions, as seen in the play *Brigadoon*.[9] Two friends are wandering in an enchanted wood where a lost city appears on one night each 100 years. They pause to rest, and a conversation ensues:

Jeff: Maybe we took the high road instead of the low road. *(Takes a flask from his inside pocket.)* Would you like a drink?

Tommy: No thanks.

Jeff: Good. That leaves more for me. *(He unscrews the top.)*

Tommy: Didn't you tell me you were going to cut down on that stuff?
Jeff: Yes, I did. But I'm a terrible liar. Besides it doesn't pay. I remember one time I was going with a wonderful girl and she used to plead with me and plead with me to give it up. So one day I did. Then we discovered we had nothing more to talk about, so we broke up.*

The game was over, the game that supplied him with care and attention, and her with a maternal gratification without the problems of intimacy. Both roles, rescuer and rescued, are required. It has been observed that the recovery of the alcoholic may herald the onset of a depressive or psychotic illness in the nonalcoholic spouse, thus reversing the roles of rescuer and rescued. Since a rescuer usually does not have overwhelming numbers to rescue, the subject must be rescued over and over again—like a child with an only toy, or the overprotective mother with an only child.

Just as revealing is the marital game playing of the addicted person, as discussing in Scott's *Struggles in an Alcoholic Family*.[10] Scott writes of the Bitter-Sweet Masquerade, the Egyptian Sphinx, Blue Ribbon Robert, the Bedroom Adult, the Scorekeeper, and the Babe in the Woods. A few words about each of these types are indicated.

In the *Bitter-Sweet Masquerade*, the person offers a sweet disposition to the outside world but a bitter one to the family. This puts the spouse in an awkward position.

The *Egyptian Sphinx* is calm and unperturbed amid the storm of problems he creates. Only when the spouse issues an ultimatum does the sphinx come to life.

Blue Ribbon Robert has given up drinking. Now the spouse had better get busy and get rid of his neuroses, or Robert will begin drinking again. This person uses sobriety as a club to beat down the mate. Having won a blue ribbon, Robert assumes no responsibility for restoring harmony to the household.

The *Bedroom Adult* establishes claim to adulthood principally through sex. The spouse's feelings are ignored. Denial of sex is an excuse for more drinking.

Babes in the Woods refer to very immature partners in a marriage. Although both husband and wife are adults from the physical point of view, each is an immature, pouting, stubborn, frightened child expecting to be supported by the other.

The *Scorekeeper* in the marital game keeps score on the other partner and seems never to forget the endless number of injustices each partner inflicts on the other.

A special word is in order at this point about the resistances related to sexual matters in the home. In the typical marriage undergoing stress, sex is frequently not the focal point of disagreement—rather it is the bargaining table. The typical husband may say, "Let's jump into bed, and this will help us solve our problems." The wife may respond, "Let's solve our problems, and then jump into bed." The alcoholic husband may complain about the lack of the wife's response to his sexual overtures. Her reply may be, "How can I be romantic and responsive to

---

*Reprinted from Lerner AJ, Loewe F: *Brigadoon*. New York, Coward, McCann & Geohegan, Inc, 1974, p 5. By permission of Alan Jay Lerner.

your advances when awakened at 3:00 A.M. on your return home from a drinking bout?" Furthermore, the alcoholic confuses priorities in sexual as well as other matters, as illustrated by the statement of a member of Alcoholics Anonymous: "When I sat down at the table I wanted to make love, and when I went to bed I was hungry and wanted to eat."

Special Problem Areas with the Spouse

Although many of the relationships and attitudes of the spouse have already been discussed, a few other areas deserve mentioning. The physician ought to have ground rules worked out for relating to the alcoholic's spouse and may prefer to work only with the alcoholic in a confidential relationship, as long as the alcoholic accepts responsibility for himself. The treatment covenant thereby exists between the physician and the alcoholic, and nothing is shared with a "significant other" as long as the agreements between therapist and patient are kept. When alcoholics demonstrate that they cannot accept responsibility for themselves, then the physician brings the spouses into the treatment picture. The physician must make known the treatment approach to both alcoholic and spouse at the beginning of therapy and let each know how relationships with the spouse will differ when the alcoholic is responsible and when the alcoholic is drinking. Another physician, equally successful in treating alcoholism, may include the spouse in many facets of the therapy from the beginning irrespective of the level of responsibility assumed by the alcoholic.

A problem seen not infrequently is a spouse's "theft" from the alcoholic of A. A. activities. The spouse attends with the alcoholic all A. A. meetings, instead of those of Al-Anon, and never lets the alcoholic really become involved in the A. A. process. The spouse gradually emerges as a competitor with A. A., thereby depriving the alcoholic of the benefits of A. A. participation. In most situations of this type, the alcoholic eventually drops out of A. A.

The physician's relationship to the spouse may be complicated at times by overt or covert attempts at seduction of the physician. Furthermore, the spouse may accuse the physician of attempting seduction, and this may relate to efforts to bolster waning self-esteem. Of course, when the alcoholic is of the opposite sex from the physician, the spouse may accuse the physician of trying to seduce the alcoholic. How and why such accusations arise in the treatment situation relate to the nature of the treatment process and emotional needs of all parties involved, including the physician.

The enabler, the spouse who takes care of the alcoholic time and time again and who seems to need this type of sick relationship, has contributed much to the psychodynamic understanding of alcoholism. A few of the spouse types discussed earlier share some similar characteristics with the enabler.

The question is often asked, should abstinence of the spouse be insisted upon? The only truly successful approach is total abstinence for alcoholic and spouse, and both should accept this goal and work toward it. Attainment of this goal means no alcohol in the house and that the nonalcoholic spouse must give up drinking entirely. The couple must be helped to plan a social and family life that encourages abstinence.

The Healing Fellowship of Al-Anon

Alcoholism is recognized as a family disease, capable of impairing the emotional and physical health of any member in the family. Al-Anon is a fellowship of spouses, relatives, and friends of alcoholics—mostly the people who are affected by living with an alcoholic. The Al-Anon Family Groups exist to help restore the family of the alcoholic to a measure of stability. Al-Anon can supplement profoundly the family's own efforts in helping each member of a family.

The physician and any other professional working with alcoholics should be aware of Al-Anon's aims, methods of operation, and accomplishments. The best way to become acquainted with the teachings of Al-Anon and the different facets of its program is to attend some of its meetings. In fact, the physician cannot comprehend the impact of Al-Anon's workings without such attendance. Furthermore, the meetings will furnish the physician an opportunity to gather some insights about alcoholism that may not be available from any other source—insights that will be gripping both intellectually and emotionally.

Al-Anon emerged from its early stages as an adjunct of Alcoholics Anonymous and incorporated in 1952 as a separate fellowship known as the Al-Anon Family Group Headquarters, Inc. The only requirement for membership is that the person has been, or is being, deeply affected by close contact with an alcoholic. Members pay no dues, and contributions are voluntary.

Local Al-Anon groups are active in educational and public relations work within their communities, cooperating with all agencies or resources involved in the treatment of alcoholism. Also, the Al-Anon groups, through regular meetings and personal contact, help the relatives of alcoholics to (1) learn the facts about alcoholism as a disease and about the treatment process, (2) benefit from the therapeutic experience of personal contact with other members who have the same problem, and (3) improve their own attitudes and personalities by the study and practice of the suggested "Twelve Steps," adopted from Alcoholics Anonymous.[11]

The basic ideas of Al-Anon, like those of Alcoholics Anonymous, are the concepts on which all spiritual philosophies are based. The working philosophy of Al-Anon forms a pattern for right living, for overcoming difficulties, and for helping persons achieve their aspirations. People come to Al-Anon to solve the specific problem of alcoholism and its disastrous effect on their lives. They apply the basic spiritual ideas by means of the "Twelve Steps." These are augmented or reinforced by the "Twelve Traditions," the "Serenity Prayer," and the concepts known simply as the "Slogans."

From experience with an Al-Anon group, the members learn about improving their own thinking and attitudes. What they need to learn varies from person to person. A woman expressed it this way:[12]

> The first thing I really learned was that I must bring myself to release my husband and my children from my direction and domination . . . The second important thing I learned

was to release myself from the need for my husband's approval and fear of his disapproval. I do what I do for free, with no strings attached; I have to be myself, and do the best I can with what I have . . . . I have learned to live by the Twelve Steps. The Fourth suggests an inventory of ourselves, and this is certainly of vital importance. There is some danger, however, of concentrating too much on digging for defects of character. Perhaps it would be more constructive to regard our defects as character traits channeled in the wrong direction. . . . I found that working the Twelve Steps helped me to rechannel those traits into constructive rather than destructive attitudes.*

This is a vivid testimony to the effectiveness of Al-Anon in helping its members learn to live through living with Al-Anon.

CHILDREN AND PARENTAL ALCOHOLISM

Probably the greatest cost of alcoholism relates to the disruption and disorganization of the family. Frightening to contemplate is the price children must pay in bewilderment, humiliation, physical neglect or abuse, and emotional deprivation. Alcoholism takes a toll in another way in the alarming frequency with which alcoholism tends to recur within families. Some authorities estimate that as many as 50 percent of alcoholics come from families where alcoholism was a problem. While a particular percentage figure may be hard to substantiate with firm data, at least it can be said that the children of alcoholics are much more likely to become alcoholics than the children of nonalcoholics. With conflicting customs and feelings about alcohol in their family and society in general, the children of an alcoholic parent have a good chance of growing up either in a broken home or in one in which they experience profound inconsistencies in their relationships with both parents. Children of an alcoholic are vulnerable to the influence of a poor or inadequate model—an alcoholic who is their parent. They see a parent coping with stress by using alcohol.

It is difficult for children of alcoholics to escape emotional problems. The severity of these will depend on factors such as the age of the children at the onset of parental alcoholism, the social class level of the parent, the sex of the alcoholic parent (emotional scarring is usually greater if the mother is the alcoholic), the quality of the relationship with the alcoholic parent, and the strength of the nonalcoholic parent. Other factors to consider in measuring the crippling impact of parental alcoholism are the inherited temperament and intelligence of the children, level of education and economic security of the family, the personality and maturity of the nonalcoholic parent, and whether or not the alcoholic parent has brought the drinking under control.

Some of the family situations that are quite disturbing to the children of alcoholics include the following:

1. The shift in or reversal of parental roles. When the alcoholic parent is drink-

*Reprinted from *Al-Anon Faces Acoholism*. New York. Al-Anon Family Group Headquarters, 1965, p. 179

ing, the nonalcoholic parent takes over his or her family responsibilities, regardless of what they may be.

2. Inconsistencies in the affection, support, and security offered by one or both parents. These inconsistencies can have a profound impact on the children's own sense of security and self-worth. The alcoholic who is often kind and considerate, sometimes overbearingly affectionate, when sober may become cruel or withdrawn when drinking. The nonalcoholic parent, responding to contrasting mood swings in the alcoholic spouse, may appear equally inconsistent and disturbed to the children while conveying to them that it is only because of her that the family is able to survive. Children may be unable to evaluate the situation in their home and unwilling to blame either parent. They often withdraw into a noncommital attitude that makes it difficult to communicate. Exposed to a fluctuating conversational level at home, ranging from morose silence to wild ravings in their parents, the children become more and more withdrawn, with a breakdown in verbal communication.
3. A disturbed nonalcoholic parent who is inadequate with the children. This parent is obsessed with the drinking of the spouse, lonely and frustrated in not having personal needs met in the marital relationship, and therefore unable to meet the emotional needs of the children.
4. Increased social isolation of the family and a sense of personal alienation. The children stop bringing friends home because of the embarrassment and humiliation when their visitors are confronted by a drunken parent. As the family turns in upon itself and feeds on the problems, the children are cut off from the support and healing of their peers.

Some children may not withdraw into their sick home setting but use a variety of methods to remove themselves from an alcoholic parent. An adolescent seen at juvenile court had been breaking into boats at the waterfront and also setting fires. Once he left his wallet, containing his name and address—in order to be caught, it must be assumed. His father had deserted the family, and the mother had begun drinking heavily. He often had to put his mother to bed or bathe her. Once when she admonished him about repeatedly getting into trouble, he replied. "Mom, I'll make a deal with you. If you stop drinking, I promise to behave and get into no more trouble." This adolescent found his home so unbearable that his antisocial behavior was a way of getting out of the family and into an institution. Nobody would interpret his removal from the family in this way as his really wanting to leave. Actually wanting to leave would carry implications of being disloyal to his family, of abandoning them in a time of great trouble.

Children of alcoholics frequently suffer from a behavior disorder with neurotic traits. The alcoholic parent is usually not a psychopath but has a conscience and feelings and shows them. After an alcoholic spree, guilt motivates the alcoholic parent to try to do better toward the children, giving them hope that he will change. The frequent swing from high hopes to shattering disappointments, owing to the inconsistent behavior of the alcoholic, may build up in the children such a basic distrust that all their later intimate relationships will be colored or distorted.

In spite of the inconsistency of the parent's overall behavior, during the periods of sobriety the children have strong feelings of identification with the alcoholic parent. This identification helps the children develop consciences. At the point at which they have to hate the parent because of the alcoholic sprees, they become guilty. They react strongly to this ambivalence and handle it by acting out. Such children do a great deal of acting out and at the same time show considerable hypochondriasis and other neurotic symptoms.

The end result in these children is a psychological disturbance composed of a reactive disorder (reactive to physical and emotional neglect) and of guilt-ridden feelings in terms of their hate of the alcoholic parent that they also love. This blend of reactive behavior and of internal conflict with guilt is diagnosed as a behavior disorder with neurotic traits.

Such a disorder will express itself in many ways. Children may cower in a corner, outwardly conforming, or they may rebel and become defiant or delinquent. Combined with their acting out, they may express the classic symptoms of the hypochondriac, as well as other neurotic symptoms. Feeding the neurotic symptoms will be the ambivalent feelings of love and hate, the sense of deep personal rejection (for example, "If my father really loved me, he would not drink"), neglect or sudden withdrawals of love produced by liquor, and so on. Guilt in its rawest form may come from what appears to the children as a betrayal of the parent. When children become old enough to be aware of persons outside their immediate family, they have also become aware of the condemnation of the alcoholic by society, and they react with shame and humiliation. They feel isolated, estranged, and different. When their alcoholic parent is jeered or laughed at, they may try to defend him out of love. Usually, however, they cannot bring themselves to make such defense, and they feel guilty over what seems to them a betrayal of their parent.

The neurotic traits of the children of the alcoholic parent often bring the children into profound conflict with the alcoholic parent. Not infrequently, the alcoholic parent goes into psychotherapy because of inability to tolerate the neurotic children.

Treatment of the Children of the Alcoholic

In the treatment of such children, the goal is to help them find a long-term relationship in order for them to develop trust and rid themselves of their acting out. Through this sustained relationship, the children are helped to work through their conflicts and guilt. This is accomplished first in relation to the therapist and in group experiences such as that afforded by Alateen or Al-Anon. Then through such therapeutic experiences, conflicts and guilt are resolved regarding the alcoholic parent.

In treatment of the children who live in an alcoholic family situation, the therapist should not forget Alateen. Alateen is for the 12–20 year-old age group and is an outgrowth of Al-Anon, the worldwide fellowship for relatives and friends of alcoholics. The first Alateen group was started in 1957 by a youth in California whose father was an alcoholic, but sober and active in Alcoholics Anonymous. His mother was a member of an Al-Anon family group, and he modeled Alateen after the Al-Anon ideas and principles. Each Alateen group is sponsored by a member of Al-Anon (at times co-sponsored by a member of A.A.) who is present at meetings but who does not participate unless invited to express an opinion or answer a question.

The purpose of Alateen is to discuss the difficulties teenagers face when they live in the destructive environment of alcoholism. The teenagers exchange experiences, encourage and help each other understand the principles of Alateen, and learn effective ways of coping with their own problems. Alateen's group therapy, like that of Alcoholics Anonymous and Al-Anon, is based on the well-known A.A. "Twelve Steps," which the teenagers discuss and apply to their own attitudes and relationships with others. The members of the group receive from each other understanding of their problems and feelings and emotional support, which facilitates change of attitude and behavior. They also receive basic information about alcoholism as a disease and the recovery process. As they gain perspective on their common problems, they change their way of thinking, and their behavior becomes more realistic. They develop feelings of security, in part because of the structuring that Alateen has brought to what had been a chaotic life situation.

In the treatment process, the therapist must remember that it is not easy to help the children unless the family cooperates in a total rehabilitation program. Assistance obtained from outside the family can be neutralized and rendered ineffectual by a continuing state of insecurity at home. Thus it is imperative that the alcoholic problem itself be tackled first, if at all possible.

In serious cases where the alcoholic is chronically drunk and repeatedly refuses to seek help, removal of the children from the home may be advisable. Drastic steps such as removal of the children from the home, separation, or divorce may be needed to awaken the alcoholic to the "eleventh hour" of the situation.

Children tolerate the family crisis better if they understand and accept the concept of alcoholism as a disease. When children understand their parent's struggle or "the dark journey of the soul," their shame can turn to pride and admiration, their defiance to obedience, their resentment to love. The feeling of hopelessness and isolation is replaced by a feeling of being needed and useful. Furthermore, upon learning of the nature of alcoholism, they may play a crucial role in persuading a parent to seek treatment. Such is the testimony of many children who have gone through this experience. For those just beginning in the work with alcoholics and their families, it is imperative to read the literature from Alateen, Al-Anon, and Alcoholics Anonymous and to attend their meetings. Also, the alcoholic, the family, and the therapist may be encouraged by the words of Francis Fenelon, 17th century French writer and cleric: "As light increases we see ourselves to be worse than we thought. . . . Bear in mind, for your comfort, that we only perceive our malady when the cure begins."

CONCLUSION

Recently, in a class in medical ethics, I asked the medical students to identify some ethical problems that are often over-looked or not identified as ethical problems in the practice of medicine. One medical student responded by saying that before coming to and during medical school he had worked, on numerous occasions, in the admission and emergency rooms of several hospitals and had noted a common response to the alcoholic—overt or covert hostility—that influenced profoundly the treatment given or not given. He also noted that if the alcoholic's family, or what appeared to be the family, brought the patient in, the response and the treatment were much better and often as humane and professional as if the problem had been other than alcoholism.

One can draw from this story many implications. It is another testimony to the value of the alcoholic's family in the alcoholic's treatment and recovery. The story also calls for a reassessment of our values in regard to our fellow humans in both sickness and health. The alcoholic is a person, belonging to a specific family and in broader terms to the family of humankind. This kinship, this relationship has been especially illuminated by John Steinbeck's *Burning Bright.*[13]

Burning Bright concerns Joe Saul, who desperately wanted a child but who did not know that his seed was dead. The desire that was strongest in him—would it go forever unfulfilled? His wife Mordeen knew he was sterile but loved him deeply, and out of her great love and without his knowledge, she turned to another man to give her husband the child he wanted. About the time Mordeen was going into labor, Joe discovered through a physician's examination of his sperm that he was sterile and unable to father a child. At that moment his joy turned to ashes, and he walked into the darkest night of his life. Then he found himself at the hospital where Mordeen had delivered. He was given a surgical mask and gown and allowed to enter the room. In the conversation that took place between them, she, although half asleep, realized that he knew the secret and understood. Her eyes were clearing now as she came from under the influence of the anesthetic. Follow carefully what took place between the two:

> "I know," he said, "I had to walk into the black to know—to know that every man is father to all children and every child must have all men as father. This is not a little piece of private property, registered and fenced and separated. Mordeen! This is *the Child.*"

Mordeen said, "It is very dark. Turn up the light. Let me have light. I cannot see your face."

"Light," he said, "You want light? I will give you light." He tore the mask from his face, and his face was shining and his eyes were shining. "Mordeen," he said, "I love the child." His voice swelled and he spoke loudly. "Mordeen, I love our child." And he raised his head and cried in triumph, "Mordeen, *I love my son*."*

This sense of family, of kinship, of community, of belonging as expressed by John Steinbeck, is the tie that binds us to alcoholics and holds them in the family of humankind. And each of us can say: my mother, my father the alcoholic; my brother, my sister the alcoholic; my husband, my wife the alcoholic; my son, my daughter the alcoholic. This is the basis of our responsibility to the alcoholic.

REFERENCE

1. McClelland D, Davis WN, Kalin R, Wanner E. *The Drinking Man: Alcohol and Human Motivation*. New York, Free Press, 1972
2. Pearson, MM, Little RB: The addictive process in unusual addictions: A further elaboration of etiology. *Am J Psychiatry* 125:8, 1969
3. Rado S: Narcotic bondage—A general theory of the dependence on narcotic drugs. *Am J Psychiatry* 114:165–170, 1957
4. Framo JL: Symptoms from a family transactional viewpoint, in Sager CJ, Kaplan HS (eds): *Progress in Group and Family Therapy*. New York, Brunner-Mazel, 1972, pp 277–284
5. Karpman SB: Fairy tales and script analysis. *Transact Anal Bull* 7:39–43, 1968
6. Sager CJ, Kaplan HS (eds): *Progress in Group and Family Therapy*. New York. Brunner-Mazel, 1972
7. Steiner C. *Games Alcoholics Play*. New York, Grove Press, 1971
8. Gallant DM, Rich A, Bey E, Terranova L: Group psychotherapy with married couples: A successful technique in New Orleans alcoholism clinic patients. *J La State Med Soc* 122:41–44, 1970
9. Lerner AJ, Loewe F: *Brigadoon*. New York, Coward, McCann & Geohegan, Inc, 1947, p 5
10. Scott EM: *Struggles in an Alcoholic Family*. Springfield, Ill., Charles C. Thomas, 1970, pp 94–97
11. *Al-Anon—Family Treatment Tool in Alcoholism*. New York, Al-Anon Family Group Headquarters, 1971
12. *Al-Anon Faces Alcoholism*. New York, Al-Anon Family Group Headquarters, 1965, p 179
13. Steinbeck J. *Burning Bright*. New York, Bantam Books, 1950

*Reprinted from Steinbeck J: *Burning Bright*. New York, Bantam Books, 1950, pp 129-130. By permission of Viking Penguin, Inc. Copyright, 1950, by John Steinbeck.

BIBLIOGRAPHY

1. Ackerman, R. *Children of Alcoholics: A Guidebook for Educators, Therapists, and Parents*. Second Edition. Holmes Beach, Florida, Learning Publications, 1983
2. Black, C. *It Will Never Happen To Me*. Denver, Colorado, M.A.C., 1981
3. Kaufman, E. Family System Variables in Alcoholism. *Alcoholism: Clinical and Experimental Research*. Vol. 8, #1, pp. 4–8, 1984

Appendix A: Sedative-Hypnotic Drugs

The drugs listed below exhibit cross-addiction and cross-tolerance with ethanol. It is uncommon to find a patient dependent upon stimulants (amphetamines, cocaine) who is not simultaneously dependent upon ethanol and/or the following substances.

Special care must be exercised to avoid the use of many muscle relaxants, cough suppressants, as well as cold and headache remedies in patients with alcohol or other drug dependencies. Many of these incorporate soporific and/or stimulant drugs not unlike those listed below. Occasionally they even include narcotic analgesics.

Barbiturates: phenobarbital (Luminal), amobarbital (Amytal), pentobarbital (Nembutal),secobarbital (Seconal), butabarbital (Butisol), and so forth; also combinations of these (Tuinal=Seconal+ Amytal) or barbiturates with other drugs (Fiorinal, Dexamyl, etc.).

Benzodiazepines ("minor tranquilizers"): diazepam (Valium), chlordiazepoxide (Librium), flurazepam (Dalmane), lorazepam (Ativan), chlorazepate (Tranzene), prazepam (Verstran), oxazepam (Serax), alprazolam (Xanax), triazolam (Halcion), clonazepam (Klonopin), temazepam (Restoril), and mixtures of these with nonsoporific drugs (Librax, Limbitrol, Menrium, etc.).

ALCOHOLISM:
A Practical Treatment Guide
ISBN 0-8089-1912-1

Others: meprobamate (Miltown, Equanil), chloral hydrate (Noctec, Somnor), glutethimide (Doriden), methaqualone (Quaalude, Sopor, Parest, Somnafac), methyprylon (Noludar), methocarbamol (Robaxin), ethchlorvynol (Placidyl), paraldehyde, bromides, and such anesthetics as nitrous oxide, ether, chloroform, and so on, and mixtures of these with nonsoporific drugs (Milpath, Pathibamate, Deprol, etc.).

Ethyl Alcohol, other alcohols, and organic solvents.

Appendix B: Criteria for the Diagnosis of Alcoholism

These criteria were compiled by a committee of medical authorities from the National Council on Alcoholism to establish guidelines for the proper diagnosis and evlauation of this disease. Criteria are weighted for diagnostic significance and assembled according to types: Physiological and Clinical (including major alcohol-associated illnesses) and Behavioral, Psychological, and Attitudinal. Because early diagnosis is helpful in treatment and recovery, manifestations are separated into their earlier and later phases. There are brief discussions of recurrent and arrested alcoholism, cross-dependence, and the types of persons at high risk of alcoholism.

The problem of alcoholism has been receiving increasing interest in the past few years. Extensive treatment programs are being mounted, hospitals are beginning to accept patients for treatment, labor-management programs are at-

---

This article by the Criteria Committee, National Council on Alcoholism, is reprinted with permission from the *American Journal of Psychiatry* 129:127-135, 1972, copyright American Psychiatric Association 1972; and *Annals of Internal Medicine* 17:249-258, 1972, copyright Annals of Internal Medicine 1972. Reprints of the "Criteria for the Diagnosis of Alcoholism" are available from the National Council on Alcoholism, 12 West 21st Street, New York, N.Y. 10010.

ALCOHOLISM:
A Practical Treatment Guide
ISBN 0-8089-1912-1

tempting to identify alcoholic employees to give them special benefits and rehabilitation, third-party payments are being afforded by insurance carriers, and courts are making special disposition for rehabilitation. Therefore, it is important to establish a set of criteria for the diagnosis of alcoholism. To this end, the National Council on Alcoholism established a committee to prepare a set of criteria, to submit it for criticism and documentation by other experts, and to publish it for the guidance of those involved in the diagnosis of alcoholism.

At the outset, it became apparent that we had undertaken a formidable task, for, despite a great deal of work in the past, much of the literature is burdened by anecdotal material and special assumptions made a priori, and there is a dearth of scientifically controlled observations on the natural course of the disease. In addition, people of many disciplines have made observations from their own points of view, which may be hard to reconcile, and there are not a few who, by their definition of disease, have eliminated alcoholism from the category of disease. But any tendency to withdraw from the field was overcome by the urgency of the task, and the committee herewith presents the results of its deliberations.

Diagnostic criteria may serve several purposes. They may be used *to ascertain the nature of a disease* from a cluster of symptoms. This was not the main goal of the committee. They may be used to promote *early detection* and provide *uniform nomenclature*, both objects of this endeavor. Criteria may be used to *prevent overdiagnosis*. This is important because of the psychological, financial, legal, and therapeutic implications in a diagnosis of alcoholism for the life of the patient. Criteria may be set for *treatment* purposes. Beyond indicating that a need for treatment exists, the committee believes that any indication of different modalities of treatment, except in broad terms, is beyond the scope of its mandate. Criteria may be set for *prognosis*; at present the prognosis for alcoholism is obscure.

Mainly, the committee expects the criteria to be used to identify individuals at multiple levels of dependence. The committee has endeavored to use objectively reproducible data that are obtainable from the patient, his immediate family, or his associates. These data have been weighted for their diagnostic significance. We have included material that would differentiate degrees of severity and that would allow for progression of the disease, where that exists, without prejudging the possiblity that cases of alcoholism may exist in which progression is not a factor. All but one consultant believed that, in alcoholism, there generally is a progression of the disease, although this might not necessarily be reflected by continually increasing drinking. Many consultants have exhorted us to concentrate more on "early manifestations." The reader will note a separation into early, middle, and late effects, which is a general guide. Our first intent, however, is that the person who is diagnosed as having alcoholism surely fits into that category.

THE NATURE OF ALCOHOLISM

The committee was unanimous in defining the disease of alcoholism as a pathological dependence on ethanol, as it is classified under Section 303.2 in the

Diagnostic and Statistical Manual of Mental Disorders, second edition, of the American Psychiatric Association [303.90 in DSM III-R].

Aside from the legal difference between the distribution of alcohol and that of other drugs, there are important scientific differences. A drug is defined in two senses: it is a substance of use in medicine, and it is a habit-forming substance. It generally produces its effect in small quantities. Although alcohol does produce an effect with small quantities, it differs from other drugs in both senses in that large quantities over a long period of time are necessary for it to become habit-forming.

Another difference between alcohol and other drugs particularly those of the optiate class, is the relative risk of addiction. Many people drink, but less than ten percent develop the psychological and physiological dependency on alcohol that can be categorized as alcoholism. With opiates, the risk of pharmacological addiction is considerably higher. Many alcoholics believe that they were alcoholics from their first drink, that their reaction to alcohol was different from that of others. These retrospective data are suspect until and unless a clear difference is established between these individuals and others. Family incidence of alcoholism and other factors may indicate a portion of the population at high risk.

Whether *anyone* who drinks a sufficient quantity over a sufficient period of time will develop alcoholism, whether a specific biochemical or psychological difference leads to alcoholism, or whether both conditions (with other as yet undertemined factors possibly turning the balance) are necessary to cause alcoholism has not been esablished. Thus, whether there is continuous or discontinuous progression from drinking alcoholic beverages to dependence on alcohol has not yet been clearly decided. Animal data suggest that anyone who drinks enought over a sufficiently long period of time will develop the signs of alcoholism. In the free state, however, neither all humans nor all animals choose the paths that lead to this condition. In establishing criteria for diagnosis, the committee wishes to avoid prejudging these issues of etiology.

On the other hand, once alcoholism is established, there is general consensus on its manifestations, and the committee thus feels it is appropriate to describe it as a disease, in agreement with the American College of Physicians, the American Medical Association, the American Psychiataric Association, and other bodies. Alcoholism fits the definition of disease given in *Dorland's Illusrated Medical Dictionary,* 24th edition:

> A definite morbid process having a characteristic train of symptoms, it may affect the whole body or any of its parts, and its etiology, pathology, and prognosis may be known or unknown.

Partial and intermittent forms of alcoholism pose some problems that will be treated separately. Isolated episodes of inebriation, even if they generate unfortunate consequences, are eliminated.

DIVISIONS OF DATA

Data are assembled according to the type of material they represent. Therefore, there are separate data "tracks"—Track I: Physiological and Clinical, and Track II: Behavioral, Psychological, and Attitudinal. The Track II data are grouped together because behavioral manifestations, the easiest to determine and most objective to recognize, imply attitudinal and psychological manifestations.

There is no rigid uniformity in the progress of the disease, but since early diagnosis seems to be helpful in treatment and recovery, manifestations are separated into "early," "middle," and "late." In addition to identifying early and late symptoms and signs, each datum was graded according to its degree of implication for the presence of alcoholism. Of course, some of the more definite signs occur later in the course of the illness. But this does not mean that people with earlier signs may not also have alcoholism.

Various terminologies for these signs have been suggested; we propose to weight them and group them into three "diagnostic levels," with those weighted as "1" being the most significant.

Diagnostic Level 1. Classical, definite, obligatory. This criterion is clearly associated with alcoholism.

Diagnostic Level 2. Probable, frequent, indicative. This criterion lends strong suspicion of alcoholism; other corroborative evidence should be obtained.

Diagnostic Level 3. Potential, possible, incidental. These manifestations are common in people with alcoholism, but do not by themselves give a strong indication of its existence. They may arouse suspicion, but significant other evidence is needed before the diagnosis is made.

DIAGNOSIS

It is sufficient for the diagnosis of alcoholism that one or more of the major criteria of diagnostic level 1 are satisfied, or that several of the minor criteria in Tracks I and II are present; see Tables B-1 and B-2. If one is making the diagnosis because of major criteria in one of the tracks, he should also make a strong search for evidence in the other track. A purely mechanical selection of items is not enough; the history, physical examination, and other observations, plus laboratory evidence, must fit into a consistent whole to ensure a proper diagnosis. Minor criteria in the physical and clinical tracks alone are not sufficient, nor are minor criteria in behavioral and psychological tracks. There must be several in *both* Track 1 and Track II areas.

Table B-1
Major Criteria for the Diagnosis of Alcoholism

Criterion	Diagnostic Level
TRACK I. PHYSIOLOGICAL AND CLINICAL	
A. Physiological Dependency	
1. Physiological dependence as manifested by evidence of a *withdrawal syndrome** when the intake of alcohol is interrupted or decreased without substitution of other sedation; ** it must be remembered that overuse of other sedative drugs can produce a similar withdrawal state, which should be differentiated from withdrawal from alcohol.	
a) Gross tremor (differentiated from other causes of tremor).	1
b) Hallucinosis (differentiated from schizophrenic hallucinations or other psychoses).	1
c) Withdrawal seizures (differentiated from epilepsy and other seizure disorders).	1
d) Delirum tremens. Usually starts between the first and third day after withdrawal and minimally includes tremors, disorientation, and hallucinations.*	1
2. Evidence of *tolerance* to the effects of alcohol. (There may be a decrease in previously high levels of tolerance late in the course). Although the degree of tolerance to alcohol in no way matches the degree of tolerance to other psychotropic drugs, the behavioral effects of a given amount of alcohol vary greatly between alcoholic and nonalcoholic subjects.	
a) A blood alcohol level of more than 150 mg/100 ml without gross evidence of intoxication.	1
b) The consumption of one-fifth of a gallon of whiskey or an equivalent amount of wine or beer daily for a period of two or more consecutive days, by a 180-lb individual.	1
3. Alcoholic "blackout" periods. (Differential diagnosis from purely psychological fugue states and psychomotor seizures.)	2
B. Clinical: Major Alcohol-Associated Illnesses. Alcoholism can be assumed to exist if major alcohol-associated illnesses develop in a person who drinks regularly. In such individuals evidence of physiological and psychological dependence should be searched for.	
Fatty degeneration in absence of other known cause	2
Alcoholic hepatitis	1
Laennec's cirrhosis	2

Table B-1
(Continued)

Criterion	Diagnostic Level
Pancreatitis in the absence of cholelithiasis	2
Chronic gastritis	3
Hematological disorders:	
Anemia: hypochromic, normocytic, macrocytic, hemolytic, with stomatocytosis, low folic acid	3
Clotting disorders: prothrombin elevation, thrombocytopenia	3
Wernicke-Korsakoff syndrome	2
Alcoholic cerebellar degeneration	1
Cerebral degeneration in absence of Alzheimer's disease or arteriosclerosis	2
Central pontine myelinolysis (diagnosis only possible postmortem)	2
Marchiafava Biomini's disease (diagnosis only possible postmortem)	2
Peripheral neuropathy (see also beri-beri)	2
Toxic amblyopia	3
Alcoholic myopathy	2
Alcoholic cardiomyopathy	2
Beri-beri	3
Pellagra	3
TRACK II. BEHAVIORAL, PSYCHOLOGICAL, AND ATTITUDINAL	
All chronic conditions of psychological dependence occur in dynamic equilibrium with intrapsychic and interpersonal consequences. In alcoholism, similarly, there are varied effects on character and family. Like other chronic relapsing diseases, alcoholism produces vocational, social and physical impairments. Therefore, the implications of these disruptions must be evaluated and related to the individual and his pattern of alcoholism. The following behavior patterns show psychological dependence on alcohol in alcoholism:	
1. Drinking despite strong medical contraindication known to the patient.	1
2. Drinking despite strong social contraindications (job loss for intoxication, marriage disruption because of drinking, arrest for intoxication, driving while intoxicated).	1
3. Patient's subjective complaint of loss of control of alcohol consumption.	2

* See Seixas.[1]

** Some authorities term this "pharmacological addiction."

Table B-2
Minor Criteria for the Diagnosis of Alcoholism

Criterion	Diagnostic Level
TRACK I. PHYSIOLOGICAL AND CLINICAL	
A. Direct Effects (ascertained by examination)	
1. Early:	
Odor of alcohol on breath at time of medical appointment	2
2. Middle:	
Alcoholic facies	2
Vascular engorgement of face	2
Toxic ambloyopia	3
Increased incidence of infections	3
Cardiac arrhythmias	3
Peripheral neuropathy (see also Major Criteria Track I, B)	2
3. Late (see Major Criteria, Track I, B)	
B. Indirect Effects	
1. Early:	
Tachycardia	3
Flushed face	3
Nocturnal diaphoresis	3
2. Middle:	
Ecchymoses on lower extremities, arms, or chest	3
Cigarette or other burns on hands or chest	3
Hyperreflexia, or, if drinking heavily, hyporeflexia (permanent hyporeflexia may be a residuum of alcoholic polyneuritis)	3
3. Late:	
Decreased tolerance	3
C. Laboratory Tests	
1. Major—Direct	
Blood alcohol level at any time or more than 300 mg/100 ml	1
Level of more than 100 mg/100 ml in routine examination	1
2. Major—Indirect	
Serum osmolality (reflects blood alcohol levels): every 22.4 increase over 200 mOsm/liter reflects 50 mg/100 ml/alcohol)	2
3. Minor—Indirect	
Results of alcohol ingestion:	
Hypoglycemia	3
Hypochloremic alkalosis	3
Low magnesium level	2

(Continues)

Table B-2
(Continued)

Criterion	Diagnostic Level
C. Laboratory Tests	
3. Minor—Indirect	
Results of alcohol ingestion: *(continued)*	
Lactic acid elevation	3
Transient uric acid elevation	3
Potassium depletion	3
Indications of liver abnormality:	
SGPT elevation	2
SGOT elevation	3
BSP elevation	3
Bilirubin elevation	2
Urinary urobilinogen elevation	2
Serum A/G ratio reversal	2
Blood and blood clotting	
Anemia: hypochromic, normocytic, macrocytic, hemolytic with stomatocytosis, low folic acid	3
Clotting disorders: prothrombin elevation, thrombocytopenia	3
ECG abnormalities:	
Cardiac arrhythmias, tachycardia, T waves dimpled, cloven or spinous atrial fibrillation, ventricular premature contractions, abnormal P waves	2
EEG abnormalities:	
Decreased or increased REM sleep depending on phase	3
Loss of delta sleep	3
Other reported findings:	
Decreased immune response	3
Decreased response to Synacthen test	3
Chromosomal damage from alcoholism	3
TRACK II. BEHAVIORAL, PSYCHOLOGICAL, AND ATTITUDINAL	
A. Behavioral	
1. Direct effects	
Early:	
Gulping drinks	3
Surreptitious drinking	2
Morning drinking (assess nature of peer group behavior)	2
Middle:	
Repeated conscious attempts at abstinence	2

Table B-2
(Continued)

Criterion	Diagnostic Level
A. Behavioral	
Late:	
Blatant indiscriminate use of alcohol	2
Skid Row or equivalent social level	2
2. Indirect effects	
Early:	
Medical excuses from work for variety of reasons	2
Shifting from one alcoholic beverage to another	2
Preference for drinking companions, bars, and taverns	2
Loss of interest in activities not directly associated with drinking	2
Late:	
Chooses employment that facilitates drinking	3
Frequent automobile accidents	3
History of family members undergoing psychiatric treatment; school and behavioral problems in children	3
Frequent change of residence for poorly defined reasons	3
Anxiety-relieving mechanisms, such as telephone calls, inappropriate in time, distance, person, or motive (telephonitis)	2
Outbursts of rage and suicidal gestures while drinking	2
B. Psychological and Attitudinal	
1. Direct effects	
Early:	
When talking freely, makes frequent reference to drinking alcohol, people being "bombed," "stoned," etc. or admits drinking more than peer group	2
Middle:	
Drinking to relieve anger, insomnia, fatigue, depression, social discomfort	2
Late:	
Psychological symptoms consistent with permanent ongoing brain syndrome (see also Major Criteria, Track I, B)	
2. Indirect effects	2
Early:	
Unexplained changes in family, social, and business relationships, complaints about wife, job, and friends	
Spouse makes complaints about drinking behavior, reported by patient or spouse	3
	2

Table B-2
(Continued)

Criterion	Diagnostic Level
B. Psychological and Attitudinal	
2. Indirect effects	
Early: *(continued)*	
Major family disruptions: separation, divorce, threat of divorce	3
Job loss due to increasing interpersonal difficulties, frequent job changes, financial difficulties	3
Late:	
Overt expression of more regressive defense mechanisms: denial, projection, etc.	3
Resentment, jealousy, paranoid attitudes	3
Symptoms of depression: isolation, crying, suicidal preoccupation	3
Feelings that he is "losing his mind"	2

PSYCHIATRIC DIAGNOSIS

After a suitable evaluation, a separate psychiatric diagnosis should be made on every patient, apart from the diagnosis of alcoholism. Patients may suffer from schizophrenia, latent or overt; from manic-depressive psychosis, obsessive-compulsive neurosis, recurrent depression, anxiety neurosis, or psychopathic personality; or have no psychiatric constellation differing from normal. The diagnosis should be made after treatment for withdrawal is complete, since alcohol is anxiety-producing and can also bring out psychological mechanisms and traits that are not apparent without alcohol. In particular, the hallucinatory behavior induced by alcohol withdrawal is not to be equated with schizophrenic hallucinatory behavior.

ALCOHOLISM WITH INTERMITTENT OR RECURRENT DRINKING

Intermittent or recurrent drinking may represent a phase in the course of alcoholism. This pattern should be noted separately. The same criteria control the diagnosis. In some individuals there are recurring episodes of inebriation that become more frequent over a period of years until a daily drinking pattern emerges. In many individuals daily drinking increases until the individual himself slowly becomes aware that physiological and psychological dependence exist. At this point periods of "going on the wagon" may occur, with a resulting intermittent or recurrent pattern of drinking. For most drinkers, there are lesser or greater periods of time when, because of circumstances or the acute effects of alcohol, drinking is not possible. This pattern is not inconsistent with other drug dependence situations, in which interruptions of use are commonplace and have been accepted without the necessity of making a separate category for them.

Even with a "steady" pattern of alcohol use, there are marked fluctuations in the blood alcohol level during each day. The patient with an alcohol problem, given free choice, does not, as one might assume, keep drinking to maintain a steady blood level of alcohol. It has been observed that men who were incarcerated for public intoxication for three-month periods had a total yearly alcohol intake and a total time available for drinking that may have been less than that of the "normal" drinker. Yet these men reported withdrawal signs and symptoms upon cessation of each drinking spree. There is also good experimental evidence for a withdrawal syndrome upon cessation of relatively short periods of heavy drinking.

Thus, where the practitioner has a patient whose drinking pattern consists of intermittent or recurrent drinking and in whom the appropriate diagnostic criteria are satisfied, the condition should be diagnosed as alcoholism (with the qualification as to pattern added if it seems important).

ALCOHOLISM: RECOVERED, ARRESTED, OR IN REMISSION

Since alcoholism is relapsing and chronic, there are very few authorities who claim a complete cure. But there are many patients who, after a time of complete sobriety, have reordered their lives in a rehabilitative way and are completely able to perform complex and responsible tasks. There are also a few patients who have returned to "social" drinking, or who have infrequent "slips" but who still function as rehabilitated persons.

Although these diagnostic criteria are not devised as a guide to prognosis, it is the opinion of the committee that a history of alcoholism in the past, followed by a significant recovery, should be taken into account as a guide to treatment, employment, and restoration of rights and privileges previously denied because of active alcoholism. Some members of the committee believed that total abstinence would not, in the future, turn out to be an absolute, final necessity for recovery from alcoholism. However, it was agreed that total abstinence, as a measure of recovery, arrest, or remission, was usually more easily measurable, definitive, and generally accepted than a change from dependence to "social" drinking. Thus, the committee agreed that the following considerations should determine the diagnosis of recovered, arrested, or remitted alcoholism:

—Duration of abstinence
—Concurrent active treatment program
—Conurrent A.A. attendance with full participation
—Concurrent self-administered and professionally guided deterrent medication

—Resumption or continuation of work without absenteeism
—No traffic violations
—No substitution of other drugs

Although the committee did not choose at this time to assign definitive time values for any of these considerations, the recovery or remission gains in its validity with a progressively longer time. For abstinence alone to be the criterion, without other therapeutic activity, there needs to be a longer time period than if abstinence is combined with other criteria.

ALCOHOL USE

Diagnostic terms that define conditions that fall short of alcoholism are necessary because of the effects of alcohol on behavior. Although the term *alcohol abuse* has wide currency, we prefer *alcohol use*, accompanying this term with a description of effect. This leaves the term "abuse" for such situations as child abuse, animal abuse, or self-abuse, where there is an animate object of the abuse, and does not anthropomorphize alcohol, which, after all, is a chemical (the "neutral spirit"). The term *misuse*, we believe, also carries an unnecessary moral implication.

ALCOHOL USE WITH INEBRIATION

Intoxication may be mild, moderate, or severe, or may lead to coma. Although alcoholics are frequently obviously intoxicated, mere intoxication is not sufficient for the diagnosis of alcoholism. Indeed the physician should be cautious in making a diagnosis of alcohol intoxication on the basis of a staggering gait, slurred speech, other neurological signs, and an odor of alcohol on the breath. In such cases, one must be sure to rule out diabetic acidosis, hypoglycemia, uremia, impending or completed stroke, and other cases of cerebral impairment. An alcohol breath test, determination of blood alcohol level, or serum osmolality measurement may assist in making a diagnosis of alcohol intoxication. A history from the patient and from family members or friends is usually helpful but must in itself be subject to evaluation. Alcohol intoxication must be thought of in any person in coma; in addition, barbiturate and other sedative intoxication must be investigated: cross-dependence and cross-tolerance are common.

ALCOHOL USE WITH PATHOLOGIOCAL INTOXICATION

In some individuals a small amount of alcohol will evoke violent, aberrant behavior. Pathological intoxication is an idiosyncratic response to alcohol and is separate from alcoholism.

ALCOHOL USE: REACTIVE, SECONDARY, OR SYMPTOMATIC

Reactive, secondary, or symptomatic alcohol use should be separated from other forms of alcoholism. Alcohol as a psychoactive drug may be used for varying periods of time to mask or alleviate psychiatric or situationally induced symptoms. This may often mimic a prodromal stage of alcoholism and is difficult to differentiate from it. If the other criteria of alcoholism are not present, this diagnosis must be given. A clear relationship between the psychiatric symptom or event must be present; the period of heavy alcohol use should clearly not antedate the precipitating situational event (for example, an object loss). The patient may require treatment as for alcoholism, in addition to treatment for the precipitating psychiatric event: one may be able to confirm the diagnosis only in retrospect.

ALCOHOL AND ANXIETY

The effects of alcohol on the rising slope of the absorption curve parallel the four stages of anesthesia, and thus excited or uninhibited behavior may be shown with mild inebriation. But it also has been documented that, with large doses over a prolonged period of time, alcohol produces anxiety. Whether this bimodal effect occurs as a regular result of any amount of alcohol is currently being investigated. The progressive rise of anxiety with continued heavy drinking is responsible for many of the effects listed as minor criteria.

CROSS-DEPENDENCE

Cross-dependence (or "cross-addiction") may begin iatrogenically or spontaneously with the use of any of the sedative class of drugs, barbiturates, or "minor" tranquilizers, in an attempt to control the anxiety generated by heavy alcohol use or in the mistaken impression that pharmacological control of the anxiety will stop the alcohol use. Such cross-dependence is so common that it must be investigated in any person suspected of alcoholism.

In addition, the life-style of persons who seek pharmacological "highs" is associated with heavy alcohol use *pari passu* with other psychoactive chemical materials. Such persons are at risk of alcoholism, and patients being investigated for the diagnosis of alcoholism should also be evaluated for use of these materials.

Treatment programs for the use of other drugs engender a significant proportion of "instant alcoholics" who, having relinquished the other drugs, turn to alcohol and experience an unusually rapid onset of dependence. Thus, patients in this category should also be screened for alcoholism, and attempts should be made to prevent its onset.

PERSONS AT HIGH RISK OF ALCOHOLISM

Epidemiological and sociological studies show that the following factors indicate high risk for the development of alcoholism. There is not complete agreement on the extent of risk for each factor.

- A family history of alcoholism, including parents, siblings, grandparents, uncles, and aunts.[2]
- A history of teetotalism in the family, particularly where strong moral overtones were present and, most particularly, where the social environment of the patient has changed to associations in which drinking is encouraged or required.[2]
- A history of alcoholism or teetotalism in the spouse[2] or in the family of the spouse.[3]
- Coming from a broken home or home with much parental discord, particularly where the father was absent or rejecting but not punitive.[4]
- Being the last child of a large family or in the last half of the sibship in a large family.[3]
- Although some cultural groups (for example, the Irish and Scandinavians) have been recorded as having a higher incidence of alcoholism than others (Jews, Chinese, and Italians) the physician should be aware that alcoholism can occur in people of any cultural derivation.[5-7]
- Having female relatives of more than one generation who have had a high incidence of recurrent depressions.[8]
- Heavy smoking; heavy drinking is often associated with heavy smoking, but the reverse need not be true.[9]

RECORDING THE DIAGNOSIS

If alcoholism as defined above is present, the diagnoses should be stated in this order:

—Alcoholism: intermittent use, recurrent use, steady use (early, moderately advanced, far advanced)
—Psychiatric diagnosis
—Physical diagnosis

If major criteria or a sufficient number of minor criteria are not met, the diagnosis should be:
—Suspected alcoholism; psychiatric diagnosis, physical diagnosis

Other diagnoses that can be made:

—Alcohol use: reactive, secondary, or symptomatic; psychiatric diagnosis; physical diagnosis.
—Alcohol use with inebriation

A description of the physical diseases associated with alcoholism and their diagnosis will be the subject of a separate communication.

REFERENCES

1. Seixas FA (ed): Treatment of the Alcohol Withdrawal Syndrome. New York, National Council on Alcoholism, 1971
2. Guze SB, Tuason VB, Gatfield P, et al: Psychiatric illness and crime with particular reference to alcoholism: a study of 223 criminals. *J Nerv Ment Dis* 134:512-521, 1962
3. Barry H, Blame HT: Birth order as a method of studying environmental influences in alcoholism. *Ann NY Acad Sci* 197:172-178,1972
4. McCord W, McCord J: *Origins of Alcoholism* Stanford, Calif. Stanford University Press, 1960
5. Perceval R: Alcoholism in Ireland. *J Alcoholism* 4:251-257, 1969
6. Whitney ED (ed): *World Dialogue on Alcohol and Drug Dependence*. Boston, Beacon Press, 1970
7. Snyder CR: *Alcohol and the Jews*. Glencoe, Ill. Free Press, 1958
8. Winokur G: Genetic findings and methodological considerations in manic-depressive disease. *Brit J Psychiat* 117:267-274, 1970
9. Pollack S: Drinking Driver and Traffic Safety Project, vol I. Los Angeles, Public Systems Research Institute, University of Southern California, 1969

Appendix C: AMA Guidelines for Alcoholism: Diagnosis, Treatment, and Referral

GUIDELINES — EXPLANATORY NOTES

I. *For All Physicians With Clinical Responsibility: Diagnosis and Referral*

A. Recognize as early as possible alcohol-caused dysfunction in the biological, psychological and social areas.

A. Manual on Alcoholism (AMA); Criteria for the diagnosis of alcoholism. (*Am J Psychiatry* 129(2):127-135, 1972; or *An Int Med* 77:249-253, 1972); and Keller, M: Definition of alcoholism, in *Quart J Stud on Alcohol* 21:125-134, 1960.

B. Be aware of those medical conditions that are frequently caused by, attributed to or aggravated by alcohol abuse.

B. Chronic tension states, vague somatic complaints, depression, cardiovascular and gastrointestinal disorders.

This article is as adopted by the American Medical Association Council on Scientific Affairs, October 8-9, 1979.

GUIDELINES	EXPLANATORY NOTES
C. Insure that any complete health examination includes an in-depth history of alcohol and other drug use.	
D. Evaluate patient requirements and community resources so that an adequate level of care can be prescribed, with patient needs matched to appropriate resources.	D. Information usually available from county medical societies, local Council on Alcoholism, and state or local Divisions on Alcoholism and Drug Abuse.
E. If there are medical needs, including severe withdrawal, make referral to a resource that provides adequate medical care.	E. Another physician, hospital or alcoholism program featuring integrated medical services.

II. *For Physicians Accepting Limited Treatment Responsiblity (To Restore the Individual Patient to the Point of Being Capable of Participating in a Long-Term Treatment Program)*

GUIDELINES	EXPLANATORY NOTES
A. Assist the patient in achieving a state free of alcohol and other sedative-hypnotic drugs, including management of acute withdrawal syndrome, which is commonly referred to as detoxification.	A. Office, hospital or clinic may be used depending on patient's condition.
B. Recognize and treat or refer all associated or complicating illnesses.	B. Both physical and psychiatric conditions.
C. Apprise the patient of the nature of his disease and the requirements for recovery.	C. Discuss issues relating to onset, nature and course of illness, as well as prognosis, if treated or untreated.

GUIDELINES	EXPLANATORY NOTES
D. Evaluate resources—physical health, economic, interpersonal and social—to the degree necessary to formulate an initial recovery plan.	
E. Determine the need for involving significant other persons in the initial recovery plan.	E. Determine clinical appropriateness, depending on ethical codes, state laws and HEW rules and regulations concerning confidentiality. Significant other persons may include families, (parents, sisters/brothers) and sexual partners.
F. Develop an initial long-term recovery plan in consideration of the above standards and with the patient's participation.	F. This long-term recovery plan would address those factors listed in the following section entitled "For Physicians Accepting Responsibility for Long-Term Treatment." At this point, the physician can assume the responsibilities delineated in the next section, or refer to another physician.

III. *For Physicians Accepting Responsibilty for Long-Term Treatment*

GUIDELINES	EXPLANATORY NOTES
A. Acquire knowledge, by training and/or experience, in the treatment of alcoholism.	A. Specialized programs: abstracts of scientific literature available from NIAAA, NCA, AMA, J Stud on Alcohol; visitation to alcoholism treatment centers and Alcoholics Anonymous.
B. The following responsibilities should be conducted or supervised by the physician:	

GUIDELINES	EXPLANATORY NOTES
1. Establish a supportive, therapeutic and nonjudgmental relationship.	1. This is the vehicle whereby the physician directs, supports, and monitors the patient over a period of years. Attempt to modify the patient's isolation, grief and guilt, and deal with other significant psychotherapeutic issues.
2. Within the confines of this relationship, establish specific conditions and limits under which the therapy will be conducted, and carefully explain them to the patient.	2. Physician and patient responsibiliies should be clearly defined.
3. Periodically evaluate and update the recovery plan with the patient's participation.	
4. Involve the patient with an abstinent peer group when appropriate.	4. At this point it is critical that referral to professionally guided or self-help groups, such as Alcoholics Anonymous, is specific and appropriate to the patient's needs.
5. Become knowledgeable about and be able to utilize various health, social, vocational and spiritual support systems.	5. i.e., vocational rehabilitation, educational advancement, skills training, halfway and recovery houses, recreational facilities.
6. Evaluate directly or indirectly significant other persons and, unless clearly contraindicated, involve them in treatment.	6. Treatment may be provided by the physician, another professional, Al-Anon or a comprehensive treatment program.

GUIDELINES	EXPLANATORY NOTES
C. Continually monitor the patient's medication needs. After treatment of acute withdrawal, use psychoactive drugs only if there is a clear cut and specific psychiatric indication in addition to alcoholism.	C. Schizophrenia or major affective disorders may be treated with psychoactive substances that are not ordinarily dependence producing or subject to abuse. However, special care should be exercised in the administration or prescribing of anti-anxiety agents, or barbiturates and barbiturate-like drugs.
D. Be knowledgeable about the proper use of deterrent drugs.	D. Specifically, disulfiram (Antabuse) in this country.
E. Throughout the course of treatment, continually monitor and treat or refer for any complicating illness or relapse.	E. Check for orgnaic and psychiatric complications, as well as for inappropriate use of alcohol or other sedative—hypnotic drugs.
F. Be available to the patient as needed or for an indefinite period of recovery.	

Appendix D: Antabuse

Almost 40 years ago, an adverse physical reaction to ingested ethanol was observed in workers whose aldehyde dehydrogenase had been inhibited incidentally by disulfiram (Antabuse). Earliest clinical thought appeared to concentrate on the possible use of this drug for aversive conditioning, a technique later abandoned by all but the most sanguine. Since 1950, knowledgeable clinicians have used disulfiram in order to achieve temporary or prolonged abstinence. Although a significant ethical change in association with improved self-understanding undoubtedly improves the likelihood of definitive or long-term recovery from alcoholism, a substantive period of abstinence (12-24 months) may, in and of itself, induce a salutory change in many patients. Since clinical experience has shown that the recommendation and use of any drug therapy—especially psychoactive substances—increases recidivism, a preferred therapeutic approach might consist of an initial opportunity to achieve sobriety by other than medicinal means. Indeed, the avoidance of any drug therapy permits patients to assume greater responsibility for their own recovery. Occasionally, disulfiram therapy may even be used by a patient to avoid commitment to group or individual psychotherapeutic involvement. On the other hand, the appropriate use of disulfiram may improve the effectiveness of an already sound treatment program. In the role of such a therapeutic adjuvant, the clinical effectiveness of disulfiram far exceeds its modest value as a sole treatment modality. A number of other drugs share with disulfiram some modest aversive symptomatology after ethanol ingestion but these have failed to achieve clinical use in this country.

The inhibition of aldehyde dehydrogenase results in little, if any, adverse effect in the absence of ethanol ingestion. Within minutes of drinking as little as 5–10 g

ALCOHOLISM:
A Practical Treatment Guide ISBN 0-8089-1912-1

of alcohol, however, such a patient may begin to accumulate enough acetaldehyde to initiate a reaction that might eventually include a flush, headache, bounding pulse, diaphoresis, nausea, vomiting, and vasomotor collapse with orthostatic hypotension. This reaction rarely persists for more than a few hours and commonly requires no therapeutic intervention other than bed rest. Occasionally, parenteral phenothiazines or even support of vital functions might be needed. The amount of disulfiram needed to inhibit aldehyde dehydrogenase rarely exceeds 250 mg/day, but is dependent upon body size, age, general health (especially hepatic function), and other drug use, especially those drugs that are metabolized by the smooth endoplasmic reticulum (SER) system (including certain sedatives, dilantin, coumadin, oral hypoglycemics, and various antirheumatic agents). Despite a fairly well defined catabolic pathway consisting of conversion to a thiol and then carbon disulfide and diethylamine, disulfiram plasma levels show marked variability from one subject to another. A slightly higher dose of disulfiram, 500–750 mg/day, may be given during the first few days in order to achieve earlier enzyme inhibition. The drug should not be started earlier than 12–24 hours after the last drink of alcohol. Since the enzyme remains inhibited for at least 4–5 days after the last daily dose of disulfiram, even modest doses of ethanol are likely to result in some untoward reaction if ingested prior to that time. By taking disulfiram each day, the patient is continuously protected, at least partially, against a return to drinking for 4–5 days. Although few physicians still use a test dose of ethanol after initiating disulfiram therapy, it is necessary to acquaint the patient with the pharmacologic information concerning disulfiram use. Patients may even be offered an identification card that would serve to alert a physician that disulfiram is being used. Patients need to know that the alcohol used in cooking fails to achieve a high enough concentration to elicit untoward symptoms. On the other hand, a few ounces of wine or beer, or even a smaller quantity of an elixir, might be adequate to result in such a reaction.

Rarely, disulfiram may result in adverse effects without the concomitant use of ethanol. The most frequent of these are somnolence and a subtle garlic-like odor on the breath. A reduction in dosage may alleviate such side-effects but rarely will it relieve the patient who experiences a hypersensitivity reaction to the drug. Occasional patients prefer to take their daily antabuse at bedtime in order to capitalize on its soporific action. Disulfiram may infrequently induce hepatic, gastrointestinal, or CNS dysfunction, but fortunately discontinuation of therapy usually results in prompt clearing of symptoms. Despite concern to the contrary, only one fourth to one third of disulfiram is eliminated as carbon disulfide. Nevertheless, this metabolite may be related to the rare organic mental syndrome or peripheral neuropathy following disulfiram ingestion. Confusion or lethargy should serve to warn of the need to reduce or eliminate the dosage of disulfiram at once. Psychosis has been described without a dose relationship but a cautious evaluation of past drug ingestion must be evaluated in such instances. It is most important to emphasize that the safety of administering Antabuse is such that the author has observed more frequent adverse reactions from salicylates than from this drug. The ratio of benefits to risk (untoward reactions) is so high that the only absolute contraindications to the use of disulfiram are: (1) hypersensitivity, and (2) the inability to understand the use of the drug (i.e., psychosis). Relative contraindications might include: (1) arteriosclerotic heart disease, especially with recent myocardial infarction or angina pectoris; (2) any severe, life-threatening illness unrelated to recent ethanol ingestion (especially cerebrovascular insufficiency); (3) pregnancy (the author prescribed disulfiram during pregnancy on two occasions, each of which resulted in a normal fetus, but there have been recent claims of teratogenicity in animals); and (4) the use of drugs such as dilantin or anticoagulants, which complicate disulfiram administration.

More important than emphasizing those rare instances in which disulfiram may not be prescribed, let us turn to the clinical indications for its use:

1. For early evaluation of patient motivation. Those patients whose level of motivation is unknown to the physician may be offered Antabuse to assist their recovery program. When the patient replies negatively and with somewhat irrational obstinency, the physician can be fairly secure in estimating a substantive likelihood for early relapse.
2. For parole or probation. Contrary to some early impressions, prolonged enforcement of abstinence may result in an increased likelihood of recovery from alcoholism. Some clinics have used a breath test for carbon disulfide in order to ensure compliance with such a program.
3. For assistance for the impulsive drinker. That patient who apparently fails to plan drinking episodes, but whose resistance to imbibing is low enough to be overcome repetitively under casual circumstances, may be significantly assisted by the use of disulfiram.
4. For the patient preoccupied with the issue of drinking. Certain patients spend most of their working hours determining whether or not to drink. The use of disulfiram each morning relieves this onerous burden and often results in considerable diminution of the associated depression. Unfortunately, such relief rarely persists for more than a matter of weeks or months.
5. For temporary assistance with critical circumstances during otherwise successful abstinence. This might result from the death of a family member or disruption of the usual support system (i.e., travel).
6. For relief of a consort's anxiety regarding the possibility of the patient drinking. The spouse's anxiety is often poorly tolerated by the alcoholic. Disulfiram therefore may reduce the tension within the family unit.
7. As an adjuvant for the patient whose continuous or periodic drinking has persisted despite the professed desire to desist and despite the use of all other modalities of therapy.
8. For increasing the duration of sobriety for the patient leaving the hospital on a pass or a discharge earlier than the physician would have preferred.
9. For assistance in a psychotherapeutic program for the patient unable to develop insight into the mechanism of his slips.

The author has found the use of Antabuse noted in point nine to be one of the most valuable to the physician conducting definitive treatment of the alcoholic. It is not uncommon for a patient to announce that he drank a few days previously. When asked for the details of this circumstance, the patient can offer no more than that he drank for only a few hours and is no longer imbibing. The patient is then offered the opportunity of taking Antabuse, and if, after the usual explanation of the mechanism by which this drug works, the patient accepts such treatment, he is informed that, during the first year of treatment, discontinuation of the Antabuse for any reason whatever will result in uncontrolled drinking within a matter of weeks or at most within three months. The patient is also informed that he might well use one of the following six rationalizations for stopping the Antabuse: (1) "I forgot to take it"; (2) "I went on a trip and forgot to take it with me"; (3) "I ran out and forgot to get the prescription renewed"; (4) "I was doing so well that I didn't think I needed it any more"; (5) "I wanted to demonstrate that I could handle it on my own"; and (6) "My daughter was getting married and I wished to be able to toast the bride." The patient is politely told that all of these rationalizations are lies and that since he would have to discontinue the Antabuse at least 5 days prior to drinking, the act of discontinuation would represent a determined plan to return to the use of alcohol.

During the ensuing therapy, it is expected that a dialogue will develop concerning the psychodynamic basis supporting the decision to return to the use of alcohol. Thus, Antabuse could be used as an integral part of a psychotherapeutic program. It may soon become apparent to the patient that alcoholic slips occur in three stages:

1. Withdrawal or reisolation. The patient stops going to A.A. meetings, fails to contact close cohorts within the recovery community, and misses appointments with the physician or clinic.
2. The patient begins to feel compromised and ill-used in the confines of a relationship that he feels powerless to change. This is usually with the consort, other family member, or employer.
3. The actual moment of drinking (the least important aspect of the slip).

Discussion of the first stage often helps to emphasize the critical nature of those empirical mechanisms whereby a return to drinking may be made less likely. Point two will commonly keynote specific psychodynamic factors with which the patient has difficulty. Recurrent review of all such aspects of slips leads to early appreciation of the compelling and self-destructive behavior patterns inherent in the drinking.

Antabuse, an adjuvant for the treatment of alcoholism, has been examined through the perspective of almost 30 years of clinical experience. It must be emphasized that viewpoints vary even among physicians with extensive experience with this drug. Moreover, no effort has been made to review the voluminous disulfiram literature since adequate reference articles are available for that purpose.

BIBLIOGRAPHY

Beaumont G (ed): The role of Antabuse (disulfiram) in the treatment of alcohol dependence. *Brit J Clin Pract* 36,38:1-37, 1984 (suppl)

Disulfiram in the Treatment of Alcoholism: An Annotated Bibliography. Addictions Research Foundation, Bibliographic Series, No. 14, 1978

Faiman MD, Jensen JC, Lacoursiere RB: Elimination kinetics of disulfiram in alcoholics after single and repeated doses. *Clin Pharmacol Ther* 36:520-526, 1984

Fried R: *Alcoholism* 1:257, 1977

Fuller RK, Roth HP: Disulfiram for the treatment of alcoholism. *Ann Intern Med* 90:901-904, 1979

Nora AH, Nora JJ, Blu J: Limb-reduction anomalies in infants born to disulfiram-treated alcoholic mothers. Letters to the Editor. *Lancet* 2:644, 1977

Paulson SM, Krause S, Wobbleton J, et al: Use of a breath test for compliance with disulfiram therapy of alcoholism in patients with and without liver disease. *Gastroenterology* 70:990, 1976

Ritchie JM: in Goodman LS, Gilman A (eds): *Pharmacological Basis of Therapeutics*, ed 5. New York, Macmillan, 1975

Index

A.A. *See* Alcoholics Anonymous
A.A. Comes of Age, 109
Abortion, 173
Abstinence, 96. *See also* Detoxification; Withdrawal.
  American Medical Society on Alcoholism and, 117-118
  antabuse and, 103. *See also* Antabuse.
  cognitive function and, 15
  early problems with, 75-77
  reasons for, 10-11, 103
  resistance to, 32-33, 42
ACA. *See* Adult children of alcoholics.
Addictive process, 168-169
Adlerian view, 192
Adult children of alcoholics (ACAs), 88
Affective disorders, alcoholism and, 90, 149-151
Aftercare, rehabilitation and, 87-88. *See also* Long-term management of alcoholism.
  short-term residential, 84
Age factor
  memory deficits and, 135
  rehabilitation and, 94
  therapy and, 169
  tolerance and, 6-7
Agitation, 5
  after detoxification, 73
  blood levels and, 7
  sedative action of ethanol and, 3, 5
  withdrawal and, 57
Al-Anon, 69, 88. *See also* Alcoholics Anonymous.
  enabler and, 112-115
  healing fellowship of, 201-202
Alateen, 88, 205. *See also* Alcoholics Anonymous
Alcohol abuse
  alcohol use vs., 222-223
  definition of, 3
Alcohol addiction, definition of, 5-8
Alcohol-associated illnesses. *See* Medical complications of alcoholism; *and specific complications*.
Alcohol dependence vs. alcoholism, 3
Alcohol-related birth defects (ARBD), 140. *See also* Birth defects.
Alcohol use vs. alcohol abuse, 222-223
Alcoholics Anonymous, 109
Alcoholics Anonymous (A.A.), 8, 15-17, 86-87, 105-110, 120
  after detoxification, 75
  anonymity and, 109
  antabuse and, 105
  clubhouse, 87
  commitment to, 16
  community education, 99
  consultation and, 79
  literature, 109-110
  low-economic-status patient and, 187
  referral to, 49
  resistance to, 16
    physician, 87
  short-term residential rehabilitation and, 83-84
  twelve steps of, 107-110
  volunteer from, 110

Alcoholism, current concept of. *See* Disease concept of alcoholism.
Alcoholism services, outpatient, 85-86. *See also specific services.*
Amblyopia, 133
American Medical Association (AMA) guidelines for alcoholism, 226-230
American Medical Society on Alcoholism, abstinence and, 117-118
Amino acid metabolism, alcoholism and, 27
Amitriptyline, prolonged withdrawal syndrome and, 146
Amnesia, alcoholism and, 25-26
Amphetamines, recovery and, 116
Anesthetic medications, alcoholism and, 139
Anesthetic use of alcohol, 48
Anonymity, A.A. and, 109
Antabuse, 231-234
  adverse reactions to, 232-233
  after detoxification, 73
  contraindications for, 104
  dosage for, 104
  indications for, 103, 233-234
  long-term management and, 103-105
  motivation and, 43-44
  protocol for, 232
  reaction, 103-104, 232
  schizophrenia and, 147
  termination of, 104-105
Anti-anxiety drugs, women and, 175
Antidepressants
  after detoxification, 73
  withdrawal and, 62
Antidisatropics after detoxification, 73
Antiemetics, 62
Antiparkinsonian drugs, 145
Antipsychotic drugs, rehabilitation and, 90
Antisocial behavior, alcoholism and, 151-152
Anxiety
  after detoxification, 73, 76
  alcohol and, 223
ARBD. *See* Alcohol-related birth defects.
Arrhythmias, alcoholism and, 131-132
As Bill Sees It, 110
Atherosclerosis, alcoholism and, 131
Autonomous self-perpetuating factor in alcoholism, 159-160

BAC. *See* Blood alcohol concentration.
Barbiturates, alcoholism and, 9, 209
Behavior, antisocial, alcoholism and, 151-152
Behavior changes as sign of alcoholism, 25
Benadryl, withdrawal and, 60
Bender Visual Motor Gestalt Test, 70
Benzodiazepines, alcoholism and, 17, 210
  schizophrenia and, 145
  sociopathy and, 151-152
"Big Book" of A.A., 118
Bipolar disorders, alcoholism and, 149-151
Birth defects, 139-140, 173-174
Blackout, 25-26
Blood alcohol concentration (BAC), 6, 55, 58
Blood disorders, alcoholism and, 136-137
Borderline personality, alcoholism and, 152-153
Breath alcohol determination, obtundation and, 55, 58
Bronchopulmonary disease, alcoholism and, 138
Burning Bright, 206-207
Burns, alcoh

Cancer, alcoholism and, 138
Cardiovascular system, alcoholism and, 130-132
Career guidance, women and, 177-179
Catabolic pathway, alcoholism and, 6
Central pontine myelinolysis, alcoholism and, 134
Cerebral degeneration, alcoholism and, 134
Cerebral dysfunction, alcoholism and, 186
Chain reaction of health, 119-120
Chest x-ray, consciousness disorders and, 58
Child-care, treatment program and, 177
Children and parental alcoholism, 202-204. *See also* Adult children of alcoholics; Family.
  denial and, 33-34
  therapy for, 204-206
Chloral hydrate, withdrawal and, 60
Chlordiazepoxide
  dosage guidelines for, 61
  outpatient withdrawal and, 63
Choice of treatment for alcoholism, 88-96
Cirrhosis of liver, 46, 127-128
Clinical presentation of alcoholism, 4, 8
  diversity in, 80-81
  psychiatric disorders and, 160-161
CNS adaptation, alcoholism and, 6
COAs. *See* Children and parental alcoholism.
Cocaine use, alcoholism and, 9. *See also* Cross-addiction.
Coercion as motivation for alcoholic, 68-69
Cognitive function, abstinence and, 15
Community mental health centers, 74
Computed tomography (CT) scan, 58, 135
Confidentiality, 119
Conflict as sign of alcoholism, 31
Confrontation with patient, 20, 37
Congenital abnormalities, alcoholism and, 139-140, 173-174

Consciousness and neurological status, intoxication and, 55-58
Consultation for physician, 79
Contract with patient, withdrawal management and, 62
Controlled drinking. *See also* Social drinking as diagnostic clue, 31-32
  long-term management and, 117-118
Coronary artery disease, alcoholism and, 131
Cross-addiction, 5-6, 6, 9. *See also specific addictions.*
  rehabilitation and, 94
  sedative-hypnotic drugs and, 209-210
Cross-dependence, 223. *See also* Cross-addiction.
Cross-tolerance, 5-6. *See also* Cross-addiction.
  sedative-hypnotic drugs and, 209-210
  variation in, 6-7
Cultural factors
  as enablers, 113-114
  low-socioeconomic-status patient and, 183-185
  rehabilitation and, 94-95
  schizophrenia and, 144
  women and, 172-173, 174-175
Cushing disease, 26, 139

Delayed withdrawal, 62-63. *See also* Withdrawal.
Delirium tremens (DTs), 63-64
Dementia, alcoholism and, 134
Denial, 9-10, 13
  dynamics of, 32-33
  family of patient and, 33-34
  motivation and, 41-43
  physician and, 19-22
Dependency
  physician-patient relationship and, 53
  psychotherapy and, 72
Depression
  clinical, 149-151
  detoxification and, 73, 76
  recovery and, 90, 116
Detoxification. *See also* Abstinence; Withdrawal.
  initial treatment after
    drugs and, 72-73
    mental status examination and, 70
    motivation and, 67-69
    problems in, 75-77
    referrals and, 74-75
    therapy and, 70
  treatment plan for, 79, 80 *(t)*
    diversity, 79-80
Diabetes, abstinence and, 25
Diagnosis of alcoholism, 8-10. *See also* Clinical presentation of alcoholism; National Council on Alcoholism; Recognition.
  amount of alcohol consumed and, 23-24
  blackouts and, 25-26
  controlled drinking and, 32
  denial and, 32-33
    family, 33-34
  general considerations for, 22-23, 37, 54-55
  general hospitals and, 27-28
  mental status examination and, 70
  obsession with alcohol and, 31
  personal history and, 23, 24, 28-29
    physician's attitude, 29
    sedative-hypnotic drugs, 29-30
  personality change and, 25
  physical examination and, 26, 55
  reasons for drinking and, 30-31
  recording of, 224-225
  secondary diseases and, 27
  withdrawal symptoms and, 24-25, 54-59
Diagnostic and Statistical Manual of Mental Disorders, second edition (DSM-II), 213
Diagnostic and Statistical Manual of Mental Disorders, third edition (DSM-III), 3
Dieting, drugs for, 116
Diphenhytramine, 60
Disease concept of alcoholism, 2-5, 4
  recidivism and, 13
  therapy and, 156-157
Distrust, low-socioeconomic-status patient and, 182-183
Disulfiram. *See* Antabuse.
Down's Syndrome, 174
Drinking
  controlled. *See* Controlled drinking.
  patterns of, 41
  secondary rewards of, 52
  social. *See* Social drinking.
Drugs. *See also* Cross-addiction; *specific drugs.*
  detoxification and, 72-73
  psychiatric disorders and, 17. *See also* Specific drugs.
"Dry Dock" A.A. groups, 120
DSM-II, 213
DSM-III, 3
DTs. *See* Delirium tremens.
Dual addiction. *See* Cross-addiction.

Early stages of alcoholism, 37-39
  history taking and, 38-39
  motivation and, 38-39
Educational factors, rehabilitation and, 95

Ego alien problems, 160
Ego syntonic problems, 161-162
Electrocardiography
  consciousness disorders and, 58
  intoxication and, 131
Elevated psychomotor activity, alcoholism and, 10
Emergency room patient, 28
Emotional reeducation, psychotherapy and, 71
Emotional support. *See also specific support groups.*
  psychotherapy and, 71
Empathy, physician and, 49-50
Employment
  long-term management and, 101, 102 (f)
  recovery and, 101
  rehabilitation and, 92
Enabler, 112-115. *See also* Al-Anon; Family; Spouse.
Encephalopathy
  portal systemic, alcoholism and, 135
  Wernicke's, 133,153
Endocrine system, medical complications of alcoholism and, 139
Environment
  rehabilitation and, 91
  withdrawal management and, 59, 60 *(t)*
Escherichia coli, 137
Ethanol, sedative action of, 3, 7
Etiologic factors in alcoholism, 21, 157-160

Family illness, alcoholism as, 29
Family. *See also* Adult Children of Alcoholics; Al-Anon; Alateen; Children and parental alcoholism; Spouse.
  crisis, motivation and, 69
  early, 194
  as enabler, 92, 112-115
  general systems model and, 194-195
  motivation and, 39-40, 51-52
  recognition of alcoholism and, 39-40
  rehabilitation and, 91-92
  role playing in, 193
  scapegoating in, 191, 197
  teenage alcoholism and, 191
  therapy for, 195-196
    children, 204-206
    couple therapy, 197
    family unit, 193
    initial approach, 196
    rehabilitation and, 88
    residential, 88
FAS. *See* Fetal alcohol syndrome.
Fee, patient motivation and, 48-49
Fetal alcohol syndrome (FAS), 139-140, 173-174
Financial considerations, 48-49. *See also* Low-socioeconomic-status patient.
Folate, 60, 136-137
Fractures, traumatic, 136
Freelance employment, isolation and, 92
Freudian view, 191
Friends
  motivation and, 39-40
  recognition and, 39-40

Gastrointestinal tract, medical complications of alcoholism and, 129-130
General hospitals, diagnostic clues and, 27-28
Genetics, alcoholism and, 29
Gingivitis, alcoholism and, 26
Glucose intolerance, abstinence and, 25
Gonadotropic defects, alcoholism and, 139
Grand mal seizures, alcoholism and, 7, 24
  cross-addiction and, 116

Haemophilus influenzae, alcoholism and, 137
Halfway house, 74, 85
Hallucinations, alcoholism and, 59, 146
Health impairment as motivation for change, 69
Heart disease, alcoholism and, 130-132
Hepatitis, alcoholism and, 127
Hip, osteonecrosis of, alcoholism and, 136
History, patient's
  diagnostic clues and, 23, 24, 28-29
  early stages of alcoholism and, 38-39
  motivation and, 36-37
Homosexuals, therapy and, 169
Honeymoon period, 75-76
Hope, alcoholism and, 13
Hospitalization, partial, rehabilitation and, 81
Hospitals, general, detection in, 27-28
Hydroxyzine after detoxification, 73
Hyperexcitable phase, alcoholism and, 159
Hypertension, alcoholism and, 131
  abstinence and, 25
  withdrawal and, 57

Illness, intercurrent, withdrawal management and, 64-65
Immunologic mechanisms, alcoholism and, 137
In-hospital detoxification, 14-15. *See also* Detoxification.
Incidence of alcoholism, 34
Inebriation, 55, 222

Infectious disease, alcoholism and, 137-138
Injury. *See* Trauma.
Inpatient rehabilitation, 81-83. *See also* Rehabilitation, inpatient.
Insurance coverage, 20
Intellectual ability, rehabilitation and, 95
Intention tremor, alcoholism and, 24
Intercurrent illness, withdrawal management and, 64-65
Intoxification, 222-223
Isolation, alcoholism and, 15-16

Job jeopardy, alcoholism and, 68
Joint Commission on Accreditation of Hospitals, 95

Korsakoff's syndrome, 133, 153

Laboratory tests, 27, 145, 217-218 *(t)*
  common changes in, 58 *(t)*
  consciousness disorders and, 58-59
  motivation and, 41
  psychiatric disorders and, 154
  withdrawal symptoms and, 24
Legal factors, alcoholism and, 68
Life threatening problems, physical examination for, 55-56
Lifestyle, alcoholism and, 31
Liver
  cirrhosis of, 46, 127-128
  laboratory tests and, 27
Living arrangements, alcoholism and. *See also* Environment.
  rehabilitation and, 91
Long-term dysfunction, alcoholism and, 17
Long-term management of alcoholism. *See also* Aftercare, rehabilitation and; Recovery.
  A.A. and. *See* Alcoholics Anonymous.
  AMA guidelines for, 228-230
  chain reaction of health and, 119-120
  concept for, 98
  controlled drinking and, 117-118. *See also* Social drinking.
  counseling and
    family, 112-115
    modes, 120-121
    pastoral, 111
    peer group, 110. *See also* Alcoholics Anonymous.
    psychotherapy, 111
  disulfiram and, 103-105
  employment and, 101, 102 (f)
  evaluation of, 120
  goals of, 99-102
  medication and, 115-117
  motivation and, 67-69
  patient education and, 111-112
  physician and, 99, 115, 121
  relapse, 118-119
Low-socioeconomic-status patient
  culture and 183-185
  distrust and, 182-183
  financial considerations and, 182 *(t)*, 186
  organizational support for, 187-188
  physician's attitude and, 182-183
  problems in management of, 182-183
  treatment planning and, 185-187

Magical thinking, alcoholism and, 17
Mallory-Weiss syndrome, 129
Malnutrition, alcoholism and, 124-126
Manic state, alcoholism and, 150-151
Marchiafava-Bignami disease, 134
Maturation arrest, alcoholism and, 137
Medical complications of alcoholism, 27, 65, 89, 215-216 *(t)*. *See also specific complications.*
  blood and, 136-137
  cancer and, 138
  cardiovascular system and, 130-132
  endocrine system and, 139
  gastrointestinal tract and, 129-130
  infectious disease and, 137-138
  life-threatening, 55-56
  liver and, 126-128
  malnutrition and, 124-126
  metabolism and, 124-126
  musculoskeletal system and, 135-136
  nervous system and, 132-135
  pancreatitis and, 128-129
  pediatric, 139-140
  perinatal, 139-140
  surgery and, 138-139
Medication
  long-term management and, 115-117
  withdrawal management and, 60-61, 62 *(t)*, 63
Memory deficits, alcoholism and, 135
Menstrual irregularities, alcoholism and, 173
Mental status examination after detoxification, 70
MEOS. *See* Microsomal Ethanol Oxidizing System.
Metabolism, alcoholism and, 124-126
Methadone maintenance, 170

Microsomal Ethanol Oxidizing System (MEOS), 6
Mineral metabolism, alcoholism and, 126
Minnesota Multiphasic Personality Inventory (MMPI), 70
Miscarriage, alcoholism and, 173
Misdiagnosis of alcoholism, 51
MMPI. *See* Minnesota Multiphasic Personality Inventory.
Mood-changing use of alcohol, 30
Mood swings
  alcoholics and, 150
  recovery and, 99, 100 (f)
Moral turpitude, alcoholism and, 8
Motivation for recovery, 12-14
  after detoxification, 67-69
  approaches to, 44-47
  denial and, 41-43
  early stages of alcoholism and, 38-39
  empathy and, 49-50
  external, 68-69
  family and, 39-40, 51-52, 69
  fee and, 48-49
  friends and, 39-40
  health-impairment and, 69
  history-taking and, 36-37
  job jeopardy and, 68
  legal considerations and, 69
  long-term, 67-69
  physical examination and, 40-41
  physician's attitude and, 49-50, 52-53
  sympathy and, 49-50
  techniques for, 13-14
  therapist and, 47-48
Motor hyperactivity, withdrawal and, 57
Munich beer heart, 130
Musculoskeletal system, alcoholism and, 135-136
Myelinolysis, central pontine, alcoholism and, 134

Nation of Islam, 187
National Council on Alcoholism
  abstinence and, 117-118
  consultation and, 79
  definition of alcoholism, 212-213, 222
  diagnostic criteria from, 34, 214-220
  recovery criteria from, 221-222
Native Americans, 184-185, 188. *See also* Low-socioeconomic-status patient.
Nervous system, alcoholism and, 132-135
Neuroleptics, prolonged withdrawal syndrome and, 146
Neurological damage, withdrawal and, 60
Nutrition, withdrawal management and, 60, 62

Obtundation of drunkenness, 55, 222
Omnipotence, psychotherapy and, 72
Organic pathology
  abstinence and, 10
  mental disturbances and, 153-154
Osteonecrosis of hip, alcoholism and, 136
Outpatient
  rehabilitation and, 85-87
  withdrawal management and, 59, 63

Pain
  detoxification and, 14
  drugs for, 116
Pancreatitis, alcoholism and, 128-129
Partial hospitalization, rehabilitation and, 81
Patient education, 14
  literature for, 45
  long-term management and, 111-112
Patterns of drinking, 41
Pediatric complications of alcoholism, 139-140
Peer group support. *See* Adult Children of Alcoholics; Al-Anon; Alateen; Alcoholics Anonymous.
Peptic ulcer disease, alcoholism and, 129
Peridontal disease, alcoholism and, 26
Perinatal abnormalities, alcoholism and, 139-140
"Periodic" status, concept of, 3
Peripheral neuropathy, alcoholism and, 132-133
Personal resources, alcoholism and, 15
Personality, premorbid, alcoholism and, 17
Personality change, alcoholism and, 25
Phenothiazines
  recovery and, 116
  schizophrenia and, 145
Phenytoin, 60
Physical dependence, alcoholism and, 3
Physical examination, alcoholism and, 55
  diagnostic clues and, 26
  motivation and, 40-41
Physical handicaps, rehabilitation and, 95
Physician
  alcoholism in, 52
  attitude of, toward alcoholism, 1-2, 11-12, 52-53
  history-taking and, 29
  long-term role of, 97, 99, 115, 121
  low-socioeconomic-status patient and, 182-183
  techniques for, 13-14
  treatment center and, 96

Physician-patient relationship, dependency and, 53
Physiological dependency on alcohol, 215 *(t)*, 217-218 *(t)*
Pontine myelinolysis, central, alcoholism and, 134
Portal systemic encephalopathy, alcoholism and, 135
Practical support, psychotherapy and, 71
Precipitating factors, alcoholism and, 158-169
Predisposition to alcoholism, 157-158
Premorbid personality, alcoholism and, 17
Primary care, 79-81. *See also* Detoxification.
Problem-solving, psychotherapy and, 71
Prognosis for rehabilitation, 50-51, 96-97
Projective Human Figure Drawings, 70
Prolonged withdrawal syndrome, 145-147. *See also* Withdrawal.
Pseudo-Cushing syndrome, 139
Psychedelics, 9
Psychiatric disorders, alcoholism and, 17, 90-91
  affective, 149-151
  children of alcoholics and, 203-204
  clinical presentation of, 161-162
  general considerations for, 142-144
  organic, 153-154
  other, 152-153
  prolonged withdrawal syndrome and, 145-146
  recovery and, 102
  schizophrenia and, 144-145
  sociopathy and, 151-152
  treatment problems with, 147-149
Psychoactive medication
  after detoxification, 72-73
  recovery and, 115-117
Psychodynamic causation in alcoholism, 191-192
Psychological dependence on alcohol, 216 *(t)*, 218-220 *(t)*
Psychological symptoms of early stages of alcoholism, 38-39
Psychomotor activity, alcoholism and, 3
Psychosis, alcoholism and, 90. *See also* Psychiatric disorders, alcoholism and.
Psychosocial plateau, 69
Psychotherapy, 70-72. *See also* Therapy.
  abstinence and, 11
  orientation for, 164-165
  phases of, 162-164
  self-help programs and, 165-168
  special needs and, 169-170
Psychotropic agents
  premorbid personality and, 17
  rehabilitation and, 90
  sociopathy and, 151-152
Pyorrhea, alcoholism and, 26

Quarterway house after detoxification, 74

Rationalizations, alcoholism and. *See also* Denial, abstinence and, 42-43.
Reactive alcohol use, 223
Recidivism. *See* Relapse.
Recognition of alcoholism. *See also* Diagnosis of alcoholism.
  early stages and, 37-39
  family and, 39-40
  friends and, 39-40
  physician's attitude and, 19-22
Recovery. *See also* Long-term management of alcoholism; Motivation for recovery.
  emotional strength and, 101
  psychiatric care and, 102
  statistics on, 102 *(t)*
Referral
  after detoxification, 73
  initial treatment phase after detoxification and, 74-75
  physician's avoidance and, 20-21
Rehabilitation. *See also* Detoxification, initial treatment after.
  aftercare and, 87-88
  age factor and, 94
  character disorder and, 90-91
  cross-addiction and, 94
  cultural factors and, 94-95
  early, intensive, 89
  educational factors and, 95
  employment and, 92
  environment and, 91
  family and, 88, 91-92
  inpatient, 81-83
    halfway house, 85
    long-term, 84-85
    physician's role, 96
    selection of facility, 95-96
    short-term, 83-84
  intellectual ability and, 95
  medical problems and, 89
  options for, 81, 83 *(t)*, 88-96
  outpatient, 85-87
  physical handicaps and, 95
  physician's role
    long-term, 97
    treatment center, 96
  previous attempts at, 92-93
  prognosis for, 96-97

Rehabilitation (*continued*)
  psychiatric problems and, 90-91
  relapse consequences and, 93
  socioeconomic factors and, 94-95
  structure and, 91
  time availability and, 92-93
Relapse, 15, 17, 46-47, 76
  antabuse and, 234
  events leading to, 119
  management of, 118-119
  physician's attitude toward, 49
  physician's role in, 102
  previous rehabilitation and, 92-93
  rehabilitation and, 93
  signs of, 16
  stages in, 234
Residential care
  after detoxification, 74
  family and, 88
  long-term, 84-85
  short-term, 83-84
Resocialization, 82
  structured programs and, 91
Respiratory rate, alcoholism and, 56
Risk factors for alcoholism, 224

Schizophrenia, alcoholism and, 144-145, 147-148. *See also* Psychiatric disorders, alcoholism and.
Secondary alcohol use, 223
Secondary diseases. *See* Medical complications of alcohol.
Secondary rewards of drinking, 52
Sedative action of ethanol, 3
  time factor in, 7
Sedative-hypnotic drugs, 209-210
  after detoxification, 73
  personal history and, 29
Sedatives, 5-6. *See also* Cross-addiction.
  prolonged withdrawal syndrome and, 146
  recovery and, 116
  women and, 175
"Sedativism," 5
Seizures, alcoholism and, 59. *See also* Grand mal seizures, alcoholism and.
Self-help recovery programs, 165-168. *See also* Adult Children of Alcoholics; Al-non; Alateen; Alcoholics Anonymous.
Self-image, alcoholism and, 13
Self-perpetuating factor in alcoholism, 159-160
Semantic problems in concept of alcoholism, 3-5
Sensory withdrawal syndrome, 60 *(t)*
Sex factor, alcoholism and, 28, 172. *See also* Women and alcoholism.
  medical complications and, 131
  tranquilizers and, 30
Sex hormone levels, alcoholism and, 173
Sexual dysfunction, abstinence and, 76
Sexual function, alcoholism and, 69
Short-term residential rehabilitation, 83-84
Skin clues, alcoholism and, 26
Skin lesions, alcoholism and, 56
Sleeping medication, alcoholism and, 62
Smoking, alcoholism and, 138
Sober alcoholic/physician relationship, 34
Social drinking, 43, 44-45, 105. *See also* Controlled drinking.
  recovery and, 117-118
Social stigma, alcoholism and, 19, 31
Sociocultural factors in alcoholism, 158
Socioeconomic factors, alcoholism and. *See also* Low-socioeconomic-status patient
  rehabilitation and, 94-95
Sociopathy, alcoholism and, 151-152
Somnifacients, 6, 209-210
Spina bifida, alcoholism and, 174
Spouse, 201. *See also* Al-Anon; Enabler.
  denial and, 33-34
  as etiologic factor, 40
  help for, 51-52
  secondary gains for, 52-53
Stereotypes, alcoholism and, 22
Stigma, alcoholism and, 37
Structure, rehabilitation and, 91
Success. *See also* Recovery.
  stress and, 158
  of treatment, 97
Sudden death, alcoholism and, 126, 131
Suicide, alcoholism and, 28, 150
Surgery, medical complications of alcoholism and, 138-139
Sympathetic confrontation with alcoholic patient, 9-10
  motivation and, 49-50
Symptomatic alcohol use, 223
Synergism, 6

TCs. *See* Therapeutic communities.
Teenage alcoholism, 191. *See also* Alateen; Family.
Temperature elevation, alcoholism and, 56
Terminology, alcoholism and, 37
Therapeutic communities (TCs), 85
Therapist, motivation and, 47-48
Therapy. *See also* Psychiatric disorders, alcoholism and; Psychotherapy.
  initial treatment phase after detoxification and, 70

withdrawal management and, 65-66
Thermal injury, alcoholism and, 28
Thiamine, alcoholism and, 60, 126, 130
cardiovascular system and, 132-133
nervous system and, 132
Thyrotoxic appearance, alcoholism and, 26
Time availability, rehabilitation and, 92-93
Time factor, sedative effect of alcohol and, 7
Tolerance to effects of alcohol, 215 *(t)*
variation in, 6-7
Tranquilizers, alcoholism and, 30, 210
recovery and, 116
Trauma, alcoholism and, 28, 55
Tremor, intention, alcoholism and, 24
Tricyclic antidepressants, alcoholism and, 17
prolonged withdrawal syndrome and, 146
Trust, alcoholism and, 76
Tuberculosis, alcoholism and, 138
Twelve Steps and Twelve Traditions, 109
Twelve steps of A.A., 107-110

Vitamin supplements, 60
Vocational rehabilitation after detoxification, 74-75
Vomiting, alcoholism and, 129

Wernicke's encephalopathy, 133, 153
Why Me?, 45
Willpower, alcoholism and, 42
Withdrawal. *See also* Prolonged withdrawal syndrome; Detoxification; Abstinence.
management of, 59-63
contract, 62
delayed, 62-63
DT, 63-64
environment, 59, 60 *(t)*
intercurrent illness and, 64-65
medication, 60-61, 62 *(t)*, 63
nutrition, 60, 62
outpatient, 59, 63
therapy, 65-66
physical examination for, 55-56
surgery and, 139
symptoms, 7, 59, 215
diagnostic clues, 24-25
initial, 55
severe, 55-58
stages in, 57 *(t)*
Women and alcoholism
career guidance and, 177-178
child-care and, 177
physiological considerations for, 173-174
sexism and, 172-173, 174-175
treatment for, 175-179
women's groups for, 175-176
Women's groups, success of, 175-176